Narcissism

Narcissism: Psychoanalytic Clinicians and Researchers in Dialogue presents current research and practice on working psychoanalytically with narcissism.

The contributors discuss a broad spectrum of approaches for understanding narcissism, from cultural-theoretical and social perspectives to clinical psychoanalytic observations and conceptual clarifications of terms, and new interdisciplinary and extra-clinical psychoanalytic research. Part I deals with the social danger posed by the close, unconscious link between pathological narcissism and extreme destructiveness. Part II is devoted to insights gained from years of psychoanalysis and long-term psychoanalytic treatment of patients with narcissistic pathology. Part III discusses how psychoanalysis tries to meet contemporary cultural challenges, and this book concludes with three chapters devoted to the important issue of narcissism in adolescence and young adulthood.

This book will be an essential reading for psychoanalysts in practice and in training.

Marianne Leuzinger-Bohleber is a professor emeritus of psychoanalysis at the University of Kassel, Germany. She is a former director of the Sigmund-Freud-Institut in Frankfurt am Main, a senior scientist at the University of Medicine in Mainz, a training and supervising analyst, and the author of numerous books and articles. She is the recipient of awards, including the 2016 Sigourney Award and the IPA's Outstanding Scientific Achievement Award.

Stephan Hau, PhD, is a professor of clinical psychology in the Department of Psychology, Stockholm University, Sweden. He is also a member of the Research Committee and a member of the Research Grants Subcommittee of the IPA, as well as a co-chair of the IPA's RTP/Sandler Conference Subcommittee. He is the editor-in-chief of *Scandinavian Psychoanalytic Review* and the author of numerous books and articles.

Rogério Lerner, PhD, is a professor at the Institute of Psychology and the Faculty of Medicine (Department of Psychiatry) of the University of São Paulo. He is also a member of the Research Committee of IPA, a co-chair of the Joseph Sandler Psychoanalytic Research Conference and Research Training Programme, and an associate member of the Brazilian Psychoanalytic Society of São Paulo.

Erik Stänicke is a professor of clinical psychology at the University of Oslo, Norway, and a training psychoanalyst. He is an experienced supervisor and teacher, and is the author of numerous books and articles.

Siri Erika Gullestad is a professor emeritus of clinical psychology at the University of Oslo, Norway. She is a training and supervising psychoanalyst, and she was awarded the Sigourney Award in 2019. She is an experienced teacher and supervisor, and is the author of numerous books and articles, including *The Theory and Practice of Psychoanalytic Therapy: Listening for the Subtext* (with Bjørn Killingmo, Routledge, 2020).

"This book provides an excellent, up-to-date psychoanalytic view of the clinical and growing extra-clinical phenomenon of narcissism. The book's collection of papers by leading psychoanalytic clinicians and researchers illustrates the complex nature of narcissistic experience and narcissistically motivated behaviours, providing a contemporary understanding of narcissism as a broad affective spectrum between the poles of a lively, realistically positive self-esteem and a possible self-aggrandizement with varying consequences for the quality of interpersonal relationships. In the course of this presentation, a fascination grows for the connection between clinical psychoanalysis and extra-clinical psychoanalytic research as well as for the inclusion of individual-centred as well as cultural-theoretical and social perspectives. Anyone who wants to know what contemporary psychoanalysis means in the 21st century will find central answers here that will stimulate their own thinking."

—Dr. med. Heribert Blass, Training Analyst, German
Psychoanalytic Association (DPV), IPA-President elect

"As pathological narcissism drives polarization, science denial, and political deception, this book provides a crucial psychoanalytic perspective on our time. Are we living in a 'narcissistic age,' where malignant, omnipotent leaders exploit unresolved vulnerabilities to manipulate the masses? Through rigorous clinical and empirical research, this work unpacks the deep entanglement of individual and collective pathologies shaping today's crises. Understanding these forces is not just necessary—it is urgent! A must-read for anyone unwilling to succumb to illusory grandiosity, regression, and the seductive pull of destructive power."

—Prof. Dr.med. Ricardo Bernardi, Training analyst Uruguayan
Psychoanalytic Association (APU), Former Dean of the Medical
faculty of Universidad de Montevideo

"This rich, timely, and vitally important book includes chapters by an international collection of sophisticated psychoanalytic theorists, researchers and clinicians presenting a much-needed broad spectrum of perspectives for understanding narcissism. Seeking a stronger interlinking between psychoanalytic knowledge of the largely unconscious individual mind and wider interdisciplinary dialogue, the chapters offer a contemporary understanding of narcissism's impact on trauma, depression, as well group dynamics, collective regression, and the role of malignant leadership. Finally and most significantly in today's turbulent times marked by autocratic turns and threats to democracy, the book sheds considerable light on powerful social issues and difficult cultural challenges. This is a book that should stimulate thinking and deepen awareness among social scientists, serious scholars, and psychoanalysts and other practitioners."

—Michael J. Diamond, Ph.D, Training and Supervising Analyst, Los Angeles
Institute and Society for Psychoanalytic Studies; Author, *Ruptures in the
American Psyche: Containing Destructive Populism in Perilous Times* and
*Masculinity and Its Discontents: The Male Psyche
and the Inherent Tensions of Maturing Manhood.*

The International Psychoanalytical Association Current Challenges in Psychoanalysis Series
Series Editor: Silvia Flechner

Narcissism

Psychoanalytic Clinicians and
Researchers in Dialogue

**Edited by Marianne Leuzinger-Bohleber,
Stephan Hau, Rogério Lerner,
Erik Stänicke, and Siri Erika Gullestad**

Routledge
Taylor & Francis Group

LONDON AND NEW YORK

Designed cover image: Getty | Cavan Images

First published 2026
by Routledge
4 Park Square, Milton Park, Abingdon, Oxon OX14 4RN

and by Routledge
605 Third Avenue, New York, NY 10158

Routledge is an imprint of the Taylor & Francis Group, an informa business

For Product Safety Concerns and Information please contact our EU representative GPSR@taylorandfrancis.com. Taylor & Francis Verlag GmbH, Kaufingerstraße 24, 80331 München, Germany.

British Library Cataloguing-in-Publication Data
A catalogue record for this book is available from the British Library

ISBN: 9781032932989 (hbk)
ISBN: 9781032932972 (pbk)
ISBN: 9781003565284 (ebk)

DOI: 10.4324/9781003565284

Typeset in Palatino
by codeMantra

Contents

Contributors

Gilles Ambresin, Lausanne, is a research lead in the research program on chronic depression at the University Institute of Psychotherapy, Department of Psychiatry, Lausanne University Hospital. He is a member in training at the Swiss Psychoanalytic Society (SSPsa). He is a psychiatrist and a psychotherapist, practicing in private practice. He is a past member of the Board of the Centre de Psychanalyse de Lausanne, a chair of the local organizing committee of the XXIst Sandler conference in Lausanne, and a member of the organizing committee of the Congrès des psychanalystes de langue française (Lausanne, 2023). He publishes in peer-reviewed journals and has authored book chapters focusing mainly on severe or chronic depression and psychotherapy.

Luciano Billodre Luiz, São Paulo, is a psychiatrist. He holds a master's and a PhD in Medicine. He is a professor and preceptor of the residency and specialization course in Psychiatry at Pontifícia Universidade Católica do Rio Grande do Sul. He is a specialist and supervisor in Psychodynamic Psychotherapy, a member of the International Society of Transference Focused Psychotherapy, and a co-founder of the Institute of Psychotherapy Focused on Transference in Brazil.

Werner Bohleber, Frankfurt am Main, Dr. Phil, is a psychoanalyst in private practice in Frankfurt am Main. He is a training and supervising analyst and a former president of the German Psychoanalytic Association. From 1997 to 2017, he was the main editor of the journal *PSYCHE*. In 2007, he received the Mary S. Sigourney Award. His research subjects and main publication themes are psychoanalytic theory; history of psychoanalysis in Germany; transgenerational consequences of the Nazi period and the war on the second and third generations; nationalism, xenophobia, and anti-Semitism; and trauma.

Nicole Cain, New York, PhD, is an associate professor in the Department of Clinical Psychology in the Graduate School of Applied and Professional Psychology at Rutgers University. Her research focuses on understanding how personality pathology and interpersonal functioning impact diagnosis, psychotherapy process, and treatment outcome. She is a past president of the Society for Interpersonal Theory and Research and is the president-elect for the Society for Personality Assessment. She served as an associate editor for *Assessment* and the *Journal of Personality Assessment*. Her research has been funded by the National Institute of Mental Health (NIMH).

Eve Caligor, New York, MD, is a clinical professor of psychiatry at the Columbia University, Vagelos College of Physicians and Surgeons; director of the Psychotherapy Division; associate director at the Columbia University Center for Psychoanalytic Training and Research; and adjunct professor of psychiatry at the Sanford Weill Medical College. Her clinical and research expertise is in the evaluation and psychodynamic treatment of personality pathology, and she has published numerous articles and books on the assessment and treatment of personality disorders.

Cristiana Castanho de Almeida Rocca, São Paulo, holds a master's and PhD in Sciences from the University of São Paulo. She is a psychologist and specialist in psychological and neuropsychological assessment and cognitive behavioral therapy, both at the Institute of Psychiatry, University of São Paulo. Also, she is a supervisor in the Psychology and Neuropsychology Service and a coordinator of the Neuropsychology and Mental Health specialization program at the Institute of Psychiatry, Hospital das Clínicas, Faculty of Medicine, University of São Paulo.

John F. Clarkin, New York, PhD, is an emeritus clinical professor of psychology in psychiatry at the Weill Medical College of Cornell University, New York City. He serves as the director of the Personality Disorders Institute (PDI) of the New York Presbyterian Hospital, the university hospital of Cornell and Columbia. His research activities have focused on the phenomenology of personality disorders and the treatment of patients with borderline personality disorder and bipolar disorder. He is the author of numerous articles and books on psychopathology, differential treatment planning and personality disorders. He has worked with Dr. Otto Kernberg and the interdisciplinary members of the PDI since 1980 to empirically investigate an object relations treatment for borderline personality organization. He is a past president of the international Society for Psychotherapy Research (SPR). He has served on study groups at the National Institute of Mental Health (NIMH) and is a reviewer for major journals such as the *American Journal of Psychiatry*, *Journal of Personality Disorders*, and *Personality Disorders: Theory, Research and Treatment*.

Stephan Doering, Vienna, is a professor of Psychoanalysis and Psychotherapy at the Medical University of Vienna. He is a psychoanalyst at the Vienna Psychoanalytic Society.

Tamara Fischmann, Berlin/Frankfurt am Main, is a professor of Clinical Psychology and Psychoanalysis at the International Psychoanalytic University (IPU) Berlin, practicing psychoanalyst DPV/IPA. She is a staff member and a scientific researcher at the Sigmund-Freud-Institut Frankfurt. Her publications mainly focus on interdisciplinary research in bioethics, dream research, attachment, as well as imaging technique studies in neuroscience. She is currently engaged in a project investigating the biological function of dreaming and in another project looking at the psychoanalytic and biological underpinnings of multiple complex traumatization in early childhood.

Siri Erika Gullestad, Oslo, is a professor emeritus of clinical psychology at the University of Oslo and a training and supervising analyst, IPA. She is a former head of the Department of Psychology and a former president of the Norwegian Psychoanalytic Association. She is the author of many articles and books within the psychoanalytic field, e.g., *Theory and Practice of Psychoanalytic Therapy: Listening for the Subtext* (with Bjørn Killingmo, Routledge, 2020). She was awarded the Sigourney prize in 2019 and is currently the chair of the IPA Research Committee.

Stephan Hau, Stockholm, Prof. Dr. Phil., Dipl.-Psych., is a psychological psychotherapist and psychoanalyst (SPAF, IPA, DPV). Since 2010, he has been a professor of clinical psychology in the Department of Psychology at Stockholm University. From 1991 to 2005, he was a research associate at the Sigmund Freud Institute in Frankfurt am Main. He serves as a member of the IPA's Research Grant Subcommittee and co-chairs both the IPA's Research Committee and the RTP/Sandler Research Conference Subcommittee. Since 2022, he has been the editor-in-chief of the *Scandinavian Psychoanalytic Review*. His research focuses on experimental trauma studies, supervision research, and nonverbal communication.

Otto F. Kernberg, New York, is a professor of psychiatry at Weill Medical College of Cornell University. He is also the director of the Personality Disorders Institute at New York Presbyterian Hospital, Westchester Division. He is additionally a training and supervising analyst at the Columbia University Center for Psychoanalytic Training and Research.

Gerd Koenen, Frankfurt am Main, is a historian and writer. He is the author of a number of books on subjects like history of Russian-German relations ("Der Russland-Komplex. Die Deutschen und der Osten", München, 2005/2023); history of Communism ("Die Farbe Rot. Ursprünge und Geschichte des Kommunismus", München, 2017); the current aggression of Russia against Ukraine ("Im Widerschein des Krieges – Nachdenken über Russland", München, 2023); and history of the New Left of the 1960s/70s ("Das Rote Jahrzehnt. Unsere kleine deutsche Kulturrevolution 1967-1977", Köln, 2001).

Rogério Lerner, São Paulo, is a professor at the Institute of Psychology and the Faculty of Medicine (Department of Psychiatry) of the University of São Paulo. He is a member of the Research Committee of IPA, a co-chair, with Stephan Hau, of the Sandler RTP Subcommittee, an associate member of the Brazilian Psychoanalytic Society of São Paulo, and a principal researcher of the Brazilian Center for Early Child Development. He has won the following prizes: 2019, Psychoanalytic Research, Exceptional Contribution Awards, IPA; 2013, Monographic award César Ades, Federal Council of Psychology; and 2012, Community and Culture Award, Psychoanalytic Federation of Latin America.

Marianne Leuzinger-Bohleber, Mainz/Frankfurt am Main, Prof. Dr. Phil., is the director in charge of the Sigmund-Freud-Institut in Frankfurt a.M., Germany (2001–2016), a professor emeritus of psychoanalysis at the University of Kassel, and a Senior Professor at the University of Medicine in Mainz. She is a training analyst of the German Psychoanalytical Association (DPV) and the International Psychoanalytical Association (IPA). She is a chair of the Research Subcommittees for Clinical, Conceptual, Epistemiological and Historical Research of the IPA (2001–2009), vice-chair for Europe of the Research Board der IPA 2010–2021; and chair of the IPA Subcommittee for Migration and Refugees 2018–2019 (since then a member of the committee). She received the Mary Sigourney Award 2016, the Haskell Norman Prize for Excellence in Psychoanalysis 2017, the Robert S. Wallerstein Fellowship (2022–2027), and the IPA's Outstanding Scientific Achievement Award 2023. Her research fields are clinical and extraclinical research in psychoanalysis, psychoanalytical developmental research, prevention studies, interdisciplinary dialogue between psychoanalysis and literature, educational sciences, and the neurosciences.

Izabella Lopes de Arantes, São Paulo, is a clinical psychologist. She holds a master's in Social Psychology from the University of São Paulo. She is a PhD candidate in Developmental Psychology at the Institute of Psychology of the University of São Paulo.

Helene Amundsen Nissen-Lie, Oslo, PhD, is a professor in clinical psychology at the Department of Psychology, University of Oslo in Norway. In her research, she has investigated what characterizes effective psychotherapists and therapy processes and outcomes across settings, patient groups, and theoretical orientations using both quantitative and qualitative methods. She is a clinical psychologist, a psychoanalyst, and a member of the Norwegian Psychoanalytic Association.

Inge Seiffge-Krenke, Mainz, Prof. Em. Dr. Phil., Dipl.-Psych., is a professor of developmental psychology at the University of Mainz; a psychoanalyst for adults, children, and adolescents (DPV, IPV); and a supervisor and training analyst. Her book publications include *Therapy Goal Identity*

(2nd ed. 2012); *Fathers, Men and Child Development* (2016); *The Psychoanalysis of the Girl* (2nd ed., 2017); *Resistance, Defense and Coping* (2017); *Adolescents in Psychodynamic Psychotherapy* (4th ed., 2020); *Young People and Their Search for the New Self* (2nd ed., 2021); and *Psychodynamic Psychotherapy with Emerging Adults* (2023).

Mark Solms, Cape Town, is a professor and director of Neuropsychology in the Neuroscience Institute of the University of Cape Town, South Africa. He is a member of the British Psychoanalytical Society and of the South African and American Psychoanalytic Associations.

Julia Sowislo, New York, PhD, is a senior research associate at the Personality Disorders Institute of New York Presbyterian Hospital. She received her PhD from the University of Basel and is licensed as a psychodynamic psychotherapist in Switzerland.

Line Indrevoll Stänicke, Oslo, PhD, is an associate professor in the Department of Psychology, University of Oslo in Norway. In her research, she has written articles and books on the treatment of adolescents, self-harm, and risk-behavior – offline and online. She is a clinical psychologist and has worked with children, adolescents, and adults at the Lovisenberg Hospital in Norway. She is a psychoanalyst and member of the Norwegian Psychoanalytic Association and a supervisor in Mentalization-Based Therapy.

Erik Stänicke, Oslo, is a professor of clinical psychology at the University of Oslo and a training analyst and former president at the Norwegian Psychoanalytic Society. He is currently the chair of the IPA clinical research subcommittee.

Series editor foreword

The International Psychoanalytic Association Publications Committee is honored to present a new book from the *Current Challenges in Psychoanalysis* series. This series delves into the evolving landscape of psychoanalytic practice, addressing contemporary issues such as trauma, cultural diversity, technology's influence, and shifts in psychoanalytical dynamics. Each volume offers concise, interdisciplinary insights from leading experts, bridging classical psychoanalytic theory with modern challenges. Designed for clinicians and researchers, this series is a vital resource for those seeking to navigate and innovate within today's complex therapeutic environment.

The Publications Committee of the International Psychoanalytical Association is pleased to present the new book *Narcissism: Psychoanalytic Clinicians and Researchers in Dialogue*, edited by Marianne Leuzinger-Bohleber, Stephan Hau, Rogério Lerner, Erik Stänicke, and Siri Erika Gullestad.

The International Psychoanalytic Association's Research Committee initiated this book based on papers presented at the Joseph Sandler Conference at the University of Vienna in September 2023. This book tries to bridge the clinical and research worlds.

Part I, Narcissism in Society and Culture, deals with the social danger posed by the close, unconscious link between extreme destructiveness and pathological narcissism.

Part II, Narcissism: Clinical Practice and Research, is devoted to insights gained from years of clinical and conceptual research in psychoanalysis and long-term psychoanalytic treatments to patients with narcissistic pathology, as well as from other forms of psychoanalytic research of these phenomena.

Part III, Confronting Contemporary Cultural Challenges, examines some current political debates and reflects on whether and in what way psychoanalysis can contribute. One controversial discussion focuses on the development of narcissism in one particular developmental phase, the so-called Emerging Adulthood.

The last two chapters of the volume are based on one central research tradition, which is closely connected to the IPA Research Committee: the attempt to combine clinical and extra-clinical research.

This book also deals with contemporary cultural challenges, such as the influence of digital age on adolescents' developmental processes, transgender, and psychoanalysis confronting the modern Zeitgeist – innovative contributions testifying to the richness of psychoanalytic thinking about our contemporary world.

This book also contributes to conceptual reflections and new integrations of interdisciplinary and psychoanalytic knowledge on narcissism, delving into the contribution of psychoanalysis to the sociocultural psychological discussion of narcissism. The authors also discuss the fact that destructive narcissism in nationalistic and fundamentalistic ideologies is gaining increased influence worldwide.

This book presents a broad spectrum of approaches for understanding narcissism, from cultural-theoretical and social perspectives to clinical-psychoanalytic observations and conceptual clarifications of terms to new interdisciplinary and extra-clinical-psychoanalytic research results.

This new book is a vital resource for psychoanalysts, researchers, and the large community of historians, philosophers, therapists working in mental health, and social workers. It allows an understanding of some of the main problems we are experiencing today.

Silvia Flechner
Series Editor
Chair, IPA Publications Committee

Preface

We are very pleased to present this book initiated by the Research Committee of the International Psychoanalytic Association (IPA). This book is based on papers presented at the Joseph Sandler Conference at the University of Vienna in September 2023, with the theme *Narcissism: Clinicians and Researchers in Dialogue*. *Narcissism* is a truly psychoanalytic concept, and the Research Committee was proud to present a conference program covering narcissism in a wide scope, e.g., basic neuropsychoanalytic research on narcissism as well as the extreme challenge of treating patients with narcissistic pathology. Specifically, however, we wanted to discuss the role of narcissism in our present-day society: The destructive narcissism in nationalistic and fundamentalistic ideologies, which – most ominously – are gaining increased influence in the world, like we see it in Putin's justification of the war in Ukraine, in the murderous narcissism of terrorist acts, as well as in the pathological narcissism of large groups. At the moment of writing this preface, we witness the destructive actions of a new American president presenting yet another grandiose, nationalistic program. Certainly, the topic of narcissism is more gloomily present than ever – even more so now than at the time of the conference. Thus, this book testifies to the relevance of psychoanalysis not only for understanding individual psychic suffering but also for grasping unconscious dynamics at play in our culture, society, and politics.

The IPA Joseph Sandler Research Conference was established during the 1990s with the specific aim of stimulating dialogue between clinicians and researchers. Since then, the conference has been an annual event, circulating between Europe, Latin America, the United States, and, most recently, China. As a chair of the Research Committee since 2022, it has been my great pleasure to witness the diversity and complexity of the psychoanalytic research presented at the Sandler – and the depth of the dialogue between clinicians and researchers that this frame allows for. While several of the contributions of this volume are based on conference papers, this book is in no way a conference proceeding.

This book comprises a section dealing with contemporary cultural challenges, e.g., emerging adulthood, the influence of the digital age on developmental processes of adolescents, transgender, and psychoanalysis confronting the modern Zeitgeist – innovative contributions testifying to the richness of psychoanalytic thinking about our modern world.

The Sandler Conference in Vienna was hosted by Professor Stephan Doering, head of the Department of Psychoanalysis and Psychotherapy, Medical University of Vienna, in collaboration with Wiener Psychoanalytische Vereinigung. Our most heartfelt appreciations go to Stephan and his staff for organizing the conference just excellently in the wonderful city of Vienna.

A very specific warm thank you goes to Professor Marianne Leuzinger-Bohleber. Marianne guarantees the continuity of our work trying to bridge the clinical and the research world. As an excellent pioneer in psychoanalytic outcome research combining in-depth psychoanalytic treatments, she embodies in her own person the very aim of the Sandler. She is to be honored for the initiative to this book.

Finally, I would like to express my sincere thanks to Ute Ochtendung for her careful and professional editing of the manuscripts.

Siri Erika Gullestad
Chair, IPA Research Committee
Oslo, February 2025

Introduction

Marianne Leuzinger-Bohleber, Stephan Hau,
Rogério Lerner, Erik Stänicke and Siri Erika Gullestad

On October 20, 2024, historian and journalist Anne Applebaum received the Peace Prize of the German Book Trade because she was one of the first international scholars who since many years recognized the enormous danger posed to Western democracies by autocrats, populists and dictators. "At a time when democratic achievements and values are increasingly caricatured and attacked, her work is becoming an eminently important contribution to the preservation of democracy and peace", the jury said in its statement on the Peace Prize.[1]

The Research Committee of the International Psychoanalytic Association and the editors of this volume share the view that Western democracies are threatened by autocratic, pathologically narcissistic leaders and their international networks. This raises the question of whether and how psychoanalytic knowledge on pathological narcissism and its individual and collective dangers might meaningfully complement the historical works of Anne Applebaum and others. Therefore, the Research Committee decided to make "Narcissism" the theme of the 23rd Joseph Sandler Research Conference, which took place from September 29 to October 1 2023 at the University of Vienna. As the conference was interesting, innovative and covered a wide range of clinical-psychoanalytic concepts and experiences, empirical-psychoanalytic research results and new neuroscientific findings on early development, the IPA Research Committee decided to make the most important conference contributions, supplemented by some additional papers on the topic, available to a wider audience in a book publication.

In a recent publication, Michel Diamond (in press) follows a similar objective. He emphasizes that psychoanalysis, as a science of the unconscious, should contribute its knowledge of irrational, "crazy" sources of human thought, feeling and action to the broad and relevant interdisciplinary dialogues on the worldwide threat to free thought and speech in Western democracies. He discusses the importance of understanding the existential anxieties of large parts of the US population caused by globalization, the looming climate catastrophe and the resulting worldwide

DOI: 10.4324/9781003565284-1

migration movements as well as the associated longing for security, prosperity, demarcation and a strong leader instead of morally condemning them. Above all, the fact that the white population will no longer be the majority of the US population in a few years seems to represent an immense unconscious threat for many and lead to a collective regression. Referring to the work of Bohleber (2010, 2024 and his contribution in this volume), Diamond discusses how populist leaders such as Donald Trump and his oligarchic supporters masterfully use social media to stimulate ubiquitous unconscious fantasies, thereby awakening nationalist, fundamentalist and xenophobic emotions and instrumentalizing them for their own purposes. In doing so, archaic mental states are actively promoted with the primitive defense mechanisms that characterize them, such as denial, splitting, projection and reversal into the opposite. Polarizing tendencies in society are not contained. On the contrary, a so-called perverse container is created.

> In the Trumpian-influenced populist groupings in which terrifying P/S^2 anxieties have been fueled and taken hold, Trump's agitating, unyielding, and captivating leadership mobilizes the group's basic assumption mentalities while serving as an external structure—a second skin (*Bick 1968*) functioning as a 'perverse' container (*Zienert-Eilts 2020*)—that promises illusory security, freedom, power, and moral superiority in an aspirational, tension-free group fantasy.[3] In *Freud's (1921)* depiction of group psychology, this process in which the collective ideal (residing in the malignant leader/group fit) replaces the individual ego ideal, unleashes a form of shameless irresponsibility unique to mass psychology.
>
> (Diamond, in print, p.13)

The matching between archaic states of the minds in a regressive large group and pathological narcissistic leadership not only characterizes current US American society but also can be observed in many autocratic systems worldwide. This volume aims to shed light on some of the irrational sources of such destructive processes from a psychoanalytic perspective.

What does psychoanalysis understand by narcissism?

Laplanche and Pontalis (1973) suggest a deceptively simple definition: "In the image of the legend of Narcissus: the love one has for one's image of oneself" (p.317, translation by authors). Over the last 50 years, the psychoanalytic understanding of normal and pathological narcissism has deepened and become more nuanced. In contemporary psychoanalysis, narcissism most frequently refers to:

1) the overall well-being of the self, including feelings of aliveness, initiative, authenticity, coherence, and self esteem; 2) self-esteem, in both

its normal and pathological forms; 3) *narcissistic pathology*, in the form of *narcissistic character* or *narcissistic personality disorder*, which exists on a continuum of severity from higher-level neurotic disorders to more-pervasive character pathology; narcissistic personality disorder includes defensive self inflation; lack of integration of the self concept; inordinate dependence upon acclaim by others; poor object relations; vulnerability to feelings of humiliation, shame, rage, and depression; entitlement; relentless pursuit of self perfection; and impaired capacities for concern, empathy, and love for others; 4) *narcissistic defenses* used to regulate self esteem, including self aggrandizement or omnipotence, idealization, and devaluation 5) *pathological narcissism*, a term describing narcissistic pathology from a specific perspective closely associated with the object relations school of the British Kleinians; 6) the clinical and theoretical emphasis of self psychology that views narcissism as a normal line of healthy development, subject to developmental arrests.

(Auchincloss & Samberg, 2021, p.162)

Freud used the concept of narcissism in many contexts to explain a variety of phenomena, such as the libidinal investment of the self, homosexuality, omnipotent thinking, hypochondria, idealization, the vicissitude of self-regard, the residue of infantile narcissism and the fulfillment of one's ego ideal. As he described in his central work "On Narcissism" (1914), he regarded the ego ideal as the legacy of infantile perfectionism. He spoke of the narcissistic libido as an energy that is released when it is withdrawn from the object and is now available for various non-sexual ego functions such as sublimation, internalization and identification. Through these mechanisms, psychic structures such as the ego ideal are built up, which then plays an important role in narcissistic self-regulation. The ego is no longer dependent on being praised by external objects, but seeks the recognition of the ego ideal (see, among others; Wurmser, 2015).

As we see, some of the conceptual confusion surrounding narcissism can be traced back to Freud himself. On the one hand, he uses the term narcissism as a metapsychological concept, but on the other hand, at a lower level of abstraction, he describes various experiences of the individual as "narcissistic". This difficulty is also reflected in future debates on narcissism. Heinz Hartmann (1939), for example, tried to distinguish between the experiential I and the more abstract self. He defined narcissism as the libidinal investment of the self (see also Balint, 1952). Edith Jacobson (1971) further developed his work and integrated the Freudian understanding of drives with ego functions, affect and object relations. She conceptualized the development of the self in connection with the internal structures of the superego, ego ideal and wishful self-image. Over time, conceptualizations of the self became increasingly important in psychoanalytic approaches to narcissism, as did greater understanding of superego and ego ideal. For example, analysts, such as J. Sandler and Joffe (1965), attempted to define narcissism in entirely non-drive terms, locating its meaning instead in terms of affective states. They defined narcissism as an "ideal state of well-being" and narcissistic pathology as an overt or latent "state of pain" (Auchincloss & Samberg, 2021, p.163).

On the basis of her analyses of very young children, Melanie Klein (1952) contradicts the Freudian view of a development state without objects. Klein states that auto-erotism and narcissism imply "a love for and relation with the internalized good object which in phantasy form a part of the loved body and self" (1952, p.51). She further asserts that in both auto-erotic gratification and narcissistic states, there is a withdrawal to the internalized object. In "Notes on some schizoid mechanisms" (1946), Klein differentiates between *narcissistic states* and *narcissistic object relations and structure*. A narcissistic state is a withdrawal to an *introjected* object. Klein relates narcissistic object relations more directly to the role of *projective identification* in the split structure of the paranoid-schizoid position. She asserts that schizoid part-object relations are narcissistic in nature. Klein writes of the projection of both good and bad parts. Good parts like the ego-ideal are projected, as a result of which the other person is loved and admired because he contains the good part of the self. Similarly, bad parts are projected so that the object is identified with this bad part of the self. Narcissistic object relations have a strong element of control because the projected parts of the self are now controlled by controlling the other person (see Bott Spillius et al., 2011, p.410, 411). Melanie Klein was therefore one of the first authors to clearly link a pathological narcissistic development with a pathology of early object relations.

Rosenfeld (1964) presented a series of key papers on *pathological narcissism*. He contradicts the Freudian view that patients with a narcissistic neurosis cannot be treated psychoanalytically. He shows that in narcissistic transference, the separateness between self and object is denied and that this serves as a defense against envy and dependency. Later, in 1971, he distinguishes between *libidinal narcissism*, in which dependency on the object and the envy associated with it is defended against, and *destructive narcissism*, in which the rejection of the object is a manifestation of the death drive. Van der Waals (1966) speaks of pathological narcissism as the result of pathological early object relations, in contrast to the conceptualization of narcissism as a fixation at an early normal point of development.

It is well known that D. W. Winnicott agreed with his Kleinian colleagues in many of his papers on the influence of the role of earliest object-relational experiences on the development of the self, of narcissistic self-regulation and of object-relational capacity. In addition, he developed a unique perspective. He was one of the first to describe that the infant can only discover its self through the shine in the mother's eye, through the early mirroring processes (see Gallese, 2023). In this sense, there is no primary narcissism independent of the object: the self is only built in and through the object "There is no such a thing as a baby!" became one of Winnicott's much-quoted sentences. He described how important the empathy of the primary object is for the development of the self and narcissism. Only a good enough, empathetic object can enable the child to develop the *early narcissistic illusion, the omnipotent phantasy*, which is within one's power to get the object to satisfy one's existential needs and bring it out of the objectively unbearable situation of total helplessness and dependency.

In this context, Winnicott speaks of primary traumatization, a human condition (see e.g. Winnicott, 1974). No infant is spared the experience of being flooded with unbearable affects, helplessness and powerlessness combined with fear of death and panic as a psychophysiological premature birth. However, if an empathetic primary object manages to end these unbearable, traumatic experiences again and again in a predictable, reliable way, this object-relational experience forms a counterweight as early embodied memories in the unconscious (see e.g. Abram, 2021, p.784f.).

Abram (2021) summarized this view concisely:

> Thus there are two Winnicottian babies: a baby who has gained from the mother's ordinary devotion in contrast to a baby who has suffered trauma because the early environment did not provide the essential psychic elements for the nascent psyche to grow (Abram and Hinshelwood 2018, 46–51).
>
> (p.779)

Winnicott pronounces that the effects of early traumatization are all the more serious the earlier they occur. *He looks at both the intrapsychic factors (subsequent interpretation of the early trauma) and environmental factors.*

> In his late work Winnicott clarified three areas on his perspective on trauma. First, it involved 'a consideration of external factors'. This refers to the inescapable fact on dependency from the very start of life. Second, trauma "breaks up an idealization of an object" because the failure of the external other causes the infant to hate the object. This refers to the infant's premature disillusionment, which indicates that the trauma is intrapsychic although caused by the psychic environment. Mother's psychic presence disappears. Third, Winnicott observed that trauma comes about because of the failure of the object's function and so its intensity and quality will be relative to each stage of the child's emotional development (Winnicott, 1965, 145).
>
> (Abram, 2021, p.779)

(See also Roussillon, 2010, for the importance of these early experiences and fantasies for the development of the self: see Bohleber, 2023.)

Kernberg (1970, 1975, 1984, 2014), who also contributes on the topic in this book, relies less on Winnicott's work, but takes up the theses of Rosenfeld and other Kleinian authors and combines them with the above-outlined ego-psychological works on narcissism. According to his conceptualization, pathological narcissism is based on early splitting processes that serve to defend against unbearable aggressive desires and lead to a disruption of the early structure of the self. Good and bad parts of the self cannot be integrated into one's own self. Instead, individuals with pathological narcissism develop a pathological, grandiose self. In the service of defense, there is often a fusion of the actual self with ideal self and ideal object representations. The grandiose self serves as a defense against unbearable feelings of dependency on the object and the envy associated with it. Unintegrated evil object and self traits are projected to external objects. As a result, external objects are experienced as malicious, unreal and mechanical. In addition, the superego cannot develop adequately.

Some narcissistic personalities function relatively well despite their paranoid fears. They try to develop an omnipotent control of their objects and flee in a *narcissistic withdrawal* if this defense fails. Other, more severely disturbed patients, develop a so-called *malignant narcissism* with a deformed superego and sociopathic personality traits (see contribution by Kernberg in this volume).

A milestone in the debates on narcissism was laid by the papers of Heinz Kohut (1966, 1977, 1984). He opposed an exclusively negative view of narcissism and emphasized the importance of "normal", well-developed narcissistic self-regulation for mental health, creativity and social behavior. Therefore, he postulated a developmental line independent of the drive development from the early, archaic forms of narcissism to a mature narcissistic self-regulation with stable self-esteem and a sustaining self-worth. Narcissistic development begins with the emergence of a bipolar self. On the one pole, he localizes the grandiose self, on the other, the omnipotent object. Through empathetic, "good enough" early object relation experiences, these archaic self-states can be gradually integrated psychically, so that the fantasies of a grandiose self can develop into mature self-regulation and stable self-esteem on the one hand. On the other hand, fantasies of omnipotence regarding the object can develop into mature respect for others and an appreciation of their achievements and merits. Kohut has also developed his own treatment technique for patients with narcissistic personality disorders.

There were fierce debates between Kohut and Kernberg, especially regarding their understanding of narcissistic rage, its treatment and its social implications. One of the most frequently put forward thesis was that the two authors had treated different groups of patients. Rosenfeld (1987), for example, differentiates between "thick-skinned" and "thin-skinned" narcissists. The first group often displays an extremely aggressive form of defense, while the second appears fragile and vulnerable. Similarly, the Psychodynamic Diagnostic Manual (PDM Task Force, 2006) differentiates between two types of narcissistic personality disorder: arrogant/ entitled (characterized by haughtiness, charisma, and belittling others) and depressed/depleted (characterized by envy and a search for people to idealize) (see also chapter by Doering in this volume).

As Leuzinger-Bohleber discusses in her contribution in this volume: In contrast to this object-relations theory view of narcissism, André Green (1998, 2001, 2007) has presented his very own theory of narcissism, in which he refers, among other things, to Freud's drive dualism between the life and death drives. According to this, Eros is always directed toward the object, toward attachment and toward *objectification*, whereas the death drive strives for the greatest possible fulfillment of a *disobjectification function* through detachment (Green, 2001, p.874). Green derives his concept of *negative narcissism* from these considerations, with which he succeeds in explaining e.g. the most severe depressive states. Severely depressed patients disobjectified their objects, themselves and even all attachment desires and libidinal and aggressive impulses in threatening states of suicidality. Such an extreme withdrawal of cathexis corresponds to negative narcissism according to Green (for further details, see Green, 2001).

André Green also developed the concept of *narcissistic moralism.* Patients with this pathology rely on moral principles to free themselves from the vicissitudes of attachment to the object and to achieve liberation from the shackles attached to the object relationship, allowing the id and ego to be loved by a demanding superego and a tyrannical ego ideal (Green, 2005). This leads to an ascetic pride and triumph over the object, but also over one's own body and the unbearable experiences of powerlessness and helplessness associated with it.

In view of these enormous conceptual differences in the understanding narcissism in contemporary psychoanalysis, Drew Westen (1990) attempts to contribute to a new clarity, primarily based on the broad findings of empirical developmental research. He distinguishes four different forms of narcissism: egocentrism, relative emotional investment in self and others, self-concept (the conscious knowledge of the self) and self-esteem (the affective evaluation of the self). He discusses that these four forms cannot be subordinated to a unified concept of narcissism, since they represent too great a variation of phenomena. Therefore, he finally postulates a broad preliminary, umbrella definition of narcissism. "Narcissism refers to a cognitive-affective preoccupation with the self" (cited in Auchincloss & Samberg, 2021, p.165). At the same time, Westen makes a strong plea for further conceptual work on the topic of narcissism that takes into account available empirically supported knowledge.

Now that theoretically and methodologically sound developmental research has become of direct relevance to theories of narcissism and object relations, it is essential that psychoanalytic thinking accommodate the findings of these studies, less we, like Narciss, become lost in our own theoretical reflections.

(Westen, 1990, p.233f.; see also Hau in this volume)

This book tries to contribute to such conceptual reflections and new integrations of interdisciplinary and psychoanalytic knowledge on narcissism.

The contribution of psychoanalysis to the socio-cultural psychological discussion of narcissism

Narcissism has repeatedly become the subject of social debates. In this context, just a few remarks:

Since the 1970s, the psychoanalytical concept of narcissism has been used in social and cultural-critical reflections on contemporary societal phenomena. Sennett and Richter (1998), for example, spoke about the "tyranny of intimacy" or the "apotheosis of individualism" in a "narcissistic age" without history or authority (Lasch, 2019). During the same decades, educators debated whether a new, no longer Oedipal, but "narcissistic type of socialization" (Thomas Ziehe, 1979) was emerging in adolescence or whether this construct merely defamed normal adolescent crises across the board (Bohleber & Leuzinger, 1981). Stänicke and Nissen-Lie take up this debate referring to the German sociologist and political scientist Hartmut Rosa (2013), Byng-Cuis Han (2015) and other authors in their chapter in this volume.

Another wave of debate was triggered by the book by French sociologist Alain Ehrenberg (1998/2016): La fatigue d'être soi (in German: Das erschöpfte Selbst, in English: The exhausted self). Ehrenberg declares the exhausted self to be the disease of contemporary society, whose behavioral norms are no longer based on guilt and discipline, but mainly on responsibility and initiative. The late bourgeois individual seems to be replaced by an individual who has the idea that "everything is possible" and is marked by the fear for his self-realization, which can easily increase to the feeling of exhaustion. The pressure for individualization is reflected in feelings of failure, shame and insufficiency and finally in depressive symptoms. For Ehrenberg, if neurosis is the illness of the individual torn apart by the conflict between what is allowed and what is forbidden, depression is the illness of the individual inhibited and exhausted by the tension between what is possible and what is impossible. Depression thus becomes a tragedy of inadequacy.

It is now undisputed that depression has become one of the most widespread diseases in Western societies. As we have discussed in other publications, empirical, clinical and conceptual research in psychoanalysis, as well as evolutionary biological considerations, have shown that *the central feeling of powerlessness and helplessness is at the center of contemporary depression* (Leuzinger-Bohleber, 2024). In the face of a globalized world with its existential threats from climate change and the resulting migratory movements, from wars and economic struggles for distribution, as well as a clash of different religious and cultural values, many people around the world feel extremely insecure and afraid (see e.g. Gullestad in this volume). As discussed in various contributions in this volume, this may lead not only to a worldwide increase of depression and other mental illnesses but also to collective regressions to early narcissistic states, which create the societal danger to be exploited by autocrats, populists and nationalists for their own purposes.

Populists, autocrats and nationalist leaders worldwide seem to have an intuitive knowledge of how to mobilize an omnipotent defense against the unbearable feelings of powerlessness and helplessness and the unconscious fantasy systems associated with them in many people. As Otto Kernberg explains in his contribution to this volume, there exists a dangerous inter-action of leaders with pathological narcissism and regressive large group phenomena. Many of the autocrats show traits of pathological narcissistic personality disorders. As discussed in detail in some contributions in this volume, they have an unconscious talent for mobilizing (early and) primi-tive defense mechanisms against powerlessness and helplessness e.g. in the way they use media and especially social media for their own purposes (see e.g. Koenen and Bohleber in this volume).

Ilany Kogan (2020) speaks of such leaders as "masters of the universe". Identification with narcissistic leaders who place themselves above the law can convey the illusion of omnipotence and immortality, which cor-responds to a primary narcissistic fantasy. As briefly outlined in this intro-duction, traces of such archaic narcissistic fantasies are present to varying degrees in all of us. One of the lessons of 20th-century German history is that, in certain societal crises, only very few individuals are immune to the seductive power of pathological narcissistic leaders.

A new need for a "Dark Enlightenment" (Whitebook, 2017)?

Of course, this volume cannot provide answers to these pressing political topics. We don't overestimate the possible contribution of psychoanalysis to the public and interdisciplinary dialogues on these complex issues. For example, Enns and colleagues (2024) have again shown that economic fac-tors, in contrast to psychological factors, were particularly decisive in the presidential elections in the USA in 2024. However, the economic factors are never the only determinants of societal crises. Therefore interdiscipli-nary analyses remain important. Therefore all the authors of this volume are trying to contribute to critical societal discourses from a psychoanalyti-cal perspective.

It seems to us that in view of the current dangers posed by populism, fake news and targeted demagogic attacks on Western democracies through social media, psychoanalysis as a science of "dark enlightenment" (White-book, 2017) that means the enlightenment of dark, unconscious sources of human feelings, thoughts and behavior is looking for new allies.

For decades, many psychoanalytic researchers of the so-called '68 generation have been primarily concerned with how empirical research in psychoanalysis can be differentiated from a positivist understanding of research. Today, in times of the global rise of populists and demagogic autocrats who combine fake news and deliberate falsification of realities as a political tool with often blatant hostility toward science, new fronts seem to be forming: Ideological distortions and media simplifications of complex realities through the deliberate distortions and falsifications on the one hand and a reality-oriented ("empirical") scientific approach to facts and truth on the other.[4]

In view of these new societal polarizations, the debate in which Freud took part in the early 1930s on the question of whether psychoanalysis was a *world view* seems highly topical, as Stänicke and Nissen-Lie discuss further in this book. Freud, as is well known, claimed that a worldview can only be an illusion, an idealization and a defense against reality, as found in religion and other belief systems. In contrast, he defined psychoanalysis as a "Wissenschaft", as a science of the unconscious (see e.g. White-book, 2017). Today, we are thinking of populist, fundamentalist and media "worldviews" and power-political rhetoricians and targeted fake news, which, as mentioned, are used diabolically by autocratic rulers to achieve their power-political goals. From a psychoanalytic perspective, these strategies are so successful because these politicians masterfully know how to play on the keyboard of ubiquitous, unconscious fantasies that are present in all of us and make us susceptible to illusory transfiguration of complex, often painful realities. It is a challenge for contemporary psychoanalysis to contribute to a deeper understanding of the irrational (unconscious) roots that make so many people in all parts of the world seducible to these populists (cf. e.g. Bohleber, 2000, 2010, 2024; Leuzinger-Bohleber & Montigny, 2021).

It is against this background that we believe a new appreciation of any form of science emerges. It is well known that all autocratic leaders have a common enemy: science and its goal of investigating and understanding complex realities in international and interdisciplinary networks, even if this leads to uncomfortable findings, as is the case in climate research. Psychoanalysis, with its specific subject of research, unconscious fantasies and conflicts, and the richness of contemporary psychoanalytic research tools, is also part of this international scientific community (see Leuzinger-Bohleber, 2021).

However, some authors in this volume discuss that in our narcissistic age, even science is not immune to misuse. As Stänicke and Nissen-Lie discuss, it can be observed, for example, in the field of comparative psychotherapy research, that narcissistic fantasies of omnipotence in science can be used to deny human vulnerability and mortality. Therapists and researchers are asked to transform into "superhuman who can quickly solve complex, mental, societal and existential life challenges" (Stänicke & Nissen-Lie, p.7 in their chapter). In contrast, the attempt not to deny one's own vulnerability and mortality in the sense of negative capability (Bion, 1961, 1962), but to keep it in mind, leads to an attitude of modesty, caution and constant critical self-reflection in both therapy and science. To achieve such an attitude seems to be a shared aim in many different forms of practice and research in contemporary psychoanalysis as we try to discuss in this volume.

Part I: Narcissism in Society and Culture deals with the social danger posed by the close, unconscious link between extreme destructiveness and pathological narcissism. As *Otto Kernberg* explains in the first chapter, summarizing his groundbreaking research of several decades, it is historical crises that lead to regressive processes in large groups and create unconscious preferences for leaders with a narcissistic personality disorder. Personalities with a malignant, destructive narcissism are often masters at seducing individuals in large groups. This leads to an extremely dangerous constellation. The atrocities committed by the National Socialists, for example, are a warning historical example of such extremely destructive societal processes.

Werner Bohleber, reflecting his years of experiences with psychoanalyses with patients with extreme destructiveness, deepens this knowledge by showing that ubiquitous, early fantasies of purity and unity, i.e. of merging with the primary object, are one source of the unconscious attraction of nationalist and fundamentalist ideologies.

Siri Erika Gullestad, asking what makes a person joining an ideology that justifies the sacrifice of innocent people by reference to a superior aim. Is it possible that the demonization of Muslims "fits" into a psychologically threatened universe and a murderous lust for revenge? Gullestad explains in detail the narcissistic, omnipotent fantasy world of the Norwegian terrorist Anders B. Breivik and its murderous effects critically reflecting on the dialectic relationship between personality and ideology.

Gerd Koenen, a historian and expert on contemporary Russia, outlines the current social situation in Russia, which made it possible for an unscrupulous, narcissistic personality like Vladimir Putin to lead his country into the war with Ukraine. Koenen's historical knowledge is a necessary addition to a psychoanalytic attempt to contribute to an understanding of the complex current situation.

Part II: Narcissism: Clinical Practice and Research is devoted to insights gained from years of clinical and conceptual research in psychoanalyses and long-term psychoanalytic treatments with patients with narcissistic pathology as well as from other forms of psychoanalytic research of these phenomena.

Rogério Lerner and colleagues make an analysis of potential underlying intrapsychic dynamics related to narcissism of two patients diagnosed with Autism Spectrum Disorders from the point of view of the Object Relations Theory using the Structured Interview of Personality Organization—Revised (STIPO-R) (Clarkin et al., 2016).

Mark Solms, representing interdisciplinary psychoanalytic research in this volume, takes up Otto Kernberg's thesis that narcissistic development cannot be separated from the development of drives and object relations. Using the neurobiological modification of Freud's theory of drives by Jaak Panksepp, he shows the narcissistic dimension in all basic emotions and drives (such as seeking, lust, care, play, fear, rage/anger and sadness/panic).

Stephan Doering summarizes the definitions and views of narcissistic psychopathologies in psychiatry and offers an overview of the diagnosis of narcissistic disorders within the framework of ICD-11 and DSM-V. The research group around John Clarkin and Otto Kernberg have been trying for years to build bridges between psychoanalytic research on narcissism and the world of psychiatry. They have conducted several studies with patients with narcissistic personality disorder and Borderline patients. *John Clarkin* summarizes the most important findings in his chapter.

Stephan Hau discusses the problems of conceptualizing personality disorders (starting with Emil Kraepelin vs. Kurt Schneider), then briefly traces the history of personality disorders in the DSM and ICD and takes the latest change in ICD-11 as an opportunity to build a bridge to psychoanalytic diagnostics (OPD), whereby the complexity of the term "personality disorder" becomes clear. This has implications for (psychoanalytic) research.

Part III: Confronting Contemporary Cultural Challenges takes up some current political debates and reflects on whether and in what way psychoanalysis can contribute. One of the controversial discussions focuses the development of narcissism in one particular developmental phase, the so called Emerging Adulthood[5].

Erik Stänicke and Helene Nissen-Lie present in their chapter critical reflections about our zeitgeist. They discuss theories with a critique of modernity, the challenge psychoanalysis faces in our time. We live in a time that praises efficiency, and they discuss if psychoanalysis affords a worldview that is an important corrective of our time but, for the same reason, may be quite unpopular.

One particularly hot social debate concerning developmental processes that is often conducted with strong emotions and ideological positions is the so-called transgender debate, as *Siri Erika Gullestad* illustrates in her article. Gullestad discusses how psychoanalysts today are faced with the challenge of encountering transgender people seeking treatment in a quickly changing and multi-polarized cultural environment. She presents some of the theoretical and epistemological questions implied in this often-polarized debate and argues that we need to integrate rapidly developing ideas of gender identity, sex and sexuality without falling back on normative models.

Line Indrevoll Stänicke will address another hot topic in this context: the influence of the digital age on developmental processes of adolescents. Online activity is discussed as having transitional qualities—an intermediate area in between the inner and outer world (Winnicott's, 1974). Engagement in self-harm content online may serve as a transitional object for illusions, play, and relational and personal exploration. However, both self-harm and the online engagement come with a risk for increased mental health difficulties.

Inge Seiffge-Krenke, one of the leading psychoanalytic researchers on Emerging Adulthood in Germany, offers an overview of empirical studies in this field, studies which add a new perspective—developmental findings, based on large investigations on non-clinical samples in many countries to psychoanalytic perspective. The narcissistic phenomena are largely temporary, as they often resolve with the transition to adulthood and the assumption of adult roles and tasks. However, there are some new aspects: It has actually been shown that some phenomena that we previously attributed to clinically conspicuous patients can now also be found in the normal population.

The last two chapters of the volume are based on one central research tradition, which is closely connected to the Research Committee of the IPA: the attempt to combine clinical and extraclinical research. *Marianne Leuzinger-Bohleber* summarizes in her chapter fist clinical findings from the MODE Study. In her short overview, 42% of the 112 included chronic-depressed, early-traumatized patients were between 20 and 30 years old, which means in the developmental phase of emerging adulthood. On the basis of a brief summary of today's psychoanalytic theories of depression, she shows the close connection between narcissism, depression and trauma and illustrates this with two short case studies (see also Bleichmar, 2010; Bohleber & Leuzinger-Bohleber, 2016). *Tamara Fischmann, Gilles Ambresin and Marianne Leuzinger-Bohleber* clinically illustrate this connection in a single case study. They summarize a psychoanalysis with a young woman who had withdrawn into a narcissistic bubble and extreme social and psychic retreat in great detail. The authors then show that the changes of dreams contain indicators for a transformation of the inner object-world of this patient, first from a clinical psychoanalytic perspective and afterward—in the sense of a methodological triangulation—with the Zurich Dream Process Coding System (ZDPCS).

Thus, this volume presents a broad spectrum of approaches for understanding narcissism, from cultural-theoretical and social perspectives, to clinical-psychoanalytic observations and conceptual clarifications of terms, to new interdisciplinary and extra-clinical-psychoanalytic research results. All of this serves to sensitize the readers of this volume to the socially and clinically highly relevant topic of the fluid transition from healthy, narcissistic self-esteem regulation to severely pathological forms of malignant, destructive narcissism in individuals, groups and in societies. It illustrates the creative potential that clinical research in psychoanalysis still has to make a contribution to interdisciplinary dialog on pressing social problems. The unique opportunity to spend hundreds of sessions studying the unconscious determinants of pathological narcissism is still one of the indispensable research paths of psychoanalysis. This is why Freud's discovery of so-called Junktim research, i.e. the inseparable link between healing and research (Freud, 1926), seems as topical as ever.

The IPA's psychoanalytic community has grown steadily over the last 100 years and now numbers around 14,000 psychoanalysts around the world. Many of them have contributed through case reports, still the core of psychoanalytic research, to a detailed understanding of the unconscious determinants underlying narcissistic personality disorders, but also that— in the best cases—psychoanalysis can help this group of patients to change their inner object world and their pathological defenses against dependencies on their own body, other people and social realities. This can help to dispense with the omnipotent fantasy of the spherical man (Aristophanes), to be able to satisfy oneself and not need anyone, but also no one, in order to be able to live. As clinically illustrated by many examples in this volume, this defense against traumatic experiences serves to cope with an unbearable flood of fear of death and panic in a situation of total dependency. As Bohleber (2010), among others, has described, this leads to a breakdown of basic trust in a helping other and one's own self-agency. As has now also been empirically shown, one of the specific possibilities of psychoanalysis is to help traumatized patients to understand the traumatization they have suffered and its consequences and thereby find a new meaning to their lives (Krakau et al., 2024). In the best case scenario, these patients don't have to cope with trauma and loss with the help of pathological narcissistic defenses anymore.

Of course, psychoanalysts are not the only professional group to have this knowledge. Writers, artists and filmmakers, in particular, impressively illustrate the close connection between trauma, depression and narcissism in their works. Let us therefore conclude this brief introduction mentioning just one single example: the recently released movie *One Life* by James Hawes, based on the novel by Barbara Winton: *If It's Not Impossible*. In the last months before the World War II, the young English banker Nicholas Winton rescues 669 mostly Jewish children from Nazi extermination in an adventurously organized transport of children from Prague to England.

Anthony Hopkins' great acting performance reminds us that he—due to his mature level of mental functioning—feels a great distance to any form of narcissistic defense against powerlessness and dependency. When he is to be honored publicly for his achievements after many years, he feels embarrassed. His memories of the terrible traumatic events are too vivid in his mind. The traumatic experience for him of not succeeding in bringing the last transport of children, the 9th train with 250 children, to London safely. Therefore, all these children were murdered in the Holocaust. In the sense of the depressive position, his gratitude for his experience that he succeeded in this rescue together with others hundreds of threatened children is inseparable connected in his mind with the traumatic experience of failure, of powerlessness, helplessness and horror at what people can do to people.

What a topical message in the face of the real danger through the worldwide network of pathologically narcissistic autocrats, described by Anne Applebaum!

February, 2025: The Editors: Marianne Leuzinger-Bohleber, Stephan Hau, Rogério Lerner, Erik Stänicke, Siri Erika Gullestad

Notes

1 "Autocracies are not controlled by a single villain, but by sophisticated networks with kleptocratic structures, a complex security apparatus of army, paramilitaries and police, and technical experts responsible for surveillance, propaganda and disinformation … The propagandists share their resources—troll farms and media outlets that spread the lies of one dictator can also spread those of another—and have common themes: the decline of democracy, the stability of autocracy, and the evil United States …" (Anne Applebaum, 2024, pp.9–10).

2 P/S is an abbreviation for Paranoid/Schizoid.

3 The *perverse* part of the psyche stands closer to the psychotic realm and is motivated by omnipotence, envy, and hatred. Perversity involves efforts to destroy reality largely through obliterating obstacles, boundaries, and differences.

4 Diamond (in print) gives a striking example for this polarization: "Populism in the American situation *turns destructive*, especially through highlighting the attacks on consensual reality and democratic ideals. The ethos of the democratic truth process—namely, a shared version of reality—have been under threat even prior to Trump's brazen lying and trading in misinformation. Trump himself, however, is not the essential problem, although he certainly expresses what originated in the 1980s, and as such Trumpism has been created over the course of several decades. Trump's rise to power and cult of personality have exposed *unresolvable* divisions that many Americans have not been particularly aware of, culminating in highly polarized media bubbles in which the question becomes "who gets to say what is true?" (p.11.) When Diamond wrote this text, he could not have imagined the extent to which his analysis would be confirmed in 2025. Donald Trump and his administration are waging an unprecedented war against all forms of science and its pursuit of objectivity and reliable knowledge. In addition, he is systematically destroying institutional structures in public administration, universities and the independent press that are committed to the educational ideal of objective facts and the investigation of complex realities.

5 Flynn and Skogstad (2006) summarize the well known close connection between narcissism and adolescence: "In adolescence, features of narcissism are ever present. Intense, self-interested or overvalued views of oneself, one's body, or ideas and capacities and so on, arise quite easily, fluidly and continuously … and they collapse equally easily, often into despair, disillusion and contradictory states of

feeling, sometimes characterized by loss of self-esteem or hope, often leaving the adolescent ridden with guilt and self-loathing. Such shifts, indeed swings, continue until some more secure sense of identity and sense of personal value is established as part of the developmental task of adolescence" (p.35).

References

Abram, J. (2021). On Winnicott's concept of trauma. *The International Journal of Psychoanalysis, 102*(4), 778–793.

Abram, J., & Hinshelwood, R. D. (2018). *The clinical paradigms of melanie klein and donald winnicott: Comparisons and dialogues.* London: Routledge.

Applebaum. A. (2024). *Autocracy, inc.* New York: Doubleday.

Auchincloss, E. L., & Samberg, E. (2021). *Psychoanalytic terms & concepts.* New Haven: Yale University Press (American Psychoanalytic Association).

Balint, M. (1952). *Primary love and psychic analytic technique.* London: Hogarth Press.

Bick, E. (1968). The experience of the skin in early object-relations. *The International Journal of Psychoanalysis, 49*, 484–486.

Bion, W. (1961). *Experiences in groups and other papers.* London: Tavistock.

Bion, W. (1962). The psycho-analytic study of thinking. *The International Journal of Psychoanalysis, 43*, 306–310.

Bleichmar, H. (2010). Rethinking pathological grief: Different types and therapeutic approaches. The *Psychoanalytic Quarterly, 79*, 71–94.

Bohleber, W. (2000). The development of trauma theory in psychoanalysis. *Psyche–Z Psychoanal, 54*(9–10), 797–839.

Bohleber, W. (2010). *Destructiveness, intersubjectivity and trauma: The identity crisis of modern psychoanalysis.* London: Karnac.

Bohleber, W. (2023). Self-agency and self-reflection – building blocks for a dual self theory. In S. Gullestad, S., E. Stänicke, E., & M. Leuzinger-Bohleber (eds.), *Psychoanalytic studies of change. An integrative perspective.* London: Routledge, 101–113.

Bohleber, W. (2024). Purity and unity: Narcissism and destructiveness in nationalistic and fundamentalistic ideologies. *American Imago, 81*, 1–16.

Bohleber, W., & Leuzinger, M. (1981). Narcissism and adolescence. In Psychoanalytic Seminar Zurich (ed.), *The new theories of narcissism. Back to paradise?* Frankfurt a. M: Syndikat, 117–131.

Bohleber, W., & Leuzinger-Bohleber, M. (2016). The special problem of interpretation in the treatment of traumatised patients. *Psychoanalytic Inquiry, 36*, 60–76.

Bott Spillius, E., Milton, J., Garvey, P., Couve, C., & Steiner, D. (2011). *The New Dictionary of Kleinian Thought.* London: Routledge.

Clarkin, J. F., Caligor, E., Stern, B., & Kernberg, O. F. (2016). *The structured interview for personality organization-revised (STIPO-R).* New York: Weill Medical College of Cornell University.

Diamond, M. (in prep). A psychoanalytic perspective on malignancies in the American Psyche: Containing destructive populism, large group regression, and cultism. Will be published in 2025 in the Special Issue (edited by M. Leuzinger-Bohleber and G. Schlesinger-Kipp), *Medea and jason: A disturbingly topical story. Psychoanalytical reflections on migration, trauma and social realities.* International Journal for Applied Psychoanalytic Studies.

Ehrenberg, A. (1998/2016). *The weariness of the self: Diagnosing the history of depression in the contemporary age*. Montreal: McGill-Queen's Press-MQUP.

Enns, P. K., Colner, J., Kumar, A., & Lagodny, J. (2024). Understanding Biden's Excot and the 2024 Election. The State Presidential Approval/State Economy Model. PS: Political Science & Politics, First View, pp. 1–8. DOI:https://doi.org/10.1017/S1049096524000994

Flynn, D., & Skogstad, H. (2006). Facing towards or turning away from destructive narcissism. *Journal of Child Psychotherapy, 32*(1), 35–48.

Freud, S. (1914). On narcissism: An introduction. *Standard Edition, 14,* 67–102.

Freud, S. (1921). Group psychology and the analysis of the ego. *Standard Edition, 18,* 63–143.

Freud, S. (1926). The question of lay analysis. *Standard Edition, 20,* 177–258.

Freud, S. (1930). Civilisation and its discontents. *Standard Edition, 21,* 57–146.

Gallese, V. (2023). From pre-natal relations to self-constitution. A neuro-behavioral perspective on primary narcissism. Unpublished paper given at the Joseph Sandler Conference in Vienna, October 2023 (will be published in the International Journal of Psychoanalysis).

Green, A. (1998). The moral narcissism. *Psyche–Z Psychoanal, 52*(5), 415–449.

Green, A. (2001). Death drive, negative narcissism, desobjectalisation function. *Psyche–Z Psychoanal, 55*(9–10), 869–877.

Green, A. (2005). Chapter 13 *The work of the negative*. Key ideas for a contemporary psychoanalysis. *Misrecognition and Recognition of the Unconscious, 49,* 212–226.

Green, A. (2007). Pulsions de destruction et maladies somatiques. *Revue française de Psychosomatique* (2), 45–70.

Han, B.-C. (2015). *The burnout society*. Stanford: Stanford University Press.

Hartmann, H. (1939). *Ego-psychology and the problem of adaptation*. New York: International University Press, 1958.

Jacobson, E. (1971). *On the psychoanalytic theory of affects. Depression: Comparative studies of normal, neurotic and psychotic states*. New York: International Universities Press, 3–41.

Kernberg, O. F. (1970). Factors in the psychoanalytic treatment of narcissistic personalities. *Journal of the American Psychoanalytic Association, 18,* 51–85.

Kernberg, O. F. (1975). *Borderline conditions and pathological narcissism*. New York: Jason Aronson.

Kernberg, O. F. (1984). *Severe personality disorders: Psychotherapeutic strategies*. New Haven: Yale University Press.

Kernberg, O. F. (2014). An overview of the treatment of severe narcissistic pathology. *The International Journal of Psychoanalysis, 95*(5), 865–888.

Klein, M. (1946). Notes on some schizoid mechanisms. *The International Journal of Psychoanalysis, 27,* 99–110.

Klein, M. (1952). Some theoretical conclusions regarding the emotional life of the infant. In: *Envy and gratitude. And other works 1947–1963.* (pp.61–93), London: Hogarth Press, 1975.

Kogan, I. (2020). *Narcissistic fantasies in film and fiction: Masters of the universe*. London: Routledge.

Kohut, H. (1966). Forms and transformations of narcissism. *Journal of the American Psychoanalytic Association, 14,* 243–272.

Kohut, H. (1977). *The restoration of the self*. New York: International Universities Press.

Kohut, H. (1984). *How does analysis cure?* Chicago: University of Chicago Press.

Krakau, L., Ernst, M., Hautzinger, M., Beutel, M. E., & Leuzinger-Bohleber, M. (2024). Childhood trauma and differential response to long-term psychoanalytic versus cognitive-behavioural therapy for chronic depression in adults. *The British Journal of Psychiatry, 225*(4), 446–453. doi:10.1192/bjp.2024.112

Laplanche, J., & Pontalis, J.-B. (1973). *Das vokabular der psychoanalyse.* Frankfurt: Suhrkamp.

Lasch, C. (2019). The culture of narcissism. In *American social character.* London: Routledge, 241–267.

Leuzinger-Bohleber, M. (2021). Psychoanalysis as a plural science of the unconscious. *General Journal of Philosophy, 46*(2), 253–267.

Leuzinger-Bohleber, M. (2024). *Depression: A Contemporary introduction.* London: Routledge.

Leuzinger-Bohleber, M., & Montigny, N. (2021). The pandemic as a developmental risk. *International Journal of Applied Psychoanalytic Studies, 18*(2), 121–132.

PDM Task Force. (2006). *Psychodynamic diagnostic manual.* Silver Spring: Alliance of Psychoanalytic Organizations.

Rosa, H. (2013). *Social acceleration: A new theory of modernity.* New York: Columbia University Press.

Rosenfeld, H. (1964). On the psychopathology of narcissism: A clinical approach. *The International Journal of Psychoanalysis, 45,* 332–337.

Rosenfeld, H. (1987). *Impasse and interpretation.* London: Tavistock Press.

Roussillon, R. (2010). The deconstruction of primary narcissism. *The International Journal of Psychoanalysis, 91*(4), 821–837.

Sandler, J., & Joffe, W. D. (1965). Depression in childhood. *International Journal of Applied Psychoanalytic Studies, 46,* 88–96.

Sennett, R., & Richter, M. (1998). *Der flexible mensch: Die kultur des neuen kapitalismus.* Berlin-Verlag.

Van der Waals, H. G. (1966). Problems of narcissism. *Bulletin of the Menninger Clinic, 29,* 293–311.

Westen, D. (1990). *The relations among narcissism, egocentrism, self-concept, and self-esteem: Experimental, clinical, and theoretical considerations.* Psychoanalysis & Contemporary Thought.

Whitebook, J. (2017). *Freud: An intellectual biography.* New York: Cambridge University Press.

Winnicott, D. W. (1965). *The maturational process and the facilitating environment.* New York. International Universities Press.

Winnicott, D. W. (1974). Fear of breakdown. *International Review of Psycho-Analysis, 1,* 103–107.

Wurmser, L. (2015). Primary shame, mortal wound and tragic circularity: Some new reflections on shame and shame conflicts. *The International Journal of Psychoanalysis, 96*(6), 1615–1634.

Ziehe, Th. (1979). *Pubertät und Narzissmus: Sind Jugendliche entpolitisiert?* Berlin: Europäische Verlagsanstalt.

Zienert-Eilts, K. J. (2020). Destructive populism as "perverted containing": A psychoanalytical look at the attraction of Donald Trump. *The International Journal of Psychoanalysis, 101,* 971–991.

Part I

Narcissism in society and culture

1 Malignant narcissism and large group regression[1]

Otto F. Kernberg

From a psychoanalytic perspective, we have to recognize that a psychoanalytic understanding only covers a limited area of the complex social forces triggered by the interaction of regressed large groups and the corresponding pathological leadership: the nature of historical determinants of the formation of social subgroups; the origin of cultural, social, political, religious and social bias; the cause of present traumatic circumstances; and the political system within which regressed large groups consolidate are important determinants that influence the development of such leadership-followers' constellations. Does psychoanalytic understanding have anything to say about whether and how we can use our present-day understanding to help prevent such calamitous situations in the future?

The purpose of this chapter is to analyze the mutual relationships between large group regression and the emergence of a particular kind of leadership related to that regressive process, namely, leaders with the characteristics of the syndrome of malignant narcissism. The main hypothesis to be explored is that the nature of large group regression translates into the search for that particular personality type—and that personalities with the syndrome of malignant narcissism are prone to aspire leadership and are very effective in achieving leadership of the regressed large group under these conditions. In turn, the mutual influence of the culture of the regressed large group and its corresponding ideological development and the characteristic behaviors of a leader evincing malignant narcissism stimulates typical behaviors in the leader. In turn, the corresponding leadership reinforces some basic characteristics of regressed large groups. To explore that linkage, we shall review briefly the concept of regression in group processes, studying group psychology both in large groups and "mass" psychology, and in small groups, reviewing the relevant contributions by Freud, Bion, Turquet, Volkan, and others. This review will be followed by the exploration of the preferred personality structures of leadership fostered by these different group structures, and the relationship between functional leadership and pathological leadership related to the requirements expressed in group regression. I then shall summarize briefly the syndrome of malignant narcissism and its derivative leadership characteristics in social institutions and the political process at large.

DOI: 10.4324/9781003565284-3

Psychoanalytic group psychology

Freud, in his 1921 text on "Group Psychology and the Analysis of the Ego" outlined what became one of the most original and tragically relevant contributions to the study of the Dynamic Unconscious, namely, the behavior of what in German is called "Masse." It refers to mass movements, or large conglomerates of people united by a common ideal, a common sense of identity related to race, religion, nationality, or a particular ideology that unifies this enormous conglomerate of individuals in an active direction or cohesive move under the direction of a particular leader. This mass psychology has to be differentiated from the situation of crowds, that is, the accidental getting together of an enormous number of people as part of usual social interactions, without any common direction or sense of a specific mutual relationship. Freud described political mass movements, particularly of fascism and communism, years before the common characteristics of mass movements and their consequences had been experienced dramatically, as it evolved in the 20th and now in the 21st centuries.

Freud pointed out that the individual who senses himself as part of such a mass movement acquires a reduced capacity for independent judgment and rational decision-making. To the contrary, what dominates the individuals within the mass movement is a sense of power by mutual identification, a sense of belonging and power derived from being part of such a large movement. It is their mutual identification that coincides with their identification with the leader of the mass movement, which provides them with a sense of shared identity, an identification with the leader who is not only powerful and idealized but also feared. At the same time, he assumes consciously and in the mind of his followers, the responsibility for the direction of the movement, and frees all the individuals from themselves having to make decisions about that movement. More generally, mass psychology induces the projection onto the leader of the individuals' ego ideal, so that moral consciousness is projected onto the leader and the individuals in the mass feel free from moral constraints. They acquire a degree of freedom that goes together with a characteristic activation of intense affective dispositions shared by the entire mass, and is particularly of an aggressive, destructive type, the target of which is directed outside the mass movement. As part of mass psychology, the participants feel powerful and secure and united in the free, unconstrained, and personally irresponsible participation in aggression against outside, feared, hated, and depreciated groups who are perceived as threatening the mass movement. The shared sense of equality, power, and freedom from moral constraints is the counterpart to a heightened suggestibility to the commands from the leader, a suggestibility enhanced by the decrease of rational, independent judgment induced by the psychology of the mass movement.

Wilfred Bion's (1961) analysis of the relation between groups and their leadership introduced a new method of psychoanalytic exploration of group psychology. As a courageous and effective tank commander in the First World War, and in his later work as a psychiatrist in military psychiatric hospitals and War Office Selection Boards during the Second World War, he developed professional experiences with both effective task groups and regressed, demoralized ones, and their leadership. He combined his psychoanalytic training and Tavistock Clinic experience, the application of Kleinian concepts of splitting and projective identification in individual treatments with his group studies and experiences in what became a new field of psychoanalytic inquiry.

Bion's (1961) studies of small group psychology provided a complementary analysis of the intimate processes affecting the regression of individuals when they are part of a group process. He described the behavior evolving in small groups of 10 to 15 members that were exclusively engaged in observing their own experiences and behavior in limited time sessions from one to two hours. He observed typical developments that he described as the "basic assumptions groups" of "dependency," "fight-flight," and "pairing." These "basic assumptions" groups emerged typically and consistently when such a small group had no specific task that would justify its existence and link it with an environment by a concrete objective that has to be accomplished. A group that gets together with a task of learning a determined subject, developing a particular project, or constructing particular objects represents "work groups" that operate rationally and with a realistic organization of the development of the particular group task. When such a task does not exist and the only group task is the observation of the group itself and the emotional consequences of such a lack of a specific task, then the basic assumptions emerge.

The basic assumption of "dependency" is characterized by a general sense of insecurity, uncertainty, and immaturity on the part of members of the group, who look for a leader who will help them understand their situation, direct the group, provide their needs, feed them with knowledge, meaning, or security, a leader who presents self-assurance and an attitude of potency and knowledge that is supportive and reassuring, provokes his idealization by the group, and the wish to depend on him. Competition for becoming the preferred "child" of that leader, mutual jealously for the amount of attention each member of the group gets from their idealized leader, illustrates the fact that this self-assured, knowledgeable, giving leader provides a sense of safety and security in being part of the group. In contrast, fear and insecurity develop if one falls outside the assured membership of such a group. If the leader does not provide the assurance of the gratification of the group's dependency needs, the members of the group experience strong disappointment or disillusionment, search for an alternative leader in the group who may replace him, idealize the new leader while attributing to him the attributes they had seen in the previous leader, and expect him to carry out the needed function of leadership of the dependent group.

The situation in the basic assumption group of "fight-flight" is completely different. Here there is a sense of tension and conflict, a preparedness to fight against out groups, and a sense of group unity as part of this fighting disposition against out-groups. Sometimes, when there is no such evident adversary out-group, a division of the very group evolves into an "in-group" who stands with the leader, and an "out-group" that fights the leader and the in-group. The search here is for a strong, self-righteous, distrustful, and controlling leader, who provides leadership in the struggle with the enemy out-group or the rebellious subgroup. In contrast to the predominance, in the dependent group, of mechanisms of primitive idealization, regressive dependency, and denial of all conflicts around authority issues, here, in the fight-flight group, there is a remarkable development of splitting operations between "us" and "them," the in-group and the out-group, a sharp differentiation between the idealization of the in-group and the projection of aggression and attacks on the out-group, and a tendency to submit to the leader as part of the psychology of a shared sense of discipline required by the fight against assumed enemies. Splitting, projective identification, and denial of aggression within the internal subgroup go hand in hand with the search for a leader who will gratify the need for this organization, usually a powerful individual with paranoid features who fits the group's demand for a sharp division between the ideal inner world of the group, and a dangerous threatening external world that needs to be fought off. In the "pairing" group, finally, a still different atmosphere prevails. Here the group selects a couple, heterosexual or homosexual, that the group perceives as united, bound together by mutual identification, love, and commitment. The group admires the couple, because it corresponds to the wish for establishing such an ideal couple love relationship, an ideal shared by all the members and expressed in this idealization but also in the related need to fight off envious feelings about this selected ideal couple. There is a sexual quality in the air, an erotized quality of relations that differs from both the regressed dependent relations of the dependent group, and from the tense, aggressive challenging and distrustful atmosphere of the fight-flight group. While the dependent group preferably selects a leader with strong narcissistic features, the fight-flight group selects a leader with paranoid features, and the pairing group a leader who tolerates the development of such a pair, helps to protect it, and conveys the assurance to the group that the erotic quality of the development of intimate relations is tolerated and welcome. The "pairing" group represents a less regressive, "Oedipal" group experience.

Within the growing interest in developing Bion's approach to groups at the Tavistock Clinic, Pierre Turquet's (1975) work stands out. With a related background in military medical services to Bion's, Turquet expanded the study of regressed group behavior to larger family groups and social institutions and, in following Bion's approach, he carried out empirical work with larger groups. He studied the behavior of large groups. These were experimental groups of 100 to 300 members, also gathered only to study the nature of their experiences and behavior over a period of an hour and a half to two hours, with the provision of a group leader. This leader, similarly to the leader provided to small groups, limits himself or herself to comment on dominant emotional experiences shared by the group, without assuming the particular leadership functions demanded by the group. The small groups establish by themselves particular expectations from the leader, once they are clearly in the dependent, fight-flight, or pairing position; the "professional" group leader will not gratify but analyze their emotional needs. Thus, the leaders that have been described for the small groups are selected and seduced into their respective leadership function in terms of the corresponding psychology of the respective small group. A similar phenomenon happens in the large group. The large group, usually, as I mentioned, composed of a membership between 100 and a maximum 300 persons, get together in concentric circles, that permit the members of still seeing each other and responding to each other—similarly as in the small group, but evidently this situation reduces enormously the possibility of the constitution of cohesive, small subgroups. All the individuals of the large group are much more isolated from each other than is the case of small group psychology.

The large group meets without any particular task except to experience and discuss its own developments. Every member has the right to speak up at any moment, and the professional group leader limits himself/herself to observing, from time to time, the dominant emotional issues affecting the group. The leader does not organize the development of any subject of the group discussions at any point. Here, again, if the large group were "structured," organized to carry out a certain task, for example, to discuss or decide about a particular subject around which it would establish an order or procedure of order and time limitations within which individuals can speak up, this would transform the group into a "work group" and become realistically focused on and occupied with such a task. The unstructured large group, to the contrary, is totally open to whatever anybody in the group may feel like saying or doing.

The typical development in such a large group situation is an enormous sense of loss of personal identity, as the individual in it cannot reliably find a commonality with anybody else. In the large group situation, efforts emerge to establish subgroups on the basis of whatever members may try to find as commonalities: needs, language, religion, profession, political views, race, or appearance of any kind; but these efforts usually fail and the group develops rapidly a collective sense of intense anxiety. While people speak freely, there is a tendency not to listen to what other people are saying. Individuals who speak up obtain no feedback. Clear efforts at projective identification fail because of the difficulty to focus on and control the reactions of others to oneself. There is a general sense of impotence and fearfulness that develops in the members, and a fear of aggression to explode in the group. At times, the group is able to identify a small subgroup within the large group or outside it, and gather around a joined, intense hate reaction against such a subgroup. This, temporarily, transforms the large group into a small mass that fights an external enemy, but even such efforts usually fail.

A tendency develops in the group for individuals to emerge that are trying to analyze rationally what is happening. It is characteristic for the large group that particularly intelligent, self-reflective, rational people are shut down immediately. To the contrary, naive, cliché formulating individuals who have a simplistic statement to make tend to be supported, with a slightly derogatory, amused attitude by the group at large, but at the same time, with a shared sense of relief, and such cliché spreading mediocrities are preferentially selected as leader of the large group. The group conveys the impression that there is a shared envy of individuals who maintain their individuality, security, rationality, and, with such a capacity, attempt to provide group leadership, while there is support of a mediocre leadership that reassures everybody and provides a calming sense of security while at the same time there is a shared subtle devaluation of that selected leader.

As an alternative development, if the intensity of anxiety and aggressive feelings is excessive, the group may veer into a paranoid direction. It selects a paranoid individual who finds a cause to fight against, a group, or an intolerable social condition, something in the external world which everybody agrees needs to be fought against and potentially destroyed. Thus, the large group, at the bottom, oscillates between the search for a narcissistic leader with a nonthreatening, simplistic quality that can be depreciated and promises a tranquilizing passivity, or else, under activation of an excessive degree of aggression, a powerful paranoid leader who unifies the group into a fighting attitude that transforms the large group into a small "mass psychology" group as described by Freud.

Vamik Volkan (2004) has expanded greatly our understanding of group psychology with what he refers to as large group regression, but what has to be differentiated from the large group as originally described by Turquet (1975) and others. Both Bion and Turquet studied artificial groups, brought together for the purpose of observing group behavior. Volkan's work focuses on the study of naturally occurring groups, especially in times of crisis. Volkan, in fact, refers to mass psychology in the sense of Freud's analysis of the psychology of large conglomerates united by a sense of mutual cohesiveness, equality, and fraternity and a common set of ideas—a common ideology—that expresses their unifying disposition, including the potential relationship to an idealized, feared, and/or direction signaling leader. Volkan studied group psychological behavior in international conflicts and conflicts between nationalistic or religious opposite political groups and, particularly, the psychological developments related to the traumatic effects of the terrorist attack in New York on September 11 2001.

In summary, Volkan proposes that, under conditions of traumatic situations, social revolutions, nature-caused disasters, economic crisis, and, generally speaking, the collapse of traditional cultural structures that regulate the daily life of the individual, the strong possibility of a large group regression develops, within which the normal social structure that assures the individual of his status—role relationships—disappears. Under such conditions, there evolves a threat to normal identity that ordinarily is reinforced by the status and role conditions of every individual within this social and cultural environment. There now evolves a search for a "second skin," a new external social structure that returns the security that had protected individual identity and sense of security. Here the emergence of a large group leader becomes important in providing to the social group in crisis a voice that reconfirms their commonality, the sense of a common ideology that assures the large group of its basic existential security, historical mission, and goodness, and differentiates it from external enemies or enemy situations that had been threatening it. The leader calls for joint action to stand up and, in short, provides the large group with a new sense of identity in terms of all the individuals belonging to that mass movement.

There is a tendency of a large group in an existential social crisis to rally blindly around such a leader, who eliminates the traditional status and role relations of individuals derived mostly from their belonging to a family, to specific relations to family members, and to the social group related to it. The leader creates a new collective "family" structure in terms of the historical importance and mission of the group. The community becomes divided into a "good" segment (the large group) that obediently follows the leader, and a "bad" segment of those perceived as opposing the leader. A sharp division between "us" and "them" is established, and "them" become enemies that need to be fought off, defended against, and attacked. The large group develops a sense of shared morality of the "good" system that becomes increasingly absolutist and punitive toward those who are in conflict with it, and the group may experience periods of massive mood swings from shared depressed feelings over the nature of the critical or dramatic situation that originated the present situation, to collective paranoid projection of aggression towards outsiders. The sense of internal goodness becomes a sense of entitlement and a gradual distortion of reality, in which unpleasant and threatening aspects of reality are denied. There evolve new cultural phenomena or modified versions of traditional social customs with particular focus on joint traumas and past triumphs of the group residing in a time collapse in which past and present are confused. The leadership feeds into this collapse of the time perspective by creating a break in the actual historical continuity of the group, and filling the gap with a "new" nationalism, a new shared sentience or a "new" morality, and a transformation of the actual history of the group.

The large group members begin to experience shared symbols as "proto-symbols," including shared images that depict enemy groups with symbols or protosymbols associated with bodily waste, vermin, dangerous, or toxic animal traits. The large group consolidates its unity by erecting sharp boundaries with the outside world, focusing on minor differences between itself and enemy groups, and searches powerfully for commonalities in its natural condition, origin, and convictions as part of their new "second skin" that protects its identity. The large group may initiate behaviors that symbolize its purification. It may change its attitude toward aesthetics, to what is considered beautiful and ugly, and there is a tendency for the large group to turn the physical environment into an amorphous gray-brown, (fecal or decomposing) structure. All these characteristics constitute an ideologically fundamented, consolidated, and expressively lived activation of the clear, separate "second skin" identity that provides the combination of security, power, freedom, moral superiority, and irresponsibility described by Freud for mass psychology. Volkan's analysis enriches and bridges the analysis of large group psychology by Turquet with Freud's analysis of mass psychology.

The combined analysis of group regression, from small group regression to large group regression and to mass psychology, illustrates some basic commonalities of these various processes. The motive for group regression, in all cases, is a loss of the functional relationship of individuals within a stable, small or large social, and cultural structure. This social and cultural structure is given by an ordinary living situation within a stable social environment not threatened by major political, international, or economic catastrophes or nature determined calamities. And, in the case of small groups, the loss of the functional tasks of the group by design or other circumstances replicates temporarily that loss of functional stability of the individual. This loss of the traditional social structure signifies a threat to individual identity and it signals the extent to which normal identity function is supported and assured by the individual's psychosocial environment. Massive loss of such a protective environment that simultaneously affects a selected group or an entire community leads to powerful anxiety and initiates regressive functions.

It is significant that the anxiety, in all cases, has to do with a threat of a definite experience of danger, the activation of negative, aggressive affect states, and correspondent defensive operations that we know from the study of severe psychopathology of individuals with primitive aggressive aggression dominated conflicts. These defensive operations, particularly splitting mechanisms, projective identification, denial, primitive idealization and devaluation, omnipotent control—all of them described by Melanie Klein (1946) as characteristic of the paranoid-schizoid position—emerge in the dependent and fight/flight group, where they structure the group within the given basic assumptions orientation, but they are ineffective for the individual in the large group situation. Here the only effective protection is an individual's isolating himself from the large group situation into the position of a "singleton" (Turquet, 1975), which will coincide with a sense of impotence and alienation and the loss of participation in the social process. The large majority caught up in the activation of massive paranoid-schizoid defenses of the large group will participate in a joint effort to compensate for the loss of individual identity by the collective search for leader-ship to replace individual identity by the "second skin" described by Volkan. In other words, it is a search for a new, shared identity linked to the dependency of a particular type of leadership. The type of leader-ship selected will oscillate between the narcissistic type of leader, as in the dependent group and the large narcissistic group described by Turquet, or a paranoid leader, as in the fight/flight group, in the mass movement, or in the large group described by Turquet when intense aggression overrides the reassuring search for a narcissistic, calming leader. I have described in earlier work (1998) how the nature of the ideology selected by the large group, particularly in mass movements, also oscillates between a narcissistic and a paranoid type. Many political and religious ideologies contain a central, humanistic core that, under different conditions of group regression may shift into a paranoid or a narcissistic distortion of the ideology. Moscovici (1981), in his sociological analysis of the effects of media and mass communication, has suggested that, while Marx described religion as the "opium of the people," the media and mass communication are the "Valium" of the people.

Leadership and malignant narcissism

In earlier analyses of the characteristics of functional leadership of social organizations, I pointed out that essential qualities of functional leadership include the following: (1) High intelligence, possibly best defined by the time span of decision making (Jacques, 1976), that is, the capacity of leadership to foresee long time developments and orient the organization he or she leads in the light of this analysis; (2) an integrated personality structure that includes the capacity for significant self-reflection and assessment in depth of other people, essential to selecting delegate leadership and the deciding about conflicts that involve technical knowledge as well as personality features; (3) a solid, autonomous moral capacity and commitment, given the unavoidable corruptive temptations of leadership functions; (4) significant narcissistic features—in the sense of solid security and self-regard that permit leadership to tolerate the unavoidable ambivalences and aggression stemming from the internal functioning of the organization as well from external sources of challenges to it; and (5) a sufficient availability of paranoid traits—in the sense of a mature distrust in contrast to naiveté that would ignore aggressive and potentially threatening developments in the work relationships of the organization.

A discrete, reasonable, and controlled amount of narcissistic and paranoid features is an important aspect of leadership, in contrast to excessive dependence needs that cannot be gratified outside the leadership function and a dangerous naiveté regarding the complexity of human relations in social organizations. Precisely these two personality features, in an exaggerated and pathological way, typically characterize the leaders selected in regressive group situations, problematic organizational functioning, and mass movements. From a different perspective, Canetti (1960) described the psychological characteristics of the "feasting mass" (Festmasse) and the "hounding mass" (Hetzmasse). These refer to the predominant behavior of respectively celebrating narcissistically or aggressively persecuting large groups under the corresponding leadership of a narcissistic and potentially hypomanic leader organizing collective feasts and orgies, in contrast to the paranoid leader of an aggressive, persecutory mob. In short, an extraordinary potential for narcissistic or paranoid leadership emerges under conditions of large group regression.

At this point, we have to explore the nature of narcissistic and paranoid character traits that are characteristic, respectively, of narcissistic and paranoid personality disorders. In fact, under conditions of social disorganization, the weakening of traditional social structures, the emergence of extremist political groups and parties, individuals with these characteristics tend to become important in providing a "second skin" to the respective groups. But there is one type of particularly relevant psychopathology that combines narcissistic and paranoid traits as part of a severe type of narcissistic personality disorder, namely, the syndrome of malignant narcissism.

I have defined the syndrome of malignant narcissism in earlier studies of severe forms of pathological narcissism (Kernberg, 1984, 2018) as characterized by the presence of (1) a narcissistic personality disorder with all its characteristic features: a pathological grandiose self, inordinate self-centeredness and a sense of superiority, strong manifestations of envy, devaluation of others, severe limitations of the capacity of emotional investment in others, and a chronic sense of emptiness that requires an ongoing search for external stimulation or the excitement derived from drugs or sexual behavior; (2) significant paranoid personality features; (3) strong egosyntonic aggression, directed against others or self; and (4) significant antisocial behavior. The basic psychopathological features of the syndrome of malignant narcissism are a dominance of unconscious conflicts around intense aggressive affect—from whatever origin, together with the development of the compensating pathology of a grandiose self. Aggressive motivation infiltrates the grandiose sense of self, leading to egosyntonic aggressivity on the one hand, and to the projection of aggression in the form of paranoid tendencies on the other. The severe deficit in the development of an internalized system of ethical values derived from the underlying basic failure in normal identity formation that affects the buildup of such an ethical structure (superego development) determines the development of antisocial behaviors.

Patients with the syndrome of malignant narcissism function along a wide spectrum of social dysfunction. The most ill patients with these characteristics suffer from a total breakdown of their capacity for social interactions, incapacity to function in work and profession, and breakdown in intimate relations, together with the development of severe affective dysregulation, and such a degree of disturbed interpersonal behavior that makes for initial confusion with borderline personality disorder. At the other extreme are patients who are able to maintain their social functions and work conditions, and only show breakdown in their personal, intimate relationships, an incapacity to significantly invest in non-exploitive behavior with others, and an extremely exaggerated concept of self and commitment to self-interests that are pursued in an aggressive way without moral restrictions. It so happens that such individuals may be perfectly adaptable to a social situation of massive group regression, in which these aspects of their personality function effectively to gratify basic needs of the regressed large group.

Under ordinary circumstances, such relatively well-functioning individuals presenting malignant narcissism possessing high intelligence, unusual technical capabilities and knowledge in some specialized area, and the capability to fulfill their ambitions to promotion within social organizations may assume leadership of social organizations in education, health, military, and religious institutions, or industry. They usually promote the institution by identifying their personal interests with that of the institution, but, over a period of time, because of their severe incapacity to assess others, their tendency to surround themselves with adulating subordinates, and their incapacity to tolerate criticism and therefore use realistic, essential feedback for institutional operations, such institutions show a typical regression. The organization evolves a sharp differentiation of levels of emotional climates. At the top of the organization, surrounding the leadership with malignant narcissism, are individuals who also present narcissistic and antisocial features. They have learned to adjust themselves to the needs of the leader to be both loved and feared while being unaffected by his interpersonal demandingness and, at times, antisocial maneuvers, so leadership with antisocial features expands corruption at the top. At a second level of organizational functioning, including the large majority of professional and institutional staff, there develops an intensely paranoid atmosphere because of the fear of a leader who is hypersensitive to criticism, who needs to be showed love and admiration, and who cannot listen to anything running against his/her will. There is a high level of institutional "paranoiagenesis" (Jacques, 1976), with frequent turnover and breakdown of staff. At the bottom level of the institution, at the periphery of its internal emotional milieu, one finds the most capable staff members, depressed and alienated, prone to be the first ones to leave the organization, sometimes depriving an organization of the most productive and creative members of its staff. So far, I summarized what happens in organized social institutions.

Large group regression and malignant narcissistic leadership

In contrast to the developments in well-structured social organizations, under conditions of social disorganization and large group regression, the emergence of leaders with the syndrome of malignant narcissism takes further socially dysfunctional and threatening characteristics. The leader's narcissistic self-centeredness and grandiosity, his self-assured signaling what he believes the large group should think and do, and his promise for a brilliant future if he is followed, powerfully reassures the members of a regressed large group against the threat of the loss of individual identity, and provides them with the second skin of an idealizing mutual identity of all in identification with the leader. The reduced cognitive level of functioning characteristic of large groups (Kernberg, 1998; Turquet, 1975) responds positively to simple slogans and clichés that the leader provides them with to confirm their value, uniqueness, importance, and power. Simple slogans replace complex thinking and correspond to the large group's need to feel that they are intimately involved with the thinking of the great leader and understand him completely, and, at a deeper, unconscious level, don't need to envy him. Everybody is equal in the pursuit of simple ideals and in the proper symbolic expression of such ideas. The well rationalized aggression against out groups is fostered by the leader's direct, crude, and sadistic expression of animosity against such out groups, devaluing and dehumanizing them while declaring the large group he directs to be the selected, ideal, morally justified, superior social group. Aggressive outburst against minorities is fostered, welcome, considered heroic and morally admirable, so that freedom to express destructive behavior excites the group and creates a contaminating festive atmosphere. Bao-Lord (1990) describes how, during the Chinese Cultural Revolution, the beating up of professors by revolutionary groups in the middle of huge public gatherings contaminated the bystanders, so that massive engagement in physical attack and murder became a welcome public spectacle.

The characteristic antisocial features of the leader with malignant narcissism are reflected in practically public dishonest behavior, matched with shameless denial of that behavior. Hitler never acknowledged his clear, indirect instructions to eliminate potentially rivalrous leaders of his S.A. troops; he never acknowledged publicly, nor in writing, his instructions for mass murder of the Jewish population under his control, in spite of being the obvious ultimate source of these orders. Stalin would invite both privileged followers whom he wished to honor for tea at his place, and also those who already had been secretly condemned to be eliminated. This was sufficiently well known in his intimate circle to cause external anxiety in the invitees, which, apparently, greatly pleased Stalin.

The leader's evident dishonesty, the self-assured expression of lies that may be easily recognized as such by an outside observer and a broader social environment or general community is perceived by the regressed large group as a courageous standing up to conventional truth, daring to say the impossible, the leader showing courage in changing his mind at any point, and shifting over, if necessary, to declaring alternative choices of who is the selected enemy at the moment. The leader's decidedly assuming moral responsibility promotes a sense of freedom from moral constraints, excitement of moving with a powerful wave of political discontent and strife as it is manipulated from the top, and cemented by the suggestibility of the large group. Repeated attacks, ridiculing, and demeaning humiliation of selected "enemies" reinforce the group's enjoyment of sadistic behavior. It was the inhumane cruelty of ISIS that exerted an exciting attractiveness to many early international followers.

Leadership by a leader with malignant narcissism within an institutional, task-oriented organization is circumscribed by the very structure of the organization; the need to carry out its technical or professional functions, the outside world that confronts the organization with consequences of failure of leadership in carrying out ordinary boundary functions, in addition to the negative effects of decreased productivity, and deterioration of human relations in the inside of such an organization. External authorities, Board of Governors, or community oversight tends to limit, in the long run, the negative effects of deficient leadership. In an open, political field, in contrast, the negative consequences of the mutual stimulation between large group regression and the emergence of leadership with malignant narcissistic personality characteristics is much more effective in its destructive consequences.

To begin with, the crystallization of a regressed social subgroup, that is, the constitution of a large group with shared feelings of threatening insecurity related to economic, cultural, or political issues, with threats to the identity or survival of that group, is experienced and shared informally by the group. A general feeling of growing tension, anxiety, and irritability initiates the search for a "second skin," that is, a longed for, decisive intervention by leadership to protect the well-being, security, and stability of the group's existence. The situation is open now to a self-assured, aggressive, powerful combative politician who spells out the generally shared feelings of dissatisfaction and resentment, and orients the group toward an external source of its troubles in the form of an external enemy power that needs to be fought off. A general paranoid orientation evolves and consolidates the large group in the active search, identification, and separation from the designated enemy group. The cultural availability of a preexisting ideology with strongly paranoid features or one that can be shifted easily into a paranoid direction may be used by a leader to establish a sense of historical continuity of this struggle with adversary forces, and include historical trauma and triumphs to provide a sense of mission in the direction of restoring such past glory or undoing historical trauma, creating a dynamic force in the pursuit of justice and right (Volkan, 2004).

The antisocial potential of the leader with malignant narcissism may manifest itself at first only in relatively discrete dishonest behaviors such as evident lies, false accusations, and circumscribed distortions of reality, all of which is expressed, however, in a courageous way that implicitly tests the extent to which the community at large may threaten the specific regressed large group with creating limits to this dishonesty or accept it. As Turquet (1975) had originally pointed out, and is also stressed by Albright (2018) and Snyder (2017), there is a "third group" constituted by the original total population that watches a combative minority—the large regressed group—enter warfare with another social subgroup, the selected victims of the attacks by the dynamic, regressed large group possessed by an extreme, paranoid ideology. If the traditional structure of society is weakened by a present traumatic situation, an economic crisis, a lost war, a natural disaster, the initial response to the provocative dishonesty that the leadership of the regressed large group propagates may be sufficiently weak, and ordinary social reactions not sufficiently alarmed to stand up against such a distortion in social communication. Now more destructive aggressive acts, distortion of reality, open encouragement of violence may develop, with an expanding affirmation and dissemination of the certainty, self-righteousness, the sense of moral justification, and superiority emanating from the revolutionary large group under the stimulation by the leader. The aggressive, paranoid, and dishonest behavior socially fostered by malignant narcissistic leadership thus evolves into an ever-growing sense of self-confirmation and power by the group. The self-assuredness of the leader and the expansion of his paranoid, grandiose, and aggressive behavior go hand in hand with the increase of a sense of power, freedom, violent behavior, and triumphant excitement of the regressed large group.

The dangers to society

Jacques Sémelin (2007) illustrates all these processes with the initial anti-Semitic ideology, work restrictions, and media attacks on Jews in Nazi Germany during the early stages of the Hitler regime, and their gradual escalation as initial resistance against social acts of violence was muted, and a gradual increase in physical violence, socially destructive behavior, and arbitrary legislation restricting Jewish life and robbing Jewish property was calmly accepted by the German population at large. In general, at this stage, relatively independent social structures, particularly, religious organizations, the armed forces, the financial elite, the judicial power, the media, the strength of bureaucratic organization, and tradition become important elements that may control this regressive process or reinforce it. The combined influence of these relatively stable social structures and powers may then determine the extent to which a regressive process evolves further into the potential extreme of the development of genocidal regimes, or is controlled in the form of an ordinary dictatorship, or ends with the eventual recovery of the civilized reaction to this social regression. An independent military that traditionally rejects its identification with a particular political orientation may counteract the establishment of a totalitarian regime, that is, an effort by the malignant narcissistic leadership to establish an obligatory indoctrination of the entire population by a determined ideological doctrine.

It needs to be stressed that totalitarian systems differ from ordinary dictatorships in their imposition of an obligatory ideological system. You don't only have to fear the leader but also must love him. The totalitarian regime established by personalities with malignant narcissism will be reinforced by such an ideology centered on the idealization and fearful submission to the leader, but an ordinary dictatorship, while less effective, also tends to achieve the same submission and destructive effects on the population. The surprising reaction of the military establishment of the Soviet Union in dropping its allegiance to the communist party happened at a point when the economic failure of the communist system interfered with the effective military competition with the United States. This development contributed fundamentally to the downfall of the communist regime. To the contrary, the German military fell rapidly into place with Nazi ideology, given its crucial role in the expansionist doctrine of national-socialist ideology geared to establish the dominance of Germany over Europe.

Social media may express an identification with a dominant traditional culture that rejects the extremes that threaten a peaceful coexistence of different ideological orientations and break the expansionist power of a revolutionary extreme group. The very fact that the Internet permits the parallel diffusion, circulation, and expansion of completely contradictory ideological investments may protect a democratic political system, but it may also be used by extremist social subgroups to organize a hidden rebellion against the status quo and facilitate communication of regressed large groups, as has been illustrated by the effective recruitment tool that the Internet has signified for terrorist Islamic groups in recent times.

In general, once a totalitarian power achieves control of the media, they become an important instrument of social indoctrination. An independent judicial system may be a significant counterweight to the aggressive assault on individual's rights and invasion of individual privacy by revolutionary groups with totalitarian ideology. But when a revolutionary government is able to control ordinary judiciary power, laws and judges may easily become corrupt. An effective bureaucracy may prevent, to some extent, social disorganization and the disruption of ordinary interactions of individuals and institutions, but a highly organized bureaucracy under state control may powerfully reinforce a totalitarian system.

A dramatic overall comparative study of genocide in three very different societies carried out by Jacques Sémelin (2007) illustrates the worst case scenarios of progression of social regression of large groups with corresponding malignant narcissistic leadership into mass murder and genocide. He compares the historical developments of Rwanda, Bosnia, and Nazi Germany leading to genocidal explosion and reaches the conclusion that similar processes occurred in all three so very different societies in terms of the historical background, culture, and socio-political situation. In all three cases, a latent animosity existed between social subgroups, Tutsi and Hutu in Rwanda, Muslims and Christians in Bosnia, the historical anti-Semitism of German culture and its rejection of the Jews. Such latent potential social splits became expressed first in all three cases, in a general ideological disposition, an extreme ideology turning one group against the other. That divisive ideology became acute at the time of social crisis derived from the complexities of decolonization in the case of Rwanda, the aftermath of the decomposition of the communist system in Yugoslavia, the consequence of the defeat of the First World War and the later economic crisis in Germany. This led to the ascent of leadership by personalities with powerful aggressive, paranoid, and antisocial features, who started out with grandiose leadership aspirations in all three cases. The end result of this process was a totalitarian situation with a socially imposed, ideologically rationalized, leadership supported political program called to exterminate the enemy group. We have more detailed information, at this point, of both Hitler's and Stalin's personalities that documents the pathology of malignant narcissism in both of them. It refers to their extraordinary grandiosity, the savage aggression, and personal sadistic pleasure in torturing their enemies, their dishonesty and paranoia, and the strange incapacity to evaluate the personality features of their immediate secondary leadership. It is no coincidence that Hitler felt closest to the two most similar personalities to himself in terms of grandiosity and dishonesty, Goebbels, Goering, and Stalin ended up trusting the psychopathic Beria more than any other member of his leadership group.

When the ascent of groups with the characteristics of regressed large group psychology, and of corresponding leadership with features of malignant narcissism is socially limited in its size, effectiveness, durability, and dramatic impact on the corresponding surrounding society, such a group may emerge as a religious or political cult that ends up in self-destruction or control by the wider social community and state. Obviously, those cults leading to murder or collective suicide represent extremes of this pathology.

In earlier work (Kernberg, 2003) discussing the prevention of socially sanctioned violence, I focused on the limited tools available from a psychoanalytic viewpoint and expertise, including a focused attention on childhood neglect and violence and the corresponding interventions at the home, in early infant and child care, in the school, and the conscious effort to combat and prevent cultural bias with active, socially fostered measures against racial, political, sexual, religious, and other ideologically tinged prejudices against social subgroups. I also questioned the concept of multi-culturalism in terms of its fostering the coexistence of sharply different subcultures within the same social environment. I stressed the need that particularly immigrants from a different culture be helped to integrate into the culture of a country in which they are making their new home.

So far, we have studied how we can contribute to reduce the burden of social prejudice against subgroups: concerted efforts of the educational approach in elementary and high school may be an important corrective. Regarding the selection of leadership, in social organizations as well as in political systems, I believe that we are progressing somewhat in the awareness of the psychological requirements of good leadership that may be considered in the selection not only of institutional leadership but, perhaps even more importantly, in the evaluation of potential political leadership. But this awareness does not assure the utilization and effectiveness of this knowledge.

The selection of good leadership in social organizations with clear boundaries, defined tasks, and correspondent administrative structures is realistically feasible. Usually, leaders are selected based on who evince appropriate technical knowledge and expertise, high intelligence, the capability to communicate with coworkers, and an appropriate background of reliable and honest work patterns. The main difficulty in the selective process lies in the area of their emotional maturity, their capacity to evaluate coworkers in depth, the presence of adequate, "paranoid" features—non-naïve critical evaluation and "narcissistic" features—the ability to stand up to criticism, and unavoidable institutional aggression. The situation is much more complex in the case of selecting political leadership. Candidates with severely paranoid and narcissistic features and even antisocial behavior may be well aware of the need to present themselves as open and friendly, attentive to others' wishes and needs, and disguise their resentful selfishness and self-absorption, and their true thinking, if the moment "is not right." Madeleine Albright (2018) has described the erroneous impression Hitler conveyed in early interviews, her own experience with Chavez (Venezuela's former president), and other political leaders that did not reveal their true personality. It is regarding newly emerging, radical movements that the danger of their so well fitting malignant narcissistic leadership be ignored—with unfortunate consequences. It is obvious that there are historical moments in which powerful social forces may operate in the direction of splitting off of social subgroups, including the unavoidable disorganizing effects of economic crises and political chaos.

Jacques Sémelin (2007) recommends international action and the responsibility of the social sciences. He believes that, in the international field, individual nations as well as the United Nations have to adopt ethical responsibility, including the responsibility to prevent social crisis that are man-made and put populations in danger. The United Nations should react in the face of situations where the protection of human beings impress the necessity of resorting to appropriate, including coercive, measures, accepting the responsibility to intervene, facilitating receiving military rescue intervention, providing assistance to resumption of reconstruction, and reconciliation. In terms of the responsibility of the social sciences, he believes that the social researcher has at least to take on the responsibility to make known our accumulating knowledge of the causes of social crisis and particularly genocide. The study of genocide is an essential, urgent need for the field of the social sciences, and that includes psychoanalysis. Psychoanalysis can contribute with the understanding of the psychology of large group regression, the psychology of the syndrome of malignant narcissism, and more generally, the interaction between leadership pathology and group regression. Psychoanalytic contributions to the understanding of optimal leadership in social institutions may be a helpful contribution to the evaluation of political leaders as well.

Here the contribution of the distinguished historian Timothy Snyder is relevant (*On Tyrany: Twenty Lessons from the* Twentieth Century [2017]). His 20 lessons include the call to institutions to distrust one party states and be wary of power militias. We must remember professional ethics, believe in truth, investigate, and listen for dangerous words. He explains the importance of establishing a private life, contributing to good causes, learning from peers of other countries. He affirms that it is important to be calm when the unthinkable arrives, be a patriot, and be as courageous as one can. He thus outlines a profile of individual courage, responsibility, independence of thinking, and public action. I think these are eminently reasonable and, in fact, essential qualities that permit the individual to stand up to the dangerous imprisonment in regressive group formations and confront dishonest, corrupting, and corrupted leadership. In the political arena, malignant narcissistic leadership should not be exposed with diagnostic psychiatrist labels, but by pointing to their public, cohesively pathological, characteristic behavior. From a psychoanalytic perspective, the development of a strong personal identity, with its related capacity to evaluate oneself and others in depth, to respect the right for privacy and individual boundaries, as well as boundaries for the couple in love and for the family, are important contributions to the achievement of the individual stance that is described by Timothy Snyder, and so are the psychoanalytic contributions to our understanding of the psychology of small and large regressed groups and their ideological consequences. And the understanding of dangerous personality formations in social leaders may help the prevention of the toxic combination of regressed groups and malignant leaders.

Note

1 The article was first published 2020 under the title "Malignant Narcissism and Large Group Regression" in: *The Psychoanalytic Quarterly, 89*(1), 1–24. doi:10.1080/00332828.2020.1685342. We have the official permission to reprint this article in our volume.

References

ALBRIGHT, M. (2018). *Fascism: A Warning*. New York: Harper Collins Publishing.
BAO- LORD, B. (1990). *Legacies: A Chinese Mosaic*. New York: Fawcett Columbine.

BION, W. (1961). *Experiences in Groups*. London: Tavistock Publications.

CANETTI, E. (1960). *Masse und Macht*. Frankfurt am Main: Fischer Taschenbuch Verlag.

FREUD, S. (1921). Group psychology and the analysis of the ego. *S.E.*, *18*, 63–143. London: Hogarth Press.

JACQUES, E. (1976). *A General Theory of Bureaucracy*. New York: Halsted.

KERNBERG, O. F. (1984). *Severe Personality Disorders: Psychotherapeutic Strategies*. New Haven: Yale Univ. Press.

KERNBERG, O. F. (1998). *Ideology, Conflict, and Leadership in Groups and Organizations*. New Haven: Yale Univ. Press.

KERNBERG, O. F. (2003). Sanctioned social violence: a psychoanalytic view. *Int. J. Psychoanal.*, *84*, 953–968.

KERNBERG, O. F. (2018). *Treatment of Severe Personality Disorders: Resolution of Aggression and Recovery of Eroticism*. Washington, D.C.: American Psychiatric Association Publishing.

KLEIN, M. (1946). Notes on some schizoid mechanisms. *Int. J. Psychoanal.*, *27*, 99–110.

MOSCOVICI, S. (1981). *L'âge des foules*. Paris: Librairie Arthème Fayard.

SÉMELIN, J. (2007). *Purify and Destroy: The Political Uses of Massacre and Genocide*. New York: Columbia Univ. Press.

SNYDER, T. (2017). *On Tyranny: Twenty Lessons from the Twentieth Century*. New York: Tim Duggan Books.

TURQUET, P. (1975). Threats to identity in the large group. In *The Large Group: Dynamics and Therapy*, ed. L. KREEGER. London: Karnac Books.

VOLKAN, V. (2004). *Blind Trust*. Charlottesville, VA: Pitchstone Publishing.

2 The return of the authoritarian

Narcissism and destructiveness in nationalistic ideologies[1]

Werner Bohleber

The return of the authoritarian

In recent decades, Western societies have been exposed to increasing dynamics of change and crisis as a result of ongoing globalization. Serious threats to pluralistic societies and modern liberal democracies have resulted in political developments that have led to a renaissance of authoritarianism and nationalism.

In its global expansion, capitalism also extended to the realm of culture and social structures. Many traditionally anchored securities of social cohesion dissolved, exposing individuals to a dynamic that the social sciences sought to conceptualize with the diagnosis "ambivalence of modernity" (Baumann, 2000; Beck, 1986/1992; Frankenberg & Heitmeyer, 2022). Paradigmatically, social individualization and liberation processes were identified, which are characteristic for the life of people in the modern age. According to them, the opportunities for planning one's own life and the variety of options for action increased. The freedom to choose and the right to individuality and self-realization became guiding ideas. But these processes had a downside: the growing options given to the individual brought with them a pressure to make decisions. Unlike in the past, when many things were more fixed, the individual now had to make more of a personal contribution, and objective freedom of choice often led to subjective inability to make decisions (Amlinger & Nachtwey, 2022, p.101). The greater equality of opportunity increased individual competitive pressure, so that feelings of envy and resentment increased. The release to an autonomous life promoted the danger of disorientation and increased the isolation of the subjects in the network of anonymous social contacts.

Christopher Lasch (1979), after all, became well-known for his diagnosis that we were living in an age of narcissism. Amlinger and Nachtwey criticize it as one-sidedly negative. With his conservative cultural critique, Lasch has misunderstood the dialectical tension of social liberalization, for in it progression and regression are interlocked and cannot be separated from each other (2022, p.96). Amlinger and Nachtwey (2022) also refuse to follow claims that narcissistic personality dispositions have increased

DOI: 10.4324/9781003565284-4

currently. The social figure of the narcissist is not an expression of a mani-fest disease of civilization, but "a smoldering contemporary experience" in which the "imaginative content of an insecure society" is embodied and gives a concrete shape to an existing normative disorder. Also, the ambiva-lent emotional world of narcissism "between self-exaltation, mortification, and rejection" has a strong tendency toward authoritarian thinking and acting (p.169).

Wilhelm Heitmeyer (2018), in turn, speaks of "authoritarian tempta-tions" inherent in a social situation in which social inequality, social disin-tegration, lack of social recognition, and feelings of political powerlessness have intensified and made individuals feel insecure about no longer being able to control their own living conditions. Feelings of powerlessness and helplessness as well as enormous anger are the result and make people with such experiences susceptible to populist and right-wing extremist ide-ologies and parties in their search for security and explanations for these social changes. This is because they offer a model of order with clear hierar-chies, and propagate traditional ways of life and dichotomous world views in which the "own" stands against "the foreign." National affiliation, like "being German," thus offers a "central identity anchor" (Heitmeyer, Süd-deutsche Zeitung 10.07.23). The authoritarian is then becoming a way to regain control over one's own identity. These social developments of the last decades have given the concept of authoritarianism a new signifi-cance. I would therefore like to briefly present the different versions of this concept.

Erich Fromm, in the studies of the Institute for Social Research on "Authority and Family" in the 1930s, described authoritarianism as a form of sadomasochistic character whose authoritarian attitude changes depend-ing on whether a stronger or a weaker person is the object. To a power-ful authority, whom he fears but also admires, he submits and represses hostility and hatred, which he then directs against weaker people. The masochistic submission frees him from fear; it not only grants protection and security but also lets him participate in the power of authority. Fromm emphasizes the double function of authority: next to the fear that results in submission, there is the idealization that leads to the willingness to follow. This dual function creates "that peculiarly irrational emotional relation-ship" that exists with authoritarian leaders and their ideological messages and makes rational argumentation recoil (Fromm, 1936, p.166).

Adorno and the Berkeley Group (1950) based their study in the 1940s on the manifestations of fascism as a "petty-bourgeois mass movement." Espe-cially with their F-scale, they were able to describe the authority-bound character and its psychological conditions in a more differentiated way. In their conception of an "authoritarian syndrome" they followed Fromm's description of the sadomasochistic character.

In the decades that followed, the social sciences moved away from the assumption of an underlying character structure of authoritarianism.

Today, it is more purposeful to expand the concept and speak of situation-dependent authoritarian reactions (Österreich, 1993) or of "readiness to follow authoritarian political offers" (Heitmeyer, 2018, p.25).

The psychoanalytically oriented Leipzig research group led by Oliver Decker and Elmar Brähler conducts representative population surveys every two years on authoritarian dynamics in German society and publishes the results in its authoritarianism studies (the most recent survey is Decker et al., 2022). They, too, no longer speak of authoritarianism as a personality trait but as a behavioral disposition. It can be reinforced by certain factors, such as a perceived threatening external situation, and can manifest itself individually in an authoritarian syndrome (the last study was Decker et al., 2022). The authors break down the authoritarian syndrome itself according to three dimensions: authoritarian aggression, aggressive submissiveness, and emphasis on convention. To this classic triad of authoritarian personality (Adorno et al., 1950) they add "projectivity," to capture the conspiracy mentality. Together, these four dimensions then form a sadomasochistic type of authoritarianism.

For all the merits that this classical explanatory scheme has acquired since Erich Fromm first conceptualized it, it has, however, only limited explanatory value for illuminating new manifestations of authoritarianism, and this for two reasons. First, the social development of recent years has brought forth a new type of authoritarianism. Heitmeyer (2018) calls it "anomic authoritarianism," while Amlinger and Nachtwey (2022) refer to it as "libertarian authoritarianism." People of this authoritarian type have abandoned conformity and identification with external social agencies. They place themselves as sovereign subjects and, in narcissistic self-exaltation, deny the dependence they experience in society. They insist on their own sovereignty and the claim to unrestricted self-development. Such attitudes lead to continued offenses because they are not fulfilled by society in the desired sense. Representatives of this type can be found recently in the movement of "Querdenker" (lateral or unconventional thinkers), COVID-19 deniers, vaccination opponents, and climate change deniers. They create an imaginary world filled with conspiracy theories, claiming knowledge for themselves with which they can explain the world to themselves and transform experienced dependence and mortification into narcissistic self-assertion.

Second, the knowledge we have gained today through the study of narcissistic phenomena concerning the relationship between narcissism and destructiveness allows us to better understand the power that narcissistic imaginaries can gain over people's minds as compared to the type of sadomasochistic authoritarianism.

In the following parts of this article, I address the narcissistic dimensions of authoritarianism. I begin with the relationship of the self to the stranger and the narcissistic dynamic that is activated in it. Subsequently, I address the narcissistic longing for a homogeneous society.

Psychoanalytical insights into the experience of the stranger

In individual development, the stranger experience is structured mentally at a very early stage (Spitz, 1965). The infant responds "to his perception that the stranger's face is not identical with the memory traces of the mother's face" (p.155). He compares and realizes that it is not the mother in front of him. In essence, therefore, stranger anxiety is not a fear of the newly appearing person, but rather separation anxiety and fear of object loss. Further development confronts the toddler with a growing sense of separateness. The need for dialogic feedback with the mother intensifies ("refueling") to gain a sense of security that helps him overcome the fear of being overwhelmed by the dissonance of the strange and the consequent fear of loss of the mother (Sandler & Sandler, 1999). A sufficient sense of security and a growing familiarity with his own self- and object-representations allows the child to perceive the stranger with curiosity and to tolerate the ambivalence associated with it. These early developmental processes show how fear of strangers is structurally related to a lack of psychological sense of security.

But how does one develop the ability to perceive another person objectively and not superimposed with projections? Here, Donald Winnicott (1969) provided groundbreaking insights with his work "The Use of an Object." At the beginning of development, the mother adjusts to the infant and his needs in such a way that he experiences the world around him in a kind of omnipotence as if it functioned according to his ideas and desires. This experience is important for the young child to build confidence in his own intentionality and self-efficacy. But at some point, the child can no longer avoid the perception of the mother as a person outside the area of his omnipotent control. This unwanted perception generates a massive aggression with which the child seeks to destroy the mother as a real Other in his (unconscious) fantasy. Normally, the mother withstands this aggression, reacting neither as upset nor compliant. In this way, she enables her child to gradually renounce his own omnipotence and to perceive her as an "objectively perceived object" (Winnicott, 1969, p.714). With this ability, the child succeeds in transcending his infantile narcissism. It is not a one-time process; rather, it must be repeated many times to become established psychologically in a relatively conflict-free manner. The recognition of the Other as a real Other beyond all projective loading by one's own ideas and intentions is one of the most difficult achievements the child has to accomplish, and it remains a lifelong mental task.

Let me briefly turn to Julia Kristeva (1991), who has elaborated an issue that is important for us here. Her conception of the stranger is based on the dialectic of self and Other: We always need the Other to understand ourselves. The confrontation with his otherness creates a certain insecurity in us, because it loosens our certainties, our unconscious gets into motion, and the Other becomes a mirror that activates the "foreigner in us." That is to say, the strange Other becomes, by way of projected perception, the bearer of our own unconscious ideas and strivings that have become "improper" to us. If we refuse to admit this inner perception, there is a danger that our narcissism will prevail and the stranger will become a victim of our authoritarian aggression. If we can change our attitude of mind and accept that in the stranger, we encounter our own unconscious as an unsettling strangeness, then we accept *difference* as an "indispensable condition for our being with others" (p.210). I elaborate more about the connection between difference and narcissism later, but first I would like to turn to social psychological issues.

Social scientific findings and their psychoanalytical interpretation

I would like to make a methodological preliminary remark. For Sigmund Freud, the evolution of culture and society was inextricably interwoven with the development of the individual. Today, we have become far more reluctant to draw direct conclusions from the individual to society. We can no longer view the two as realms that mirror each other, but must take into account the abstract control mechanisms that are operative in social processes. As they are anonymous, these mechanisms intervene in the life-world of the individual in very different ways from how other people do it. Exceptions are mass ideologies as well as ethnic-nationalistic phantasms, where psychoanalysis can make a direct contribution when it comes to explaining the power they can gain over people's imaginations.

With the so-called Mitte (Center) studies of 2021 and 2023, the Bielefeld Institute for Interdisciplinary Research on Conflict and Violence conducted representative population surveys on right-wing extremist and democracy-endangering attitudes in Germany (Zick & Küpper, 2021; Zick et al., 2023). The results show that democratic and anti-democratic positions are mixed in the population. It is true that 72% describe themselves as convinced democrats and agree with the view that "different cultural groups enrich our society." But the ambivalence of these attitudes is then reflected in anti-pluralist views: 25% (in 2023, 26.3%) of respondents hold the opinion that "too much consideration is given to minorities"; more than 30% go further and believe that the Federal Republic is "over-alienated to a dangerous degree by the many foreigners" (Zick & Küpper, 2021, p.88). Likewise, 25% (2023: 33%) of respondents clearly identified as populist, and 41% (49%) indicated that they "tend to be" populist (Zick et al., 2023, p.120). Populist-leaning respondents are significantly more likely to be authoritarian, xenophobic, anti-Semitic, and conspiracy-minded (Zick et al., 2023, p.128). The boundaries to right-wing populism and right-wing extremism are also proving to be fluid. For example, the percentage of respondents who classify themselves as politically right of center has increased from 9% to 16% in the last two years (p.99). The acceptance of a single right-wing extremist ideological fragment can attract other fragments in the individual attitude pattern, a transfer that is often mediated by affect and leads to radicalization. In the most recent Bielefeld study of 2023, the percentage of respondents exhibiting a far-right worldview increased from 2%–3% to 8% (Zick et al., 2023, p.70). In this fluid mix of populist and extreme right-wing ideas, the phantasm of a "völkisch homogeneity," or the idea of the "true people," plays an underlying driving factor that has been massively reactivated in the current social situation with its manifold crises and the reception of many refugees.

The phantasm of homogeneity

The idea of homogeneity is not always consciously advocated; it often remains latent, but can be identified as a motive behind other statements. Although many of the respondents agree with an open society and cultural diversity, the idea of a homogeneous community with its emotional appeal does secretly come into play in contexts of conflict. Right-wing populist and New Right ideologies, on the other hand, openly advocate the restoration of a national homogeneous Volksgemeinschaft under the label of "ethnopluralism." It is the core element of the New Right. This ideological concept obviously develops an appeal that should not be underestimated and can explain why 28% of the population tends toward New Right attitudes and as many as 40% of respondents believe that German society is being infiltrated by Islam (Zick et al., 2016, p.155ff.).

The separate statistical analyses of the Bielefeld researchers revealed a surprising finding. The idea of homogeneity exerted an independent influence on the respondents' statements. Statistically, it represented an independent factor that could not be explained by factors such as authoritarianism or social dominance orientation, nor by the fact of one's own social disadvantage (Zick & Küpper, 2012, p.171).

I examine this finding more closely from the perspective of psychoanalysis and explore the question of what makes the idea of a homogeneous national society so attractive. In clarifying this question, I refer to social science analyses of nationalism. Exceptionally influential has been the work of the American political scientist Benedict Anderson (1983), who conceptualized the nation as an *imagined community*. In doing so, he relied on the fact that members of a nation will never know, meet, or even hear from most of their fellow members, but that the image of their national community is alive in the minds of each of them. This mental image of the nation is always a mixture of fact and fiction, and for that very reason, it can have a powerful emotional impact. Just think of the associative meaning of terms like "fatherland" and "motherland." These familial symbols, and the body and its limbs, form a fund of symbols that every society uses to represent its political and social identity problems, the relationship between inside and outside, borders, purity, homogeneity, and mixing.

Now, it is important to recognize that these symbolic formations of national ideas are not only emotionally charged, but that *collectively shared unconscious fantasies* are also attached to them, because without them, their enormous emotional appeal, but also the often violent enforcement of political positions based on them, could not be explained (for more details, see Bohleber, 2010. Methodologically and conceptually, I rely on a concept of "ubiquitous unconscious fantasies" (similar to Bendkower, 1991). They are ubiquitous because they are about the basic facts of life. They relate to bodily needs and to stages of development, especially a mother's provisioning and dependence on her, sibling rivalry, the primal scene, and the Oedipus complex. Narcissistic fantasies of grandiosity, omnipotence, and fusion may also be associated. In their striving for fulfillment, these fantasies can projectively attach themselves to the perception and formation of social events, institutions, and cultural value patterns. On the other hand, they are pressed into service from outside—that is, from social agencies—and are shaped and thus channeled by objective structures, by institutions, communicative conventions, and linguistic traditions. In earlier work (Bohleber, 1992, 2010), I have psychoanalytically examined the imaginative world of nationalism and encountered three groups of unconscious imaginative complexes; they revolve around: care-taking fantasies and sibling rivalry, purity and the idea of the Other, and the fantasy of a sheltering whole.

a   Provision Fantasies and Sibling Rivalry

I will only briefly go into the first unconscious fantasy complex. Refugees and asylum seekers are often accused of: "They only come to exploit our social system." Or one gets to hear: "They get everything immediately and we get nothing." In the minds of these accusers, an idea is activated that there is provision without any effort on the refugees' part. Jacob Arlow (1992) was the first to draw attention to a connection of this idea with a primitive hostility against siblings in his analysis of anti-Semitism. The associated childhood conflicts revolving around greed and murderous aggression are repressed, but form a universal unconscious fantasy that can be used socially. The conflicts are regressively acted out on a level of archaic aggression as a claim to sole possession and participation in and fusion with a collective mother-imago. The useless devourer is the sibling rival and the disruptive intruder who must disappear or be destroyed. The dehumanization and the fantastic voracity attributed to the strangers and refugees turned into parasites is thus projectively kept away from the ideal harmonious community.

b   Ethnically Closed Identity and Purity Phantasms

Behind ideas of purity lies the fear of dirty drives, bodily fluids, excrement, smells, and so on. They arouse disgust and revulsion, are rejected as animalistic, and are often projected onto Jews, Africans, refugees, women, and sexual minorities, who are attacked or persecuted. These are well-known, psychoanalytically well-studied connections. One reflects oneself in narcissistic purity, dirty are the (foreign) Others.

However, there is another aspect that is important for our topic. Purity has a close connection with identity at the large group level. As the ethnologist Mary Douglas (1966) has pointed out, dirt is something that is out of place in a definition that is culturally old. Thus, dirt is judged as something that should not belong if a symbolic system is to endure. Uncertainty, insecurity, and ambivalence cannot be tolerated but must be eliminated as impure in order to create a homogeneous, symbolically consistent national collective free of fissures and distortions.

When notions of homogeneity are virulent in a population, the sense of being a member of the nation activates a narcissistic identification in which individual differences from others are blotted out (Freud, 1921). Individuals then assure themselves of their attachment to the nation and their identity by narcissistically identifying with each other and experiencing themselves and others as being the same. The unavoidable difference and ambivalence toward the others, which nevertheless cannot be faded out, is experienced as disturbing and threatening and leads to aggressive charging of differences, which are projected outward for inner relief. Otherness and strangeness then emerge as the polluting thing that must be eliminated.

Such a world of narcissistic mirroring and purity carries with it a massive persecutory aggressiveness against those who are different, who threaten the inner cohesion. This self-centered narcissism cannot tolerate anything different or deviant from itself and, if it persists or is politically functionalized, has the dangerous tendency to become progressively radicalized. Then, belonging to an idealized community and persecuting violence are mutually reinforcing. This connection between collective narcissism and violence has been demonstrated time and again in the social sciences on the basis of individual socio-political developments. Theodor Adorno et al. (1950), for example, characterized the inner dynamics of fascist characters as "psychic totalitarianism," and Mortimer Ostow (1996) wrote of a "pogrom mentality."

In several research projects, the Indian anthropologist Arjun Appadurai (2006) has investigated the aspects of globalization that are disturbing in their novelty and has focused on the new potential for violence that this development has produced, especially the attacks on cultural or political minorities that take place worldwide. Minorities are suitable for many states as a projection screen for their own fears of real or fantasized inferiority or marginalization. The insecurity and mortification of being more exposed to global developments than being able to influence them leads to a lack of tolerance toward any kind of collective foreignness and gives rise to fantasies of purity, which can discharge into violence against minorities. Appadurai's (2006) thesis now is that, behind the modern nation state lies the idea of the "national ethnos," which haunts societies like an ethnic phantasm and creates a "fear of not being whole and complete." Such a notion of fear can be politically instrumentalized against minorities and lead national majorities to adopt an aggressive and murderous attitude, because the existence of minorities prevents them from expanding "their status as a majority to that of an immaculative community, to a comprehensive pure ethnos" (p.21). But the aversion and violence against the minority is merely the symptom. At the center is the intolerability of *difference*. Appadurai emphasizes that it is not about the Freudian "narcissism of small differences," but about eliminating difference itself. If the idea of pure ethnos gains power over people's minds and they are completely immersed in it, the Other as the stranger is perceived only as a threat.

c   Globalization and the Fantasy of a Sheltering Whole

Psychoanalytic group research (Anzieu, 1975; Jacques, 1981; Money-Kyrle, 1951; Turquet, 1975) has revealed that regression in a group or mass goes far beyond the Oedipal level described by Freud; thus, other deeper narcissistic identifications are still operative. As members regressively merge into the group, it becomes an illusory substitute for the first lost object, the mother of infancy (Foulkes, 1975). This research is of considerable relevance to fantasies about the nation. Thus, at the core of national identification is an illusionary omnipotent elation to merge with each other in a great whole. The result is an inflation of narcissistic feelings that undermines the realistic image of one's own nation.

This symbolic world is gaining renewed appeal today in a situation in which the idea of an ethnocultural nation state is gaining renewed popularity in Europe. Isaiah Berlin (1990) spoke of an "ideology of organicism." In it, complexly composed cultural nations are ethnically appropriated. Values, goals, and purposes receive their legitimation only from their organic integration into the nation. The foreigner does not fit in and is supposed to live out their uniqueness elsewhere. Politically, "ethnopluralism" is propagated; each ethnic group should live in its historically evolved territory. Such a collective world of ideas activates fantasies and longings for organic unity in the individual. The individual members of the nation identify narcissistically with each other. Freud (1921, p.113) made it clear that identification is an emotional bond. It is the affects of the individuals that combine with the phantasmatic representation of the national as the "whole" and produce an experience of equality (Balibar, 2022, p.983). The individuals then no longer belongs to themselves but are a member of a great whole. Their own small self can phantasmatically dissolve into the great whole and revel in an illusionary omnipotent elation. The idea of the whole creates a "totalization effect" and triggers an enormous aggressiveness in the individuals as soon as something foreign comes into play. If everything is supposed to be white and one feels oneself to be part of it, then the colorful disturbs, because it causes the state of a narcissistic self-assurance and the feeling of uniformity to collapse. A sense of security and belonging is lost and triggers fear of "losing one's own completely" (Jongen, Journal "Die Zeit," No. 23, 25.5.2016). This psychological state of affairs makes it understandable why mixing is the main fear of all right-wing extremists. Taguieff (1988/2000) speaks of "mixophobia," a fear that has a tendency to escalate to the paranoid idea of the "Great Exchange" of populations, which the New Right insinuates into European governments as a secret program. The result is massive resentment that easily turns into open violence.

d Summarizing Remarks on Difference and the Attractiveness of Fantasies of Homogeneity

Difference, otherness of the Other, and ambivalence are anthropological facts that permeate social relations and personal relationships. They all make demands on the psychic processing of each individual. But what is the reason that we find this so hard to bear and are tempted to want to escape into homogeneous imaginary worlds of narcissistic unity and purity?

Freud had asked himself why undisguised antipathies and aversions can arise in humans toward strangers. He recognizes in it an expression of a self-love and of narcissism, which

works for the preservation of the individual, and behaves as though the occurrence of any divergence from his own particular lines of development involved a criticism of them and a demand for their alteration. We do not know why such sensitiveness should have been directed to just these details of differentiation; but it is unmistakable that in this whole connection men give evidence of a readiness for hatred, an aggressiveness, the source of which is unknown.

(Freud, 1921, p.101)

Today we know more about this issue of narcissism, which can trigger such aggressive and destructive reactions when experiencing difference. If we follow Winnicott, narcissism is based on the recurrent longing and desire for omnipotent control of the object. But this desire cannot be fulfilled because it brings with it unremitting mortifications that are grounded in the objectivity of the object. To escape this vicious circle, the subject has to give up ("destroy") this omnipotently controlled object desired in their fantasy to be able to perceive it objectively in its own characteristics. The refusal to recognize the difference of the Other involves a narcissistic rage that becomes destructive. On the collective level, this wishful scenario, which remains unconscious, can be projected into the phantasm of a perfect and homogeneous homeland and can be integrated into a corresponding political ideology. If such a collective narcissism is not tamed, it unleashes processes of stigmatization and exclusion of others, resulting in hatred and violence. The stranger is then not recognized in their difference, but is "just a bundle of projections" (Abram, 2013, p.327; Winnicott, 1969, p.712).

I would like to close with a quote from Zygmunt Bauman (2000), which sums up my own thoughts excellently:

> The ability to live with differences, let alone to enjoy such living and to benefit from it, does not come easily and certainly not under its own impetus. This ability is an art which, like all arts, requires study and exercise. The inability to face up to the vexing plurality of human beings and the ambivalence of all classifying/filing decisions are, on the contrary, self-perpetuating and self-reinforcing: the more effective the drive to homogeneity and the efforts to eliminate the difference, the more difficult it is to feel at home in the face of strangers, the more threatening the difference appears and the deeper and more intense is the anxiety it breeds.
>
> (p.106)

Note

1 The article was first published under the title "Purity and unity: Narcissism and destructiveness in nationalistic and fundamentalistic ideologies" in: *American Imago, Vol. 81*, No. 1, 1–16, 2024. We have the official permission to reprint this article in our volume.

References

Abram, J. (ed.) (2013). *Donald Winnicott today*. Routledge.

Adorno, T. W., Frenkel-Brunswik, E., Levinson, D. J., & Sanford, R. N. (1950). *The authoritarian personality*. Harper and Row.

Amlinger, C., & Nachtwey, O. (2022). *Gekränkte Freiheit. Aspekte des libertären Autoritarismus* [Offended freedom. Aspects of libertarian authoritarianism]. Suhrkamp.

Anderson, B. (1983). *Imagined communities: Reflections on the origin and spread of nationalism*. Verso.

Anzieu, D. (1975). *The group and the unconscious*. Routledge & Kegan Paul.

Appadurai, A. (2006). *Fear of small numbers. An essay on the geography of anger*. Duke University Press.

Arlow, J. A. (1992). Aggression und Vorurteil: Psychoanalytische Betrachtungen zur Ritualmordbeschuldigung gegen die Juden [Aggression and prejudice: Some psychoanalytic observations on the blood libel accusations against the Jews]. *Psyche–Z Psychoanal, 46*, 1122–1132.

Balibar, E. (2022). Massenpsychologie und Ich-Analyse. Das Moment des Transindividuellen [Group psychology and the analysis of the ego. The trans-individual moment]. *Psyche–Z Psychoanal, 76*, 969–991.

Bauman, Z. (2000). *Liquid modernity*. Polity Press.

Beck, U. (1992). *Risk society. Towards a new modernity*. Sage. (Original work published 1986)

Bendkower, J. (1991). *Psychoanalyse zwischen Politik und Religion* [Psychoanalysis between politics and religion]. Campus.

Berlin, I. (1990). *Der Nationalismus* [The nationalism]. Hain.

Bohleber, W. (1992). Nationalismus, Fremdenhass und Antisemitismus. Psychoanalytische Überlegungen [Nationalism, xenophobia and anti-Semitism. Psychoanalytic considerations]. *Psyche–Z Psychoanal, 46*, 689–709.

Bohleber, W. (2010). *Destructiveness, intersubjectivity, and trauma. The identity crisis of modern psychoanalysis.* Karnac.

Decker, O., Kiess, J., Heller, A., & Brähler, E. (eds.) (2022). *Autoritäre Dynamiken in unsicheren Zeiten. Neue Herausforderungen – alte Reaktionen?* [Authoritarian dynamics in uncertain times. New challenges – old reactions?]. Psychosozial-Verlag.

Douglas, M. (1966). *Purity and danger: An analysis of concept of pollution and taboo.* Routledge.

Foulkes, S. H. (1975). Problems of the large group from a group-analytic point of view. In L. Kreeger (ed.), *The large group. Dynamics and therapy* (pp.33–56). Karnac.

Frankenberg, G., & Heitmeyer, W. (eds.) (2022). *Treiber des Autoritären. Pfade von Entwicklungen zu Beginn des 21. Jahrhunderts. [Drivers of the authoritarian. Paths of development at the beginning of the 21st century].* Campus.

Freud, S. (1921). *Group psychology and the analysis of the ego. Standard edition* (Vol. 18, pp.69–143). Hogarth Press.

Fromm, E. (1936). Studien über Autorität und Familie. Sozialpsychologischer Teil. *Erich Fromm Gesamtausgabe. [Studies on authority and family. Social psychological part. Erich Fromm Complete Edition].* Deutsche Verlagsanstalt, Bd. 1, 139–187.

Heitmeyer, W. (2018). *Autoritäre Versuchungen. Signaturen der Bedrohung* [Authoritarian temptations. Signatures of the threat]. Suhrkamp.

Jacques, E. (1981). Social systems as a defense against persecutory and depressive anxiety. In G. S. Gibbard, J. J. Hartmann, & R. D. Mann (eds.), *Analysis of groups* (pp.277–299). Jossey Bass.

Kristeva, J. (1991). *Strangers to ourselves.* Columbia University Press.

Lasch, C. (1979). *The culture of narcissism.* Warner Books.

Money-Kyrle, R. E. (1951). *Psychoanalysis and politics.* W. W. Norton.

Österreich, D. (1993). *Autoritäre Persönlichkeit und Gesellschaftsordnung. Der Stellenwert psychischer Faktoren für politische Einstellungen – eine empirische Untersuchung von Jugendlichen in Ost und West* [Authoritarian personality and social order. The significance of psychological factors for political attitudes – an empirical study of young people in East and West Germany]. Juventa Verlag.

Ostow, M. (1996). *Myth and madness. The psychodynamics of antisemitism.* Transaction.

Sandler, J., & Sandler, A. M. (1999). *Internal objects revisited.* Karnac.

Spitz, R. (1965). *The first year of life. A psychoanalytic study of normal and deviant development of object relations.* International Universities Press.

Taguieff, P.-A. (2000). *Die Macht des Vorurteils. Der Rassismus und sein Double* [The power of prejudice. Racism and its double]. Hamburger Edition. (Original work *La force du préjugé*, published 1988).

Turquet, P. (1975). Threats to identity in the large group. In L. Kreeger (ed.), *The large group: Dynamics and therapy* (pp.87–144). Constable.

Winnicott, D. W. (1969). The use of an object. *The International Journal of Psychoanalysis, 50*, 711–716.

Zick, A., & Küpper, B. (2012). Zusammenhalt durch Ausgrenzung? Wie die Klage über den Zerfall der Gesellschaft und die Vorstellung von kultureller Homogenität mit *Gruppenbezogener Menschenfeindlichkeit* zusammenhängen [Social cohesion through exclusion? How complaints about the disintegration of society and the idea of cultural homogeneity are linked to *group-focused misanthropy*]. In W. Heitmeyer (ed.), *Deutsche Zustände. Folge 10 [German conditions. Volume 10]* (pp.152–178). Suhrkamp.

Zick, A., & Küpper, B. (eds.) (2021). *Die geforderte Mitte. Rechtsextreme und demokratiegefährdende Einstellungen in Deutschland 2020/21* [The challenged center. Right-wing extremist and anti-democratic attitudes in Germany 2020/21]. Dietz.

Zick, A., Küpper, B., & Krause, D. (2016). *Gespaltene Mitte – Feindselige Zustände. Rechtsextreme Einstellungen in Deutschland 2016* [The split center – hostile conditions. Right-wing extremist attitudes in Germany 2016]. Dietz.

Zick, A., Küpper, B., & Mokros, N. (eds.) (2023). *Die distanzierte Mitte. Rechtsextreme und demokratiegefährdende Einstellungen in Deutschland 2022/23* [The distanced center. Right-wing extremist and anti-democratic attitudes in Germany 2022/23]. Dietz.

3 Murderous narcissism in a terrorist act

A psychoanalytic perspective[1]

Siri Erika Gullestad

On July 22, 2011, Anders Behring Breivik, a 32-year-old white Norwegian man from one of Oslo's well-to-do neighborhoods, set off a bomb at the Norwegian Government Headquarters in the center of Oslo, killing seven people and crippling many more. Dressed as a policeman, he then drove to Utøya, a small island about 40 kilometers from Oslo, to the summer camp of 600 young people from the Social Democratic Party.

During one hour he, killed—in cold blood—69 youths and children, one by one, shot in the chest and in the head, through hands helplessly trying to protect the face. Pretending to be a policeman who was there to protect them, Breivik induced them to leave their hiding places. Groups of children hiding under rocks or behind their leaders were massacred. Breivik's original plan was to execute Gro Harlem Brundtland, former prime minister of Norway and a symbol of the victories of modern feminism. She had given a political speech at Utøya earlier that day. The decapitation of Brundtland was to be videotaped and put on the Internet, modeling al-Qaeda operations. The plan had to be changed, however, because Breivik was delayed.

The shock in Norway was total. How was this possible? How can we understand these acts of evil? In his own view, Breivik was motivated by extremist right-wing ideology. The bomb and the massacre were intended to be a wakeup call: Breivik wanted to save Norway. Just before the massacre he sent out a manifesto of 1,500 pages to more than a 1,000 recipients, the key message of which was that a revolution was necessary to save Norway from Eurabia—a Europe dominated by Muslims. The manifest speaks about the Nordic race and Grand National values, and is full of contempt for multiculturalism, feminism, and the dissolution of authority in our modern society. All through the ten-week trial, Breivik—immovable—maintained that he realized that what he did was "horrible." It was,

---

1 The chapter is a shortened and revised version of Gullestad, S. E. (2017). Anders Behring Breivik, master of life and death: Psychodynamics and political ideology in an act of terrorism. *International Forum of Psychoanalysis*, 2(4), 1–10.

DOI: 10.4324/9781003565284-5

however, "necessary." The destructiveness was, according to Breivik's understanding, ideologically motivated.

Experts on terror also regard ideology as the explanatory factor (Hagtvet et al., 2011). The question is, however, what makes a person join an ideology that justifies the sacrifice of innocent people by reference to a superior aim? Is it possible that the demonization of Muslims "fits" into a psychologically threatened universe and a murderous lust for revenge? Can we understand Breivik's ideological attitudes as expressing inner, dynamic forces? This is the main question I will discuss here.

Breivik's ideological universe

An astounding aspect of Breivik's manifest is the strong defense of a traditional form of society, resting on patriarchal values. This seems to be the deepest root of his attack on multiculturalism and fear of Eurabia. He is intensely concerned about the demography of modern Western societies, with declining birth rates of "valuable," white, Christian people. He vehemently rages against feminism and cultural Marxism. He despises the "feminization" of the whole society, and also of himself. In the school he was attending as a child he was, he says, "forced to learn to knit and sew." Breivik's hatred is also directed against the dissolution of sexual morality: Quote: "An alarming number of young girls in Oslo, Norway, start giving oral sex at the age of 11 and 12." It comes as a paradox that, during his teens, he was attracted to masculine boys from minority cultures, like the Muslim culture of Pakistani people, characterized by codes of honor. These boys were not "feminized." Indeed, when I read Breivik's manifesto, I was struck by the affective intensity in describing the threat of feminism. In the manifesto text, this threat comes forward as deeper than the threat posed by the Muslims. Paradoxically, Breivik's contempt of women's liberation parallels that of the Muslims he hates.

Psychiatric illness?

How did Breivik come to feel this way? And what is the relationship between his way of thinking and his actions, i.e., between his ideology and the massacre? Immediately after Breivik was imprisoned, it was decided that he should be subjected to forensic psychiatric observation, to determine whether he was mentally ill, i.e., psychotic. In that case, he could not, according to Norwegian law, be held accountable for his deeds. The first forensic report (Husby & Sørheim, 2011) concluded that Breivik suffered from paranoid schizophrenia and that he was not accountable. In this report, Breivik's ideological ideas are regarded as delusions resulting from psychosis—indeed, the two experts decided to totally disregard the manifest as irrelevant for understanding the case. The report considers Breivik's use of terms like "suicidal Marxist"/"suicidal humanist" as neologisms indicating "bizarre delusions" (Husby & Sørheim, 2011, p.225). Neglecting Breivik's ideological universe means that there is no *motive* in the psychological sense of the term, the deeds are caused by illness, and there is in fact nothing to *understand*.

Professionals within the psychiatric field heavily criticized this first report. The victims and survivors from Utøya, who had experienced the mass murderer as rational, cold, and manipulating, and not at all as "mad," also met it with disbelief. On the other hand, many people felt that the atrocity of his acts *must* mean that Breivik was "ill" (contrary to evidence that mental illness is usually *not* the explanation of terrorist acts [Bhui et al., 2016]). An intense public debate followed. Consequently, and contrary to Norwegian tradition, the court decided to demand a second forensic assessment. This second evaluation concluded with the diagnosis of narcissistic personality disorder, no sign of psychosis. Assessments by medical doctors and psychologists treating Breivik in prison supported this second report. After a ten-week trial, the court concluded that Breivik was not psychotic and that he was to be held accountable for his actions. The verdict was prison and not treatment in a psychiatric institution. The judge, a woman, went against the pleading of the prosecution, and came forward as an autonomous and independent voice. Norway was relieved!

Mother and son

How can we understand Breivik's personality in a dynamic perspective? Two sets of data are of particular interest here (Borchgrevink, 2012; Seierstad, 2013). Firstly, interviews of friends of Breivik and of people who knew the family during his childhood. Secondly, information conveyed by the case records from the psychiatric institution that observed and evaluated the family when Breivik was four years old.

Breivik was born into an extremely conflict-ridden relationship between his mother, a nursing assistant, and his father, who had a master's degree in business administration and worked as a diplomat. Both parents had children from previous marriage. After a short, turbulent marriage, living in London due to his father's job, his parents got divorced. Little Anders was then 18 months old. After the divorce, he continued to live with his mother and half-sister in Norway, seeing his father only seldom. According to family friends, his mother perceived her ex-husband as a "monster," whereas he saw her as "mad" and "impossible to talk to."

When little Anders was two years old, his mother sought official help, asking for a weekend home for Anders. She was worn out both physically and psychically, and because Anders was a demanding child. Close acquaintances of the family witnessed a mother-son relationship full of violent conflicts followed by emotional reconciliations. Anders' mother was extremely unstable in her attitude toward the little boy, furious at one moment, treating him as if he were a prolongation of the hated father, and then showering him with caresses.

The mother sought help once more, when Anders was four, and this time was referred to a well-known child psychiatric unit, where the small family was admitted for observation for about three weeks. A team of eight persons, including a psychologist and a chief psychiatrist, observed the family, providing assessments of both mother and Anders and of the interaction between the two of them. According to the case record, his mother had wished for an abortion when pregnant with Anders, but was indecisive. Already during pregnancy she experienced her baby as difficult—from the moment she felt him kicking, she knew her baby boy was "evil." The mother experienced her son as "aggressive, clinging and extremely demanding."

The clinic's observational team describes a mother alternately drawing her little son tightly toward herself, "symbiotically," and then pushing him aggressively away. She said that she wanted to "peel him off" herself. According to the clinic, the interaction pattern was characterized by "double communication." The mother's relationship to her son was described as "sexualizing" and as "projecting primitive aggressive and sexual fantasies, everything that she feels as dangerous and aggressive in men" (case record, cited from Borchgrevink, 2012, p.341). After the divorce Anders slept in his mother's bed at night. His mother had made some half-hearted efforts to break this habit. However, unclear boundaries between mother and son remained. According to the police interrogations, Breivik—"for a joke"—gave his mother a vibrator when her relationship with a boyfriend ended in 2004. A fact that, indeed, cries out for an explanation! As for the psychiatric evaluation, Anders's mother was regarded as having weak mentalizing ability—everything was the fault of other people. The mother was diagnosed as functioning on a borderline level.

The psychologist assessing Anders at the age of four, partly through the method of play therapy, reported that Anders was an "anxious, passive child warding off contact, with a manic defense with restless activity and a put on, averting smile" (Borchgrevink, 2012, p.42). Anders was unable to play, and was characterized as "pedantic" and "extremely orderly." There was a "complete lack of spontaneity and appearance of joy and pleasure."

The report of the psychiatric clinic concluded that Anders ought to be placed in a foster home. After reading the reports, Anders's father claimed custody over the boy. As his mother refused, the case was brought to the court, which decided in favor of the mother. After this verdict, Anders only occasionally visited his father and his new wife, then living in France. From when Anders was 15 years old there was no more contact between father and son.

Growing up: Oslo West in the 1980s

Anders Behring Breivik grew up in a time of great social and cultural changes—Oslo West was at this moment confronted with multiculturalism for the first time. During the 1980s the subway between Oslo West and Oslo East became connected for the first time, allowing for easy transportation between different regions of the city. This was a time of child robberies, i.e., gangs of immigrants coming from the east to rob "naïve" children living in white neighborhoods, taking their money, expensive jackets, etc. I myself at this time had children attending the same school as Breivik—my own son was robbed, as was the son of my best friends. This was the context of Breivik's adolescence.

At the age of 13, Anders began identifying himself with the hip-hop milieu of Oslo East, becoming friends with an immigrant Pakistani boy belonging to one of the "cool" gangs. At the same time, he started tagging, soon trying to become the toughest, most fearless in the gang. His signature was "Morg," a name taken from a cartoon, known as the executioner with a double-headed axe used for the execution of Morg's own people. Morg was the first of Anders's "doubles"—later, he created different fictitious characters playing Internet games, among them Justiciary Knight Andrew Berwick, the avatar that would eventually carry out the Utøya massacre.

When reading interviews with Anders's schoolmates (Borchgrevink, 2012; Seierstad, 2013), one is struck by the fact that Anders never became fully integrated in any group. Although apparently a member of a gang—sooner or later he was somehow left behind. Indeed, it is heartbreaking to realize what intense efforts he made to become a member of the hip-hop gang, of the tagging milieu and later of the right wing *Progress Party*—and how he always remained—somehow—an outsider, experienced by many as somewhat strange. Also his romantic relationships failed. For a short period, he dated a mail-order bride from Belarus. His mother was delighted that at last her son had found a girlfriend. But it came to nothing. Some of Anders' friends were convinced that he was secretly gay. His appearance was somewhat feminine, he liked to dress elegantly and wear makeup, and also he had been observed visiting gay bars. However, he angrily denied being gay—he would rather boast that he was quite a brothel man.

A psychoanalytic perspective

First a caveat: What I say about possible dynamics in the mother-father-son relationship has the status of hypotheses. I can have my thoughts about unconscious patterns, but I cannot know. In psychoanalysis, the validity of an interpretation lies in the *dialogue* with the patient—and here there is no such dialogue. Indeed, there is a need for humility.

As concerns the relationship between Anders and his mother, what particularly needs to be emphasized, is the symbiotic quality of a strikingly ambivalent mother-son relationship. Certainly, the expression of wanting to "peel him off" testifies to the mother's experience of boundlessness in relationship to her son—as do her difficulties in denying him access to her bed at night. As described in the case record, the mother drew Anders close to her, then violently rejecting him. This pattern seems to be repeated by

Anders—as an adult he would suddenly "throw" himself into his mother's lap and embrace her, only to withdraw and ignore her completely. The most striking example of an atypical relationship between mother and son, however, is the vibrator gift that Anders gave his mother in 2004 when the relationship with her boyfriend had ended. Undoubtedly, this is a gift that testifies to the lack of normal boundaries between mother and son.

On a conscious level, Anders Behring Breivik experienced his mother as a nuisance. Interestingly, he did not want his mother to be present in court or to see her during the trial, stating that she was his "Achilles' heel" and the only person that could make him "emotionally unstable." It seems warranted to speculate that on an unconscious level the mother might have been experienced as symbiotically engulfing—a powerful figure endangering the core of his masculine identity. She seems to represent a threat of e-masculinization and castration. The mass-murderer's rage and contempt toward the feminized society seems to conceal a deep fear of the feminine mode—and conceivably of female sexuality. Probably, unclear boundaries may result in a need to protect oneself against inner chaos and confusion. In this context, the loss of the father—a potentially protecting figure, able to assist a son caught in a symbiotic relationship—is certainly most significant.

Self identity

From the clinical context, we know that a response to an engulfing mother may be intense aggression: What is at stake for the child is the protection of his very self. In this context, the formation of a *personal myth* (Kris, 1956; Green, 1991; Gullestad, 1995) may have a purpose. A personal myth refers to an autobiography that has a defensive function and at the same time represents something cherished. It implies mythification and heroization of the self, protecting against underlying feelings of weakness and worthlessness. Breivik's picture of himself as a "savior of Europe" may be regarded as a personal myth of this kind. It represents a blown up self-image shielding against the experience of being a loser—the self-image is organized in an either-or-manner: the person feels either invincible or like "nothing," the self-state oscillating between extremes (Gullestad & Killingmo, 2020).

A main function of a personal myth is to help overcoming anonymity and becoming *special* (Gullestad, 1995). Also, the myth may serve as a liberation from a mother figure experienced as seductive and destructive (Green, 1991; Gullestad, 1995). Through heroization of the self, the original dependency on the mother is denied. The heroic fantasy of being Justiciary Knight Andrew Berwick also may serve to deny the feminine, weak (gay?) side of him.

Surely, it seems that Breivik's enormous aggression was primarily directed against females and the feminine element. After all, Breivik's main plan for 22 July was to execute Gro Harlem Brundtland by decapitation. Gro—Norwegian people call her by her first name—symbolizes what Breivik hates more than anything, namely the liberation of women and the creation of a society with equal rights for men and women. The image of guillotining certainly seems to represent the ultimate revenge.

As we know from psychoanalytic developmental theory, lack of emotional feedback that affirms the child's feeling of being a separate self in his own right will inevitably affect the formation of a coherent self (Kohut, 1971). To my mind, Winnicott's concept of "false self" (Winnicott, 1965) seems to well describe Anders Behring Breivik—a false self, built to comply with the demands of other people. Remember how the psychologist described Anders—a four-year-old boy lacking ability for "expressing himself emotionally," unable to play, with a complete lack of spontaneity. One might think that the self that Breivik presented to peers as an adolescent lacked authenticity to a degree that made normal friendships difficult. According to Winnicott, for a more authentic self to develop, the mother's "mirroring face" is crucial—mother's specific emotional feedback lets the child experience a kind of omnipotence, which is a prerequisite for the spontaneous creative capacity of the child to develop. At some point, however, the child has to perceive that the mother is outside the area of his omnipotent control—which engenders aggression. In this context, I would like to emphasize Winnicott's seminal paper "The use of an object" (1969). Winnicott, in this chapter, underlines the child's need for mother's survival of his aggression. Anders' mother apparently did *not* survive what she imagined being her baby's attacks on her: Already in pregnancy she felt his kicking inside the womb as an expression of evil. Her response was a wish for abortion. And she stopped breastfeeding him because she felt that his sucking was destroying her. When a mother is not able to withstand her child's aggression, the child will get no help to experience the mother as an *other* person, i.e. as a subject in her own right. This means that the child will be assisted in gradually renouncing his own omnipotence and transcending his infantile narcissism.

> the recognition of the Other as a real Other beyond all control and projective charging by one's own ideas and intentions, is one of the most difficult achievements the child has to accomplish and it remains a lifelong mental task.
>
> (Bohleber, 2023)

It is this task that failed in Anders Behring Breivik's development.

Oedipal catastrophe

On the background of what we know about the sexualizing relationship Anders' mother drew her son into, it seems warranted to speculate that the son somehow—at an unconscious level—may have replaced his father in the position as mother's partner. Such boundary transgression entails breaking the incest taboo, with unconscious fulfillment of wishes that in their very nature are outlawed. Gaining access to a privileged position that should have been reserved for an adult, male partner would seem to stimulate an omnipotent state of mind. Indeed an Oedipal triumph!

However, the triumph is not a real one. The negative side of narcissistic omnipotence is the experience of failure—of being too little, too weak. Breivik never succeeded in the competition with other men, whether it be in adolescence groups (hip-hop, tagging) or, later, in business or politics. In Breivik's case, the fantasized omnipotence would seem to represent a compensation for an underlying feeling of failed masculinity. On this background, the vibrator gift comes forward as multi-determined, condensing different motives. For one, it may suggest an almighty position—the giver is the one able to provide satisfaction. In my view, however, the gift first and foremost conveys contempt: The receiver of the present—the mother—is reduced to a sexually unsatisfied woman probably comprising the image of a whore. Most likely, she is a representative of the dissolution of sexual morality that Breivik so intensely despises.

Master of life and death

In the case of Breivik, we witness not only a lack of consolidation of masculinity, but also—most importantly—a deficiency in the formation of superego. The superego comprises the double dictum of the precept "ought to be" and the prohibition "may not be" (Freud, 1923, p.34). For Breivik, no prohibitions seem to have been internalized. On the contrary, he seems to have identified with an imagined almighty paternal authority, expressed in his pretending to be a policeman during the massacre. He comes forward as invincible—he has the right to act as a judge and to decide over life and death, with a license to kill. Breivik is all-powerful, also as concerns moral judgment. Justice is done, thanks to him.

The self-appointed position of being the "savior of Europe" clearly testifies to the almighty, narcissistic, godlike mindset of the mass-murderer. Indeed, breaking the incest taboo means placing oneself above the laws that constitute human society. One cannot be held to account, thus entering the realm of the inhuman. Although the price of exclusion from the life of ordinary mortals is deep loneliness, the outlaw position would seem beyond guilt—maybe providing a right to realize the forbidden. On this background, the concept of *narcissistic omnipotence* comes forward as condensing several aspects of Breivik's inner world. His relationship to his mother—condensed in the vibrator gift—as well as his moral stance is characterized by an all-powerful, condescending attitude.

Sadism at Utøya

One of the most conspicuous features of the killings at Utøya was how machinelike Breivik appeared, like a robot. According to survivors, he was utterly calm and composed. The expert psychiatrists (Husby & Sørheim, 2011) comment on Breivik's special, introverted, and frozen smile when he talked about details linked to the massacre—a smile we also repeatedly witnessed in court. His smile conveyed the distanced attitude of an outside observer, not affectively present in what he talked about. Whereas many murderous acts are the result of an affective breakthrough—of "warm" aggression—the massacre of July 22 was the outcome of Breivik's thorough planning over several years and instrumental preparation for the moment of killing. Through the use of drugs and of meditation-like techniques Breivik "de-emotionalized" (his own expression) himself. Breivik described that after having crossed "a border" through the first murder, he experienced the rest of the massacre like a video game. The killing was in cold blood. It would seem the *quality* of the aggression unfolding at Utøya can be understood as a result of a splitting mechanism: The killings were, so to speak, committed by an alien, split-off self. As Breivik's manner of being was usually pleasing and "up to" other people, it would seem that the split off, grandiose self could express feelings of rage and aggression that normally were warded off and dissociated.

There is more to the aggression than cold distance, however. Breivik went about killing with an exhilarating grin. Survivors of Utøya also tell about excited shouting—"You will all die today, Marxists!" This kind of excitement would seem to be a sign of *pleasure* in murdering, thus indicating a *sadistic* component. The way the mass murderer seduced the children to emerge from their hiding place also bears the mark of sadism, meaning that inflicting pain and humiliation provides instinctual satisfaction.

Ideology and personality

Psychodynamic hypotheses of narcissistic omnipotence cannot in itself explain actions like those we witnessed on July 22. It may be a *necessary*, but certainly not a *sufficient* condition in explaining the massacre. The main problem in explicating July 22 is the passage from thought to action. After all, many right-wing extremists *think* like Breivik without endorsing his action. Psychology, in my view, provides no definite answer to this question. At the same time, psychological knowledge may shed some light on the topic. As is well known from social psychological studies (Zimbardo, 2007), belonging to a group represents a mighty driving force for evil deeds. Executioners and torturers do not act as individuals, but rather as members of a collective identity. The killings of Utøya, however, apparently are the work of a loner. Yet, is there a group involved in this case as well? Here, we need to consider the role of ideology.

In his twenties, Anders gradually became more and more politically engaged. Formation of a personal identity takes place through interaction with peers and the social world. Ideological worldviews are often endorsed precisely in young adulthood, at a point of time when it is expected that the individual separates from his parents and establishes an independent social identity through occupation and choice of a partner. Maybe identification with the grand national values and a "pure" people represents a "solution" when the individual identity project appears too complicated?

Psychoanalysts have, since the 1930s tried to analyze the authoritarian, destructive ideologies that came forward in the 20th century, Nazism and fascism, and what type of personality is drawn to these ideas (Reich, 1933; Fromm et al., 1936; Adorno et al., 1950). The studies also demonstrated an authoritarian longing, i.e. many people *wish* to be part of hierarchical, authoritarian structures, an escape from freedom (Fromm, 1941). This motive is elaborated in recent psychoanalytic studies seeking to identify unconscious dynamics of contemporary extreme ideologies (Bohleber, 2010). In adhering to an ideology, the question of "Who am I?" may be replaced by "Where do I belong?" Bohleber, states. Belonging to a group, the young adult is spared the challenge of forming a separate, individual identity—in a world of rivalry, competition, and plurality. The same search for identity seems to apply for Muslim radicalization.

Recent studies underline that we need to grasp how the young adult's feeling of displacement and frustration, as well as her dreams and longings of a better society, may be at the basis of radicalization (Leuzinger-Bohleber, 2016; Seierstad, 2013; Vestel, 2016).

Loss of traditional privileges in relation to women, family, and society, experienced by a lot of white, Western men, may be a stronger motive than we would like to think (cfr Trump's influence in US and the rise of right-wing movements in e.g. France and Germany). Grand national values, belonging to a "pure" people—certainly, these are forceful psychological motives, also substantiated by social science research. A most important finding from recent surveys in Germany is the emphasis informants put on *homogeneity*—the idea of a homogenous national society. Surely, this idea is at the core of Breivik's ideology.

In 2006, five years prior to the massacre, Breivik moved back to his mother's flat to live in his childhood room. For the next years, he would spend most of his time playing Internet games. Within this fictional world grandiose self-images and myths are acted out. Games like *Call of duty* replace real trials of strength—and Breivik became a master in this illusory world. His first question to his defense counsel the day after the massacre was, "How many did I kill?" The answer to the question probably gave the basis for imaginary heroic deeds. This pretense world also makes possible the making of a group needed for feeling connected, not through the encounter with a real "you," but through mirroring from anonymous fellow partisans, in an echo room. In this room, ideology is created, which, in turn, inflames actions. While being founded in personally motivated hatred and vindictiveness, the subjective war scenario is projected and justified with reference to a war "out there." In this perspective, the individual generates the ideology that in the next round makes action "necessary."

The relationship between psychological motives and ideology becomes dialectical: one seeks an ideology that "fits" partly unconscious intentions; the ideology, however, is indispensable to legitimate actions.

Given this background, we need to underline the connections between psychological dynamics on the one hand and the ideological world of the terrorist on the other. The feeling of being threatened by invasion as well as hatred toward an annihilating object—these seem to be themes on the psychological as well as on the ideological level. On the psychological level: Being threatened by an engulfing mother. On the ideological level: Being threatened by immigrants implying loss of the traditional privilege of being a white man.

This line of understanding is in sharp contrast to the first forensic report. Through psychiatric "glasses" focusing on illness, there is no link between the diagnosis and Breivik's manifesto—the ideological ideas are seen as delusions resulting from psychosis. In contrast, a psychoanalytic perspective opens up for comprehending *why* the mass murderer felt threatened and called on for defense and revenge. In this view, there are links between psychological explanations on the one hand and Breivik's self-understanding and values on the other. At the same time, connections to the cultural, social, and political Norway that has also formed Breivik's personality are established. In this analysis, ideologies are interpreted in a dialectical movement, both through what the French philosopher Paul Ricouer (1965) calls a "hermeneutics of suspicion," with a view to grasp psychological causes, and in a "teleological" frame (1965), with a view to the values and intentions that the individual identifies with.

Concluding remarks

Psychoanalysis, with its potential for highlighting unconscious dynamics, certainly is a powerful theory. In the clinical situation, the hypotheses that the analyst has about patients' inner motivations are validated in the dialogue with that patient. Thus, the patient is the final "judge" on the validity of interpretations. To analyze a person that we do not have a dialogue with is quite another matter. Indeed, it should be emphasized that our thoughts here have the status of being hypothetical. Should we for that reason abstain from thinking psychoanalytically about cases like July 22? To my mind, the horrendous nature of a massacre of this kind calls for all attempts at understanding. We need multifactorial explanations—sociological, political, cultural, ideological—and psychological. The psychoanalytic contribution in this multifactorial field is to highlight possible unconscious dynamics. In the eyes of Breivik, the terrorism perpetrated against the government building and the Utøya massacre carried a message: the violence should introduce a manifesto and an ideology, conveying the message of a threatened Europe and the mass-murderer as a savior. The killer wants us to look at him, and it is as a rescuer that he wants us to see him.

However, the director does not control the stage. In an imaginary reality he might, within a relational scenario without a real "you," without friction, but not so in the real world. Here we do not control the eye of the other. One of Sartre's (1947) fictional figures says, "Hell that is the others"—a hell because we do not control how other people see us. The terrorist wants us to perceive his actions as he himself does. For those of us trying to understand his actions, however, the explanation of the ill deeds is not to be found in his self-understanding and his ideology, which cannot be taken at face value.

Philosophers have criticized psychoanalysis for its "disclosing" attitude, which does not take the person at his word but sees through the reasons given by the person himself. Confronted with unspeakably extreme actions like Breivik's, a "disclosing" look is not only advisable, but also difficult to avoid. The mass-murderer has staged a scene, with uniforms, medals, and specific bodily postures. As I have argued earlier (Gullestad, 2013), he wants us to look at him in a specific way, but what we see is someone who wants to be looked at in this specific way. Anders Behring Breivik does not have it his own way! What the world notices, confronted with his ill deeds, is not what he wants us to see. What we see is unfathomable evil.

References

Adorno, T. W., Frenkel-Brunswick, E., Lewinson, D. J., & Sanford, R. N. (1950). *The authoritarian personality*. New York: Harper.

Bhui, K., James, A., & Wessely, S. (2016). Mental illness and terrorism. *BMJ, 354*, i4869.

Bohleber, W. (2010). *Destructiveness, intersubjectivity and trauma: The identity crisis of modern psychoanalysis*. London: Karnac Books.

Bohleber, W. (2023). *Purity and unity—Narcissism and destructiveness in nationalistic and fundamentalistic ideologies. Paper to be presented at the Joseph Sandler Psychoanalytic Research Conference in Vienna, 2023*.

Borchgrevink, A. S. (2012). *En norsk tragedie: Anders Behring Breivik og veiene til Utøya*. [A Norwegian Tragedy. Anders Behring Breivik and the Roads to Utoya]. Oslo: Gyldendal.

Breivik, A. B. (2011). *2083. A European declaration of independence*. Retrieved from: https://norskgoy.wordpress.com/2011/07/23/anders-behring-breivik-manifest/

Freud, S. (1923). *The ego and the id. Standard edition* (Vol. 19, pp.2–66). London: Hogarth Press.

Fromm, E. (1941). *Escape from freedom*. New York: Farrar & Rinehart.

Fromm, E., Horkheimer, M., Mayer, H., & Marcuse, H. (1936). *Autorität und Familie*. Paris: Felix Alcan.

Green, A. (1991). On the constituents of the personal myth. In P. Hartocollis, & I. D. Graham (eds.), *The personal myth in psychoanalytic theory*. Madison, CT: International University Press, pp.63–89.

Gullestad, S. E. (1995). The personal myth as a clinical concept. *International Journal of Psychoanalysis, 76*, 1155–1166.

Gullestad, S. E. (2013). Ideological destructiveness: A psychoanalytic perspective on the massacre of July 22, 2011. *Division Review, 7*, 29–36.

Gullestad, S. E. (2017). Anders Behring Breivik, master of life and death: Psychodynamics and political ideology in an act of terrorism. *International Forum of Psychoanalysis, 2*(4), 1–10.

Gullestad, S. E., & Killingmo, B. (2020). *The theory and practice of psychoanalytic therapy. Listening for the subtext.* London and New York: Routledge.

Hagtvet, B., Sørensen, Ø., & Steine, B. A. (2011). Ideologi og terror, totalitære ideer og regimer [Ideology and terror, totalitarian ideas and regimes. Oslo: Dreyer.

Husby, T., & Sørheim, S. (2011). *Rettspsykiatrisk erklæring avgitt den 29.11.11 til Oslo Tingrett i henhold til oppnevnelse av 28.07.2011* [Forensic report].

Kohut, H. (1971). *The analysis of the self. A systematic approach to the psychoanalytic treatment of narcissistic personality disorders.* New York: International Universities Press.

Kris, E. (1956). The personal myth. A problem in psychoanalytic technique. *Journal of the American Psychoanalytic Association, 4*, 653–681.

Leuzinger-Bohleber, M. (2016). From free speech to the IS – Pathological regression of some traumatized adolescents from a migrant background in Germany. *International Journal of Applied Psychoanalytic Studies, 13*(3), 213–223.

Reich, W. (1933). *Massenpsychologie des Fascismus* [The mass psychology of fascism]. Copenhagen: Verlag für Sexualpolitik.

Ricoeur, P. (1965). *De l'interprétation*: *Essai sur Freud.* Paris: Edition du Seuil.

Sartre, J.-P. (1947). *Huis clos* [No exit]. Paris: Éditions Gallimard.

Seierstad, Å. (2013). *En av oss. En fortelling om Norge. (One of us. The story of a massacre in Norway – and its aftermath).* Oslo: Kagge.

Vestel, V. (2016). *I gråsonen. Ungdom og politisk ekstremisme i det nye Norge.* Oslo: Universitetsforlaget.

Winnicott, D. W. (1965). *The maturational processes and the facilitating environment.* London: Hogarth Press.

Winnicott, D. W. (1969). The use of an object. *International Journal of Psychoanalysis, 50*, 711–716.

Zimbardo, P. (2007). *The lucifer effect: Understanding how good people turn evil.* London: Rider.

4 Putin is not the answer, but the question[1]

On neurotic fears and collective narcissism

Gerd Koenen

If I had quite a hard time with this lecture, then partly because of the over-abundance of questions and aspects that I have always come across anew in my previous, extensive, historically grounded "Reflecting on Russia—in the Flashes of the war" (to cite the title of my last book), an unprovoked campaign of annihilation against Ukraine, whose destructive, but also auto-destructive furor is not easy to explain (Koenen, 2023). In addition, there are the difficulties that it constitutes for me, as a trained historian and at best half-read layman in the field of psychoanalytic theories, to link the perspectives, approaches and vocabularies of both disciplines.

Psychoanalytic theorizing—in my layman's reading and perception—infers from the instinctual conflicts of individuals described as models that can be anthropologically generalized and from there unfolds a specific cultural and social critique. A special, contemporary focus was already in Freud's writings but also in later psychoanalytic theories of society, on the relationship of modern "masses" to their "leaders". In these, societies embody and exalt themselves "narcissistically", forming an idealized "Super-Ego" in the literal sense. It is precisely through this act of idealizing identification that it becomes possible to suspend all ethical "Super-Ego" commandments that are otherwise valid in private life and to unleash uninhibited destructive energies against real or alleged enemies (Freud, 1974).

The phenomena of such individual or collective destructive narcissism can certainly be deciphered to some extent from the side of the pleasure and aggression instinct of individual people and modern masses. But when I read an author like Franz Neumann (1954), for example, in the analysis of democracy and dictatorship, one also gets quite far with the concept of "fear", as it arises from "alienation" as a kind of modern condition (in the philosophical sense), which—according to Freud—can be divided into real fear and neurotic fear. Neumann arrives at a political science categorization of the kind that a repressive, dictatorial system uses depressive fear and fear of persecution and perpetuates it itself, while a democratic and liberal system "institutionalizes real fear" (Neumann, 1954, p. 39), precisely in order to cope with real problems and frightening challenges, including warlike aggression.

DOI: 10.4324/9781003565284-6

This idea can perhaps be linked to the concept of "narcissism" in such a way that a sense of reality that overcomes fear and successfully faces existential challenges enables democratic societies to develop a constructive, collective narcissism. And without romanticizing, one can probably say that the thoroughly warlike, but not militaristic, rather civil heroism of Ukrainian society in the face of aggression aimed at destroying its self-chosen way of life and political sovereignty is also bringing to light the other, more positive side of the otherwise more pejorative term "narcissism". Particularly of a "collective narcissism", as it has found a thoroughly meaningful embodiment in the figure of the little comedian Volodymyr Zelensky, who forcibly and unexpectedly became a war president (Koenen, 2023, pp. 33–38; p. 66).

These different forms of collective narcissism, as they are presented in the appearances, the ways of speaking and the identifications with these two antagonistic war presidents, could of course also be described very well with Max Weber's concept of "charisma". Max Weber's "charisma" is an analytical category that focuses primarily on the sociological form and the objective historical conditions of "extra-everyday rule". However, the description of the various "charismatic followerships" is also difficult without a certain amount of social psychology (Weber, 1976 [1921/1922], pp. 179–182).

Or let's take another term with a great scientific tradition: that of "mentalities", which in the tradition of the French "Annales" school differs fundamentally from older attributions of "national characters" in that it does not seek the causes in quasi-natural, innate characteristics of the respective groups of people—in our case, for example, "the Russians" (see Ariès, 1994). Instead, he tries to understand how "mentalities" from a "longue durée" of very specific, rather material, e.g. geophysical or civilizational and socio-historical prerequisites have been reflected in empirical patterns of action or social formats. In this sense, "mentalities" are first and foremost the products, only then the causes or driving forces of historical developments. Through socio-economic transformations or violent, disruptive events, they are always subject to new, repeated transformations, so they are not fixed, unchangeable—but they tend to be something very long-lasting, not easy to strip off (Braudel, 1977). In a similar vein, Norbert Elias has thought about how the "process of civilization", which is fed by many objective, material circumstances that create a "social compulsion to self-compulsion", then perpetuates itself in processes of "psychologization" or "habitualization" (Elias, 1976, p. 312 ff.).

These are also theoretical approaches that would have to play a major role in any deeper "Reflecting on Russia". However, these mental imprints must be understood as the result of a "long" historical sequence of sometimes extraordinarily violent experiences, in which political and social eruptions and repressions have dialectically detached and conditioned each other. In these historical cycles, and especially in extreme experiences such as the Stalinist "Great Terror" but also the "Great Patriotic War", which was waged without regard for own and others' losses, forms of a peculiar affective bond between power ("Vlast") and the people ("Narod") have developed, which could also tip over into their opposite overnight in the event of the power apparatus being shaken by the death of the dictator or by external defeats.

If the history of Russia in its "longue durée" has indeed shown circular features, then it is by no means in the sense of a return of the same, but in the sense of dramatic evolutions that require each a precise description. That is why attempts to put in an essentialist way a "Russian mentality" (a term which is used almost inflationary, even in the singular) in fixed formulas have rightly fallen into disrepute, because mental dispositions appear as something static, almost "eternal". Incidentally, they fatally coincide with the enthusiastic propaganda narratives about an "eternal Russia". Even better (or worse): This Russia is attributed the mystical quality that, according to a 19th-century poet's words, "cannot be grasped with the mind, but can only be felt with the soul" (Koenen, 2017).

In contrast to other historians, I have always found that it is hardly possible to adequately grasp and describe real historical processes and events without taking psychological elements into account. However, the focus of our disciplinary attention as historians is first and foremost on the objective, the structural, the contemporary historical circumstances from which political actors act, and at the same time, the conditions that enable them, for example, when it comes to totalitarian rulers or warlords, to exercise such power over their subjects and to commit such crimes against them or others.

The title I have chosen, "Putin is not the answer, but the question", is intended to direct the view beyond the biographical educational elements, the characteristics or even abilities of Vladimir Putin as a person (as interesting as they are) primarily to the enabling conditions of the position of power that he now holds. And this currently also applies to the question of how it was possible for him, as a lonely, unadvised final decision-maker, to plunge his country and the whole world into this insane and self-destructive war of conquest; and how and why, despite the catastrophic failure of his invasion, which was designed as a blitzkrieg, he was nevertheless able to persuade the majority of his society to follow him and the relatively small power cohort gathered around him further into this criminal adventure.

His personal motives are more than clear: he wants to go into the history books. The fact that he is already one of the country's longest-reigning rulers, with a constitutional entitlement to a lifelong, quasi-monarchical position of power, is obviously not enough for him: what is needed is the great, the decisive, the "historic" deed. He does not want to be just the moderately successful administrator of a stagnating rump empire, but the savior and rebuilder of a great empire and a quasi-natural world power. In this spirit, he has repeatedly fantasized in embarrassing obviousness about a "thousand-year" historical continuity, ranging from Vladimir the Holy (nomen est omen), to Ivan the Terrible, and Peter the Great, to Joseph Stalin, the victor in the Great Patriotic War and World War II, up to him, Vladimir Vladimirovich Putin.

This war now unleashed is therefore to become Putin's "Great Patriotic War" against a world of enemies, namely against a "collective West" which—this was already an old Soviet theory—makes use of fascist and other evil forces. At present, this is said to be a "satanic" horde of sexually degenerate people under the rainbow flag, and also Nazi-Emblems, who are supposed to undermine the great Russia from within as well as from without, in order to ultimately divide and destroy it. So, exactly that, what Putin now intends to do to Ukraine is said to have been intended by a hostile world conspiracy for Russia. But this is more than a mere demagogic distortion. Rather, in this projective reversal, there is a core of neurotic fear, which Putin may even share with his subjects, but in any case wants and must inculcate in them in order to put the country completely on a war footing.

From an individual psychological point of view, this ambition can certainly be called a malignant super-narcissism or downright megalomania. But malignant narcissists with delusions of grandeur can be found on every corner of the World Wide Web. An analysis of the character or even the eclectic self-fabricated ideologies of Vladimir Putin alone explains little. Rather, the historically analytical view must first be directed at the contemporary circumstances or the social and power structures, and from there at the socio-psychological or mental state of those who have raised him to the shield and follow him, both in the oligarchic power and property elite grouped around him and in the broad masses of "his" people. Then it will become clear, as I would like to explain in the following, that in the midst of the neurotic, depressive collective fear that Putin creates and at the same time acts out, there is actually a grain of truth, i.e. a piece of real fear. Except that their actual sources and reasons do not lie in the external world, for example an "advancing NATO", but in the interior, in the current constitution and the historical way of existence of Russia itself.

The situation in which Putin entered the stage of Russian politics already contains some keys to understanding this connection. Of course, I cannot provide more than a few highlights in this short presentation.

Who was this Putin anyway—whose name had only been heard by 2% of Russian citizens in 1998, when he was still quite shy on the public stage? A former officer of the Soviet secret service from the second rank, who allegedly quit his service in 1991 of his own free will and became head of the office of the democratically elected St. Petersburg mayor Sobchak, who was soon shrouded in corruption allegations, responsible for administration and economy. In 1998, Putin was found (coincidentally or not) in the

Kremlin's asset management. Whether and to what extent, as Catherine Belton (2022) and others believe to have found out about "Putin's network", he was already active in Dresden, later in Petersburg, and finally in Moscow, above all in a shadow world of unofficial and informal or even mafia-like financial and asset transactions. Whether and to what extent these transactions were built up and conducted in the footsteps of the old, conspiratorial KGB networks at home and abroad—all this is quite relevant, but it does not provide the decisive key to further developments: namely, the question of how Putin came to be in this position of an almost absolute sovereign and charismatic leader.

When Yeltsin, who was almost unfit for office and deeply unpopular, appointed this pale, unknown intelligence officer from the Kremlin administration in quick succession, first as supervisor of the new FSB secret service, then as prime minister and shortly afterward in early autumn 1999 as his designated successor in the 2000 presidential election, this was probably at the instigation of a backroom camarilla of economic oligarchs, high-ranking intelligence officers, military and officials, who all believed that they could control this young ambitionist and, in case of doubt, saw him off again.

For Putin himself, all this should have been a heavy political burden. Instead, his popularity rose exponentially—from 31% to 80% between August and November 1989. Initially, there were several, even understandable reasons for this.

On the one hand, there were the attacks on large residential complexes in Moscow and elsewhere with hundreds of deaths, which were immediately attributed to Islamist Chechens and led to Putin terminating the peace agreement sealed by a handshake in 1997 and unleashing a new war against the semi-independent republic of "Ichkeria", which was waged with devastating violence and terror. So he was already running for president as a wartime prime minister. That it could have been, as not a few indications indicate, the secret service (FSB) itself, and then presumably Putin himself, who carried out these monstrous attacks for exactly this purpose, is a thought that one hardly dares to think through to the end—despite the long stretch of political opponents who have since been infamously eliminated with poison, pistol or other proven means, from Anna Politkovskaya (2005) to Boris Nemtsov (2015) to Alexei Navalny (2024), to name only the most well-known.

To the electorate of 2000, which had recently experienced the shock of hyperinflation and had been expropriated a second and third time, this pale intelligence officer, even if he was Yeltsin's candidate, could at least appear as an energetic and young centrist. All that was needed was the ambiguous promise of a "restoration of statehood and legality" in the midst of a state of anomie and everyday lawlessness. When Putin—as can be seen in an impressive documentary by Vitaly Mansky (*Putin's Witnesses*, 2018)— moved into the headquarters of his freshly created party on the evening of the presidential election in March 2000, with a noisy, relatively young troop of political technologists (as they actually called themselves) to celebrate the incoming results, the nearby Kremlin was shrouded in darkness, like most of the time in Yeltsin's long absences. To put it bluntly: The place of power that Putin and his squad entered as homini novi in order to never give it up again was empty.

Putin almost immediately filled this place with some talent and instinct for the historic opportunity that was offered to him. All those who believed they could use him were dismissed or taught better in a very short time, until all of them, the economic oligarchs, the representatives of the organs of power and the high officials, kowtowed to him—if they did not want to be paraded in a tiger cage in the courtroom and end up in the camp, like the smart oil boss Khodorkovsky, who had dared to contradict Putin in front of the camera.

What was officially supposed to serve the fight against corruption actually served to form a new power and property elite around the center that Putin and his inner "family" now occupied. This followership system of the old Soviet nomenklatura with its rope teams or of the tsarist hereditary, court and service nobility and the civil servants ranks now became all the more a system of completely unvarnished enrichment, but above all a corrupt system of favoritism for political loyalties and services rendered. At the same time, the show trial against the oil tycoon Khodorkovsky also fit into Putin's concept of turning Russia or Russia Inc. into an (almost) pure energy and raw material exporter that used the industrial expansion of the world economy and the upswings of the others (the Europeans or the Chinese) to create a foreign cash fund for the purpose of a new rearmament campaign in order to become a world power again.

This concept also proved to be quite realistic, not least because the USA and the West wore themselves out in their "War on Terror" after September 11, were hopelessly involved in the Middle East and remained dependent on Russia and China as the veto powers in the UN Security Council. Thus, the entry of the new Eastern European NATO member states, which could no longer be postponed, was flanked by multiple offers of a "strategic partnership" to Russia, which was also included in the G-7, now G-8 meetings. In fact, Putin was by no means particularly worried about a "NATO advance" at the time; rather, as he vividly lamented at the Munich Security Conference in 2007, he found himself not equally involved in the decisions of American world politics, such as in Afghanistan and Iraq (Koenen, 2023[2005], p. 477 et seq.).

But the deeper reasons for the popularity and the continuing vassal loyalty, which Putin knows how to mobilize and coin with a large part of his voters again and again in plebiscitary ways, do not simply lie in the unscrupulous efficiency and fortune of his politics. Rather, they touch on other motives and sensitivities that have to do with the chaotic, gone awry history of Russia as the heartland of a global empire. It has left behind a historical, socio-economic and mental void that attracts forced meanings, hypertrophic fantasies of grandeur and megalomaniac self-images.

What do I mean by that? First of all, there is the void left behind by the disappearance of the USSR as an imperial megastate and a superpower that was unique in its kind, with all its elements a transnational culture of life that had developed under this umbrella and had even extended into the vassal states of Eastern Europe, for example the GDR. Putin's superlative of the "greatest geopolitical catastrophe of the 20th century" used in his inaugural speech in 2005 struck a deep chord in Russian self-esteem, precisely where there was a blank space. (Remember Michael Gorbachev's often cited word of the "white spots" in Soviet history.)

In doing so, the sympathetic formula of the "imperial phantom pain" of the Russians fails to recognize that this was about more than just the overdue disappearance of the penultimate, still existing multi-ethnic empire. In view of the hysterical outbursts of hatred and rampant, often anti-Semitic conspiracy theories that circulated in Russian politics and journalism in the early 1990s, some observers, including myself (Koenen, 1991), have spoken of a "Russian Versailles complex" in analogy to German history, in the sense of the collapse of a world power supposedly "undefeated in the field" and stumbled by a stab in the back from behind. In reality, however, it was precisely the relatively peaceful and democratic character of the shipwreck of 1989 that was the real deep sting, the core of the alleged "humiliation" and revanchist bitterness fed by it, which has become the leitmotif and maxim of action of the Putinist era.

Secondly, there is the emptiness of the own history of Russia proper, especially if one wants to reopen it in a Russo-centric way. Russia, as none other than the great Russophile Alexander Solzhenitsyn once said in the 1980s, has inflicted the biggest wounds in its recent history on itself (cf. Koenen, 2023, p. 214). Not foreign aggressors or occupiers, but their own, Soviet government killed its country's children en masse or sent them to camps. This corresponded to a perspective that had also immediately forced itself on me when I was in Moscow for the first time in 1989 for a report on the historical debates, which raged at that time in the Russian public. Most of the German mass crimes had taken place outside their own national borders—in Poland, Ukraine or Belarus—and the majority of the victims were Jewish or "Gypsy" people or citizens of the occupied countries who had been excluded from the German "Volksgemeinschaft". In 1989, on the other hand, mass graves were found and opened in the Russian heartland, as well as in other Soviet republics, and sometimes near or in the suburbs of Kiev as well as Moscow or Leningrad, i.e. right on their own doorstep, in which tens of thousands, hundreds of thousands of victims of the Great Terror of the 1930s lay, while at the same time, the vast archipelago of camp complexes emerged like an ante-diluvian fossil (Koenen, 2023[2007]).

This was and is a history that is infinitely more difficult to understand and "process" than German history was for us as "afterborn" (in the words of a famous poem by Bertolt Brecht). The German mass crimes were exposed to the whole world in 1945. The Soviet, and since the new Russia had taken over the legal succession, the "Russian" mass crimes, on the other hand, had remained hidden for over half a century, were never really allowed to be addressed or revealed. Every second family, it is said, had to mourn victims of Stalinist mass terror; and in this, the Russians hardly differ from the non-Russians among the former Soviet citizens—but very clearly, for example, from the Germans, for whom this does not apply in the same way.

I will quote Alexander Etkind, who made this difference, but above all its psychological consequences, clear with great precision:

> The Holocaust was about the extinction of the others. Soviet terror was self-destructive. This has complicated the unfolding of three important forces that restructure the world after a disaster: the cognitive aspiration to learn from a disaster, the emotional need to mourn the victims; and the active desire to establish justice.
>
> (Etkind, 2013, p. 8 f.)

In addition to these phenomena of a state-enforced "inability to mourn" (to cite a famous book by Alexander and Margarete Mitscherlich from 1967) and the feelings of derealization that the implosion of the Soviet universe has left behind, especially in the Russian heartland, there is also a void left by the decades of an ideologically and artistically bred lie about one's own country and about one's own history. This was coupled with the systematic suppression of many modern sciences and bodies of knowledge in Soviet times, which would have made awareness not only about the world but also about one's own country, possible at the height of time—gaps that were not really filled afterward, except with set pieces of postmodern Western theory production, which contributed significantly to the post-truth cynicism of Putin's "managed democracy" and his spin doctors and ideologues.

In her pitch-black book *The Future Is History*, Masha Gessen (2018) has repeatedly talked about how not only large parts of the theoretical knowledge of the 20th century but also a language in which one's own history and present could have been adequately grasped were missing. One of the people Gessen presents is the Moscow psychoanalyst Marina Aruntyanyan, who in the 1990s tried to discuss her knowledge and practical clinical experience obtained from accessible specialist literature by means of training seminars and teaching analyses in the West (including Germany)– and often had to struggle with nagging feelings of narcissistic insult. At the same time, she often felt helpless (I refer to Gessen's report) in the face of neurotic disorders of her clients, who lived in a situation of constant anxiety and subliminal fear that they shared with the country as a whole. Many of the Western mentors with whom she discussed her cases declined to characterize these disorders as "traumatic". They considered all the fears and feelings of powerlessness of their clients to be projections without external, real reference. Aruntyanyan "wished she had been able to think like that herself". Instead, she began to delve into Freud's concept of a "death drive": "Could it be that this city and this country were about to bury themselves? (…) Everything alive (…) evoked aggression here. The life energy of this society had become unbearable (…) Life was a foreign agent" (Gessen, 2018, p. 571).

I don't know whether these are the words and thoughts of Aruntyanyan or of Gessen, who had to leave Russia in 2013. As an external observer, I would neither trust nor concede such a conclusive judgment to myself, and certainly not as a German historian. But what Aruntyanyan and Gessen accentuate is the real burden of traumatic experiences that have remained unprocessed for two or three generations, which in this case are not a run-of-the-mill word or a fashionable term, but a psychological reality of its own kind that can hardly be dealt with individually.

On the other hand, a number of very tangible geophysical, climatic, socioeconomic, communicative and other factors can also be found for the notorious powerlessness of Russian society in the face of its respective autocratic rulers and oligarchic elites. If the history of the USSR can be described, for example, as a forced attempt at imperial space development, infrastructural penetration and ethnic and cultural amalgamation (in the sense of the production of a "Soviet people" and a "Soviet culture"), then the failure of this multi-victim enterprise has led to large-scale desertification and disintegration, especially within the Russian heartland. These phenomena of a withdrawal from large areas of the country include, in addition to all the uncompensable human losses due to civil war and war, hunger, forced labor and mass terror, as well as a demographic decline that has been going on for decades, in which many historical and current, material and psychological factors come together.

It was and is Putin himself who repeatedly invokes this fear of emptiness and disintegration, as when he said in 2012 on his third or actually fourth inauguration that Russia would "simply dissolve" if it did not return to its "traditional values". But what should these "traditional values" still be? Since then, they have been reinvented again and again in elaborate media mass productions, in a politics of remembrance artificially trimmed to "patriotic pride" in monuments, mausoleums, museums and history books. And as manipulative and often primitive as these forms of mass education are, it is precisely the real empty space of land, history and society that attract such meanings like a physical vacuum.

Putin gave this double syndrome of fear of loss and self-aggrandizement an offensive turn when, in his speech on the annexation of Crimea in the spring of 1914, he apostrophized the Russians as "the largest divided nation in the world" that had the right to live in a country again. This also is called to become the natural center of an even larger "Russian world" shaped by language, culture and religion, which extends "from Kamchatka to the Carpathians", from the Baltic Sea to the Black Sea—and ultimately must encompass, it was not difficult to deduce, the entire geopolitical sphere of the old Russian multi-ethnic empire (Schmid, 2015).

Here in Crimea, which he named in a bold analogy to a "holy place" in the Russian Orthodox world comparable to Jerusalem, Putin also paid homage to "Saint Vladimir" (actually the Varangian prince Voldemar or Volodymyr) as the founder of "Holy Rus", in whose succession he placed himself—I already said: with embarrassing over-ambiguity—and to whom he had a larger-than-life statue erected on one side of the Kremlin in 2016, which was supposed to neutralize the much older Kiev statue of St. Volodymyr, as it were.

For Putin, however, it was and is not only a temptation to tailor such a "historical role" (in the sense of a role-play) to himself; rather, such a role is offered to him again and again by a many-headed, bustling, surpassing or outdoing each other crowd of eulogists, propagandists and ideologues (including some prominent women). The first to do so was his spiritual mentor and personal confessor, Metropolitan Tikhon (Shevtunov), a former film student who still runs a large and lucrative media corporation in addition to his official duties and once praised Putin as a "God-sent" savior and restorer of Russia as early as 2010 and recommended his deeds to the intercession of the faithful (Snyder, 2018, p. 64).

In a way, Putin could hardly help but enter this role of savior, leader, but also preceptor of his country and people—a role that he has then filled since 2012 with a growing self-confidence that can without hesitation be qualified as megalomaniac narcissism. Whereas it is unclear whether or what he believes or does not believe himself. It is just the old, insoluble story of the leader, whose charisma is produced by his entourage or by the disoriented and "fatherless" masses themselves and is offered and ascribed to him (Weber, 1976).

To conclude: Russia, the "Russian Federation" of today, is itself a completely new state that—like Ukraine, like Kazakhstan and the others—emerged from the collapse of the Soviet Union and in this process must first reinvent itself as a nation—like all other new nation-states of the 20th century had to do. It is quite true that the old Russian Empire and the Soviet Union already bore traits of a colonial empire, as the Ukrainians in particular claim today, partly following Western "post-colonial discourses". But this was also true of internal Russia itself in a certain way. As early as the 19th century, the term "self-colonizing empire" (Etkind, 2011) appeared, which was related to the undeveloped expanses as well as to the serfs of Russia. Neither the Tsarist Empire nor the Soviet Union were "Russian" in any strict sense, and the Russians were as much and as little a ruling people as the Turks were in the Ottoman Empire. Both of them, however, were more closely fused with their imperial superstructure than the other peoples of their empire and were prevented from becoming modern nations precisely because of this. And both of them felt naked and defenseless as a result, reacting hysterically and aggressively as the imperial superstructure flew away in the winds of history—in the case of the "Young Turks" to the half-finished genocide of the Armenians in World War I and the mass expulsion of the Greeks after defeat.

Ukraine has now become embroiled in a war of existence and liberation, which it must wage out of sheer self-preservation and by which, with Western support, it will hopefully be able to decisively frustrate Russia's ambitions. Such a defeat would also be a historic opportunity for Russia to finally find itself, to use its productive potentials and abilities for its own development, to become a large but "normal" nation among other nations. It could become the economic, communicative, cultural bridging land between West and East, North and South that it is actually called to be. The neurotic caricature of "Russophobia" in which his enemies supposedly indulge can then be omitted. And this would release Russian society itself from the compulsion to compulsively design itself as a virile, warlike, morally strict, homophobic, pious country, in contrast to the effeminate, degenerate, materially greedy, disintegrating West—as a kind of fantasy Sparta, which it is not at all. Hopefully, this would also be the final implosion of the hypertrophic narcissistic self-aggrandizement in which its elites, its ideologues and, to some extent, its masses have always indulged—precisely because they lacked a clearly defined, positive self-image as a society and community.

Note

1 *Presentation at the IPA Sandler Conference, 29.9.23 in Vienna.*

Literature

Ariès, P. (1994). Die Geschichte der Mentalitäten. In J. LeGoff, R. Chartier & J. Revel (Hg.). *Die Rückeroberung des historischen Denkens. Grundlagen der Neuen Geschichtswissenschaft.* Frankfurt a.M.: Fischer-Taschenbuch-Verlag, 138–165.

Belton, C. (2022). *Putins Netz. Wie ich der KGB Russland zurückholte und dann den Westen ins Auge fasste.* 9. Auflage. Hamburg: HarperCollins.

Braudel, F. (1977 [1958]). Die longue durée. In M. Bloch, F. Braudel & L. Fèbvre. *Schrift und Materie der Gesellschaft. Vorschläge zu einer systematischen Aneignung historischer Prozesse.* Hg. von Claudia Honegger. Frankfurt am Main: Suhrkamp.

Elias, N. (1976 [1969]). Über den Prozess der Zivilisation. *Soziogenetische und psychogenetische Untersuchungen. Zweiter Band: Wandlungen der Gesellschaft. Entwurf zu einer Theorie der Zivilisation.* Frankfurt am Main: Suhrkamp.

Etkind, A. (2011). *Internal Colonization. Russia's Imperial Experience.* Cambridge-Malden: Polity.

Etkind, A. (2013). *Warped Mourning. Stories of the Undead in the Land of the Unburied.* Stanford: Stanford University Press.

Freud, S. (1974 [1921]). Massenpsychologie und Ich-Analyse. In S. Freud. *Fragen der Gesellschaft. Ursprünge der Religion.* Band IX, Studienausgabe, hg. von Alexander Mitscherlich, Angela Richards, James Strachey. Frankfurt am Main: S. Fischer, 61–134.

Gessen, M. (2018). *Die Zukunft ist Geschichte: Wie Russland die Freiheit gewann und verlor*. 2. Auflage. Berlin: Suhrkamp.

Koenen, G. (1991). Die russische Neue Rechte zwischen Nationalbolschewismus und Neofaschismus. In K. Hielscher & G. Koenen. *Die schwarze Front. Der neue Antisemitismus in der Sowjetunion*. Reinbek: Rowohlt, 14–43.

Koenen, G. (2017). Die Farbe Rot. Ursprünge und Geschichte des Kommunismus. *Drittes Buch: Warum Russland? Teil VIII: In Oriente – Der Osten wird rot*. München: C.H.Beck.

Koenen, G. (2023[2005]). Der Russland-Komplex. *Die Deutschen und der Osten. (Aktualisierte und erweiterte Neuauflage 2023)*. München: C.H. Beck.

Koenen, G. (2023). *Im Widerschein des Krieges: Nachdenken über Russland*. München: C.H.Beck

Neumann, F. L. (1954). *Angst und Politik*. Tübingen: Mohr.

Schmid, U. (2015). *Technologien der Seele. Vom Verfertigen der Wahrheit in der russischen Gegenwartskultur*. Frankfurt am Main: Suhrkamp.

Snyder, T. (2018). *The Road to Unfreedom*. Russia, Europe, America. New York: Tim Duggan Books.

Weber, M. (1976 [1921/1922]). *Wirtschaft und Gesellschaft: Grundriß der verstehenden Soziologie*. 5.Auflage, bearbeitet von J. Winckelmann. *Tübingen: Mohr. Erster Halbband, Erster Teil: Soziologische Kategorienlehre*. Drittes Kapitel: Die Typen der Herrschaft. 4. Charismatische Herrschaft.

Part II

Narcissism

Clinical practice and research

5 Challenges in understanding narcissism in patients with autism spectrum disorder

Consequences for psychoanalytical work and research

*Rogério Lerner, Izabella Lopes de Arantes,
Cristiana Castanho de Almeida Rocca,
and Luciano Billodre Luiz*

Introduction

Autism spectrum disorders (ASDs) are neurodevelopmental disorders of multifaceted aetiology with a strong genetic influence. Although it is not a personality disorder, many of its characteristics can affect the personality development of individuals with autism, a matter that has been raising concern lately.

Strunz et al. (2015) conducted an assessment study involving four groups of patients: individuals with ASD, individuals with Narcissistic Personality Disorder (NPD), individuals with Borderline Personality Disorder (BPD), and a nonclinical control group. ASD individuals scored significantly higher on the dimensions of neuroticism (a characteristic associated with narcissism) and emotional dysregulation compared to nonclinical controls. Consistent with lower levels of extraversion, ASD patients also scored significantly higher on the inhibitedness dimension compared to both NPD patients and nonclinical controls. Among all groups, ASD individuals exhibited the lowest scores in openness to experience, particularly in the subscales of aesthetics (appreciation of art and beauty), feelings (openness to inner feelings and emotions), and actions (openness to new practical experiences).

Rinaldi et al. (2021) conducted a literature review highlighting the limited number of studies evaluating personality disorders—a clinical condition often associated with significant narcissism-related difficulties—among individuals diagnosed with ASD. The authors identified only 22 studies involving adults with autism without intellectual disabilities. These studies reported the following personality disorder diagnoses with their respective minimum and maximum prevalence rates: paranoid personality disorder

DOI: 10.4324/9781003565284-8

(0% to 25.9% among patients with ASD and comorbid ADHD), schizoid personality disorder (13% to 36%), schizotypal personality disorder (0% to 23.4%), antisocial personality disorder (0% to 18.5% among patients with ASD and comorbid ADHD), borderline personality disorder (0% to 14.8% among patients with ASD and comorbid ADHD), avoidant personality disorder (2% to 34%), obsessive-compulsive personality disorder (17% to 42.6%), and dependent personality disorder (0% to 22.2% among patients with ASD and comorbid ADHD). Although the comorbidity with narcissistic personality disorder (0% to 6.4%) was low, difficulties associated with narcissism-related processes were evident in other diagnoses. Across all studies using personality assessment tools based on the Big Five model, the Neuroticism trait— possibly reflecting difficulties in narcissistic development—was elevated in individuals with autism compared to comparison groups.

May et al. (2021) conducted a meta-analysis exploring the overlap in the frequency and presentation of ASD and BPD. They found a low combined prevalence of BPD in ASD (4%) and of ASD in BPD (3%) along with inconsistent findings in studies comparing symptoms and related challenges between the two conditions. The prevalence of dual diagnoses (BPD in ASD cohorts and ASD in BPD cohorts) was similar to the general population prevalence of each disorder.

Broglia et al. (2024) carried out a study using the Pathological Narcissism Inventory (PNI) in a sample of 87 adults diagnosed with ASD without intellectual disabilities. The results indicated that individuals on the spectrum demonstrated elevated expression of vulnerable narcissistic traits. However, no significant scores were observed on scales measuring grandiose narcissism. *These findings suggest that comorbidities between ASD and narcissism might be more common than currently recognized in the literature.* This discrepancy may stem from reliance on the diagnostic criteria outlined in the *Diagnostic and Statistical Manual of Mental Disorders* (DSM), which predominantly emphasizes grandiose narcissistic traits while potentially overlooking vulnerable narcissism. The study also posited that individuals with ASD might exhibit narcissistic vulnerability in managing internalizing symptoms such as anxiety and depression. Nonetheless, the authors emphasized the urgent need for further research with larger and more diverse samples to produce more robust findings on this topic.

All studies mentioned above are evidence of impairments in the development of personality of individuals with ASD, even if they do not receive a diagnosis of a personality disorder.

Being affected by autism may be a challenging condition for the development of the personality as psychoanalysis conceives this process. Here, we briefly discuss this subject from the perspective of Kleinian and post-Kleinian contributions, highlighting the role of aggression as a formative element in object relations and in the development of the ego and the inner world.

The infant reacts in different ways to the libidinal investment with the primordial object. Positive emotions serve as favourable valences and negative ones as unfavourable valences for their experiences and qualify their sense of the self and of the object that are under construction in their mind. This libidinal investment, the care received, and the satisfaction of the infant's needs lead to a gradual loving appreciation of the sense of the primordial object by the infant and, through its introjection, of the ego. However, this loving appreciation of the object competes with the baby's omnipotence and the retaining of all libidinal investment, mobilizing hatred and aggression directed towards both the ego and the object. The demands of the id for full and immediate satisfaction are diverse, leading to frustrations experienced by the infant interpreted by him as attacks by the object, which feed the cycle of aggression.

The baby's aggressiveness is projected into the object, which installs itself as a threatening and cruel core in the superego through introjection. The binary construction of the inner world results from splitting both the ego and the object as good or bad, idealized or persecuting. The constant and fluid occurrence of introjections and projections between ego and the object is the basis of the identification and diversification of emotions, mobilizing different defences that serve psychic development. This process enables the increase in complexity of the capacity for emotional representation of lived experiences. Loving experiences must predominate to lessen the intensity of aggression and the imperative demands of the id.

This increased complexity leads to the integration of good and bad aspects of both the ego and the object, advancing the conception of the inner world from binary to triadic, giving way to the ability to forgive, to think and to transform envy into regret for attacks and into jealousy due to the fear of losing the object. The demand of the ideal over the ego can then be negotiated between reality, the id and the superego, which starts to develop a dimension of authority, ensuring limits that protect against the excesses that threaten the mind with fragmentation as well as life itself, favouring a more integrated and realistic view of the self, others and the world. Throughout life, there is a non-reductionist mutual influence between the intrapsychic domain described above and intersubjective experiences, with consequences to the ability to love oneself and others.

The ways adults care for the baby influence this process. The infant relies on the minds of those who care for them to transform their emotions in association with attitudes that mitigate their discomfort, gradually enriching their experiences with thoughts and words. This bonding is responsible for developing emotional regulation as internalized by the baby.

Important difficulties between mothers and babies can occur for several reasons: the baby may have difficulties in processing and expressing their emotions or in introjecting the product of their transformations by the ones who take care of them. Furthermore, those who care for the baby may have difficulties perceiving the baby's needs and discomfort.

The baby's aggressiveness, an important factor in the search for a relationship with the caregiver and in connecting with the world to internalize it, plays also a key role in the gradual separation between the initial care and the caregivers so that the baby can achieve greater autonomy and feelings of self-effectiveness. Those who take care of the baby may have difficulties tolerating the manifestations of aggression, which can be an obstacle to the baby expressing their exploratory capacity and creativity with spontaneity, potentially affecting their ability to love themselves and the object.

The two primary characteristics of autism that form the basis for diagnosis, as outlined in the *Diagnostic and Statistical Manual of Mental Disorders* (5th edition; DSM-5, American Psychiatric Association, 2013), are impairments in communication and interpersonal relationships, alongside the presence of restricted or repetitive interests and behaviours. Additionally, sensory, motor, and emotional regulation difficulties are common in individuals with autism. These challenges become evident at an early age, particularly through motor skills, as observed by Fulceri et al. (2019). Such difficulties pose significant challenges for the infant's capacity to process and express emotions.

Parents of infants who are on the autism spectrum often react to their child's difficulties, even when they are not consciously aware of the neurodevelopmental trajectory. Studies, such as those by Garcia Durand et al. (2019), report higher rates of anxiety and depression among parents of children with autism compared to the general population, potentially due to the emotional and practical demands of caregiving.

Difficulties in emotional processing experienced by infants with autism may significantly impair their ability to experience satisfaction and feel cared for and loved. These deficits can disrupt the process of introjecting a "good object," a crucial developmental milestone. This disruption, coupled with an impaired capacity for satisfaction, may lead to heightened levels of despair and aggression in the child. Consequently, there may be a reinforcement of the introjection of a "bad object" as the core of the superego and heightened demands from the id for immediate gratification.

This disrupted process can obstruct the fluid exchange of introjections and projections between the ego and the object. Such impairments may compromise the autistic individual's ability to identify and differentiate emotions, a deficit frequently observed in clinical practice. These challenges often limit the capacity for emotional representation of lived experiences, resulting in a concrete and literal interpretation of emotional and relational phenomena.

Moreover, these impairments can affect the integration of good and bad aspects of both the ego and the object, fostering rigid fragmentation and splitting. The inability of the ego to negotiate between the demands of the ideal, the id, and the superego may result in the superego becoming overly punitive and sadistic. This dynamic can lead to feelings of persecution, shame, hopelessness, humiliation, and despair.

Parental interactions with autistic infants are often shaped by the characteristics of the disorder. Impairments in emotion regulation, motor skills, and language development are often noticed by parents, even if they are not explicitly aware of them. Parents frequently report feelings of confusion, despair, guilt, and anger. Despite these challenges, most parents persist in their efforts to capture their child's attention and foster communication, often struggling to elicit responses.

However, the parents' role in supporting their child's emotional development may be compromised. Difficulties in helping the child transform emotions into adaptive responses and behaviours can hinder the enrichment of their experiences through thoughts and words. This, in turn, affects the child's development of emotional regulation as an internalized process.

Parents of autistic children often describe the challenges of interpreting their child's needs and discomforts. These difficulties may exacerbate their struggles to tolerate aggressive manifestations, with cascading consequences for the child's exploratory capacity, creativity, spontaneity, and ability to form a loving relationship with themselves and others. This dynamic may be one of the contributing factors to the impaired autonomy observed in individuals with autism as they grow older.

The hypothesis we aim to explore is that autism may increase the likelihood of developing pathological narcissism, a construct described by Kernberg (1975, 1984) as a personality disorder characterized by grandiosity or vulnerability, diminished empathy, exploitative tendencies in relationships (whether dominant or submissive), reliance on primitive defence mechanisms, and superficial relational dynamics.

Vulnerability is an internal state in which a person's self-esteem is significantly fragile and extremely dependent on the assurances of others, in front of whom the person feels despised, humiliated or like a failure, fuelling hopelessness, revolt and emptiness. Vulnerability can be defensively covered by grandiosity, which is the pretence of superiority, or it can manifest itself explicitly in the face of any frustration or difference between the person and others.

Failure in empathy involves disregarding the feelings of others and expecting one's own interests to prevail over those of others. When feeling frustrated, failure in empathy leads people with pathological narcissism to feel attacked and then to counter-attack explicitly or implicitly by means of contempt.

People with pathological narcissism utilize more primitive defence mechanisms due to difficulties in integrating their representations of themselves and others. Consequently, their connection with reality is unstable, and their bonds tend to exhibit emotional superficiality.

The most severe manifestation of pathological narcissism is malignant narcissism, which is a combination of narcissistic, paranoid, and antisocial tendencies. In addition to the self-image marked by grandiosity and lapses in the ability to feel empathy, these individuals also exhibit an important sadistic element. These traits can manifest themselves in violent behaviours that colour the feeling of triumphant control with deleterious consequences concretely imposed on others, gaining prevalence or even exclusivity as a source of self-esteem and satisfaction.

This chapter discusses aspects of narcissism from the psychoanalytic perspective using data previously collected of two patients with ASD. The data was collected when they were referred by their psychiatrists to seek psychological evaluation because of having ASD. The clinical records of these two patients were selected for the current study for being the only two patients with ASD of the clinic who were above 18 years of age and were not intellectually impaired.

Methods

In this exploratory study, 11 items that assess the construct "narcissism" in the Structured Interview of Personality Organization-Revised (STIPO-R) (Clarkin et al., 2016; Brazilian version established by Luiz, 2020) were applied a posteriori to the results of the Thematic Apperception Test (TAT) (Murray, 1967) completed by the two autistic patients during a comprehensive psychological evaluation.

Subjects

Patient 1: Female, approximately 50 years of age at the time of evaluation. The patient was diagnosed with ASD level 1 (DSM-V).

The score on the Social Responsiveness Scale, Second Edition (SRS2, Constantino & Gruber, 2015), was 65, indicating significant impairments in reciprocal social behaviour.

The result of the Personality Factorial Battery (Nunes et al., 2013) was very high (percentile > 90), with low self-esteem, fear of abandonment by significant people, insecurity, extreme dependence on close relationships and difficulties in making decisions even in trivial day-to-day situations.

The scores on the version of the Wechsler Intelligence Scale for adults (WAIS-III, Nascimento, 1997) adapted and standardized for a Brazilian population were as follows: global intellectual score, 124, in the upper performance range; verbal score, 112, in the higher average of performance; and execution score, 127, with above-average performance.

Patient 2: Female, approximately 18 years of age at the time of evaluation. The patient was diagnosed with ASD level 1 (DSM-V).

The SRS2 score was 53, within the normal range. Patients with very mild autism may have scores at the upper end of the normal range if they are well adjusted and their adaptive functioning is relatively intact.

The most significant results of the Factorial Personality Inventory-II (FPI-II) (Leme et al., 2013) were extremely high scores in assistance (indicating great desires and feelings of pity, compassion and tenderness), intraception (indicating a high tendency to be guided by feelings, fantasy, imagination and introspection), cuddling (suggesting a strong desire for support and protection and a hope of their desires being satisfied) and deference (indicating reverence and desire to admire and support a superior).

The scores on the Brazilian adaptation of the Wechsler Abbreviated Intelligence Scale (Trentini et al., 2014) were as follows: global score, 103, indicating average performance; verbal score, 115, indicating upper average performance; and execution score, 90, indicating average performance.

Measures

1 **STIPO-R**

The STIPO-R is a semi-structured interview with 55 items from 6 fundamental domains used to diagnose the level of personality organization according to psychoanalytic precepts. The 6 domains are identity, object relations, primitive defences, mature defences, aggression and moral values. This interview is consistent with the new dimensional model for assessing personality proposed in Section 3 of the DSM-V and ICD-11.

The interview includes a narcissism subscale, which has 11 questions distributed across 6 domains, which are listed below.

Narcissism 1, Question 3: Identity, Investment capacity, Satisfaction: Assesses satisfaction with work or study and pride in considering that one is doing a "good job".

Narcissism 2, Question 9: Identity, Sense of self, Need for admiration: Assesses the importance given to the need for approval from other important people, the need to be the centre of attention and the sadness when approval is not received.

Narcissism 3, Question 9: Identity, Sense of self, Fluctuation of self-esteem: Evaluates the intensity and frequency of variations in self-esteem.

Narcissism 4, Question 25: Object relations, Investment in others, Egocentrism: Assesses egocentrism.

Narcissism 5, Question 26: Object relations, Investment in others, Boredom: Assesses loss of interest in people over time.

Narcissism 6, Question 29: Object relations, Investment in others, Economic view: Evaluates the frequency and intensity of rivalry and the feeling that people are obtaining advantages.

Narcissism 7, Question 30: Object relations, Investment in others, Empathy: Evaluates the difficulty in offering support and comfort to close people in emotional distress.

Narcissism 8, Question 32: Primitive defences, Idealization/Devaluation: Assesses the frequency and intensity of idealization and devaluation.

Narcissism 9, Question 36: Primitive defences, Narcissistic fantasies: Assesses frequency and intensity of fantasies of grandiosity.

Narcissism 10, Question 46: Aggressiveness, Directed at others, Envy: Assesses the frequency and intensity of reactions of envy and self-depreciation resulting from the success of others.

Narcissism 11, Question 55: Moral values, Exploitation: Assesses the frequency and intensity of exploiting other people for one's own benefit.

2   TAT

The TAT involves the presentation of a set of images (displayed on different standardized boards) from which the examinee will construct narratives. The objective is to indirectly access ideas about how the external and internal worlds are perceived and what emotions or feelings are mobilized in certain situations. The responses of the patients also allow for the consideration of various aspects of issues related to the narcissistic organization of the personality.

Board 1: "The boy and the violin": The most common narratives related to this board include themes about authority, ways of dealing with responsibilities and the self-ideal.

Board 3: "The young woman at the door" (female version): Feelings of guilt and despair may appear; in this version, both the sex and age of the character are more easily identified, which may limit the likelihood of projection.

Board 6: "Surprised woman" (female version): This picture explores the relationship between the daughter and father figures. The narrative usually describes the woman being surprised by the man, who is generally understood as a father but can also be described as a romantic partner.

Board 7: "Girl and doll" (female version): This picture explores the relationship with the maternal figure, which can be perceived as a source of support or impediment to the person's achievements.

Board 11: "Primitive stone landscape": This picture is one of the most abstract pictures of the test. The narratives commonly include themes related to the way in which the person faces new challenges. The narratives can involve fantastic and primitive elements that favour the perception of a person's attitudes towards unconscious issues.

Board 16: "Blank": This board is blank, and owing to the absence of a drawing to precipitate the narrative, the person tends to project themselves, often appearing as current issues or even transference issues at the time of the test (Murray, 1967).

Ethical issues

Resolution No. 510/2016 of the National Health Council of Brazil states that material collected from patients during clinical appointments that are not originally intended for research may be used without the need to sign a consent form, provided that their identity is protected. Additionally, measures are taken to disguise each report abstract so that it cannot be recognized by its author.

Discussion

Summaries of the narratives produced by each patient for the TAT boards are described below, followed by a discussion of aspects of narcissism based on STIPO-R items, analysis of the TAT responses and interviews with participants that took place at the time of evaluation.

Patient 1

Board 1: A boy who did not like to study would go to school and just play without paying attention. His father, who was a violinist, told him to learn to play the instrument, but the boy got angry because he couldn't play and decided to pay attention in class, so he wouldn't have to take violin lessons.

Narcissism 1, Question 3: The boy in the narrative who does not take pleasure in studying may reveal low capacity of investment by the self because of difficulties in the identification of the ego with a good internalized object. His inability to learn to play the violin as his father wanted may indicate the introjection of this object as an impediment to the growth of the ego, leading to an avoidant submission (deciding to pay attention in class) for fear of the paternal cruelty owing to the frustration of his representation as an ego ideal (playing the violin).

Narcissism 2, Question 9: The boy in the narrative becoming angry can represent a shock to his self-esteem due to his need for approval from other important people who represent an idealized object, such as his father.

Narcissism 4, Question 25: Playing at school to avoid studying may reveal an egocentric defence of the boy against negative feelings towards the ego. The father imposing his interest as a punishment on the son who does not share the same appreciation for the violin may reveal an egocentric imposition of his own ideal, disregarding the boy's needs.

Board 3 RH: The woman has had a tough life and always worked hard to provide education for her three children. Currently, she is crying because everyone has gone their own way, and she is alone with her husband.

Narcissism 2, Question 9: The woman's crying can represent the impact of her need for approval from other important people who represent an idealized object, such as her children, on her self-esteem. This need may be a defensive effort of compensation for the feeling of impoverishment of the ego.

Narcissism 5, Question 26: The withdrawal of the children from their mother may reveal a tendency to withdraw from people who were once close, losing interest in the despised and abandoned maternal object as a massive projection of the ego felt as unattractive, helpless and victimized by the harshness of life, representing a cruel superego. The children represent the triumphalist superego aspect that deprives the maternal object of value.

Narcissism 6, Question 29: The woman crying because she misses her children while in the company of a husband who is not valued as an object capable of providing comfort may reveal a rivalry between husband and children for the mother's preference. This rivalry may be the splitting of the maternal ego and the projection of the ideal aspect into the children and the devalued one into the husband.

Narcissism 7, Question 30: The husband and children not supporting the female character in her sadness may represent difficulty in offering support, consolation and comfort to people close to them who are experiencing emotional distress because they feel that the ego itself is impoverished and has not been sufficiently valued by the maternal object.

Board 6 MF: A secretary who liked to be alone was arranging her things in the office while thinking about her life, and her boss came into the room smoking, knowing that she did not like this habit.

Narcissism 1, Question 3: The secretary taking pleasure in being alone thinking about life instead of work may indicate a defence against the low investment capacity of the self caused by difficulties in identifying the ego with a good internalized object in face of the boss being characterized as a superego object that despises her preferences (smoking in the room), imposing a relationship of submission.

Narcissism 4, Question 25: Both the secretary thinking about her life and the boss imposing himself by smoking are characterized as egocentric. The resort to egocentrism can be considered a defence against feelings of ego inferiority represented by the secretary, who is submissive to the boss.

This hypothetical analysis is consistent with the fact that this patient left work many years ago and does not feel motivated to resume any productive activity. She felt hopeless, perceiving her life as monotonous and emotionless.

The patient reported being afraid that people who are emotionally important to her would withdraw as a result of her attitude. In an attempt to control this type of situation, she adopts attitudes that go against her will, with the sole objective of submissively pleasing others. She feels insecure and very dependent on the attention of people close to her.

The analysis of her narratives that was done by the clinician during the assessment suggested that she fears having aggressive reactions when she feels insecure and despised. In addition, she exhibited a melancholic way of dealing with losses and felt sadness because of the distance of her children, tending to isolate herself in pain.

The patient reported being very suspicious and fearful that people might have bad intentions. She tries not to express herself in public because she feels embarrassed in situations of greater exposure.

The patient reported being critical and harsh with male authority figures, resisting the affection she might otherwise obtain. In contrast, female figures are perceived as fragile and in constant need of help, unlike male ones, who are endowed with power.

Patient 2

Board 1: A boy sadly observes his violin. He broke the instrument because he played too hard. He does not have the money to fix it. He was angry because he could not play well.

Narcissism 3, Question 9: Being angry can reveal a cruel superegoic attack against the ego that is experienced as a failure (expressed as not being able to play well). As a defence against this internal attack on the ego, the boy turns his violence outwards, ruining the violin. Given that these defences are inconsistent and eventually fail, the sad look can signify a projective identification of the damaged ego with the damaged object. Not having money to repair the violin may indicate a feeling of ego impoverishment due to massive projections into the object, followed by discouragement, represented by the inability to repair the instrument.

Board 3RH: A woman was very sad with the direction her life had taken. She had lost her dog to an illness and was very lonely because he was her only friend. The woman was married but had divorced her husband.

Narcissism 5, Question 26: The woman having the dog as her only friend after the divorce may indicate a tendency to despise the expendable object (husband), massively projecting her experience that her ego is despicable into him.

Narcissism 6, Question 29: If the relationship with the dog as her only friend is viewed as a triumph in a rivalry with the husband whom she despised by divorcing, sadness over the dog's death can represent an experience of defeat in the face of the object of rivalry (the husband) instead of the loss of a loved object (the dog). The defeat may be inflicted by the disease or by the course of life, which can be perceived as cruelly vengeful owing to the projection of women's superego aspects that are prone to rivalry.

Board 6 MF: A man looks angrily at a woman, who feels scared, because he believes that her attitude in fighting for female independence and the right to work in a sexist society is inappropriate.

Narcissism 2, Question 9: The man becoming angry can represent a shock to his self-esteem caused by his need to be the centre of attention of other important people as a compensation for the feeling of impoverishment of the ego.

Narcissism 4, Question 25: The man's anger towards female independence may have more than one emotional meaning. It may result from the frustration of his egocentric need to control the woman as an object in which there is a massive defensive projection of his ego, which is felt as inferior, weak and submissive, identifying the protagonist (the man) with the cruel superego that denies the emotional value of the female object.

Narcissism 10, Question 46: In addition to the above consideration, the narrative can represent that valuing the woman for entering the workforce may impact the man in terms of his weakened ego capacity in the face of his ego ideal: the woman achieves what he feels unable to. By becoming independent, frustrating the man's need for superego control and gaining a value that is envied by the weakened male ego, the woman may receive a projection of the cruelty of this superego so that her autonomy is experienced as an attack on the male protagonist, which reinforces his anger. The woman may feel frightened by the aggressiveness of the man's superego as himself does deep inside.

Board 7: A teenager who feels lonely holds her newborn brother, who was having a crying fit, in her arms, while the mother reads poems to try to calm him down. The girl becomes upset because she wanted to go out with her friends, but she loves her brother very much.

Narcissism 2, Question 9: The loneliness of the adolescent can reflect the impact on her self-esteem because of her need to be preferred by other important people who represent an idealized object, such as her mother, as a compensation for the feeling of impoverishment of the ego.

Narcissism 4, Question 25: The crying baby may represent a feeling of helplessness in face of objects experienced as egocentric and unfit for caring, since the mother reads to the baby without having him in her lap; he is held by his sister, but she has her friends in mind instead of him. Despite loving her brother very much, the girl experiences a defensive split, in which the girl's expectation of going out with her friends prevails, making her feel lonely when frustrated. This split impedes that the love for her brother softens her. The friends she wanted for herself can be viewed as a triumph over the mother and baby around which the girl's experience is ego-centred as a defence against helplessness. The mother who does not hold her crying baby in her arms and reads instead of addressing him directly may also represent an egocentric attitude.

Narcissism 6, Question 29: Through the projection of the superegoic rivalry, the girl may feel that the baby and the mother triumph over her; she seeks revenge by longing for her friends and by not satisfying herself with the emotional value of her brother, on whom the girl projects her despised ego.

Feeling spoiled by the mother-baby pair, the girl may project this feeling into her brother, who continues to cry, feeling spoiled of the calm that the mother could offer him. The sister feels that she has to submissively lose what she wanted (visiting her friends) to take care of her brother. He gains her presence, but she loses what she wants.

Board 11: A seven-year-old girl is very sad about having lost her parents while walking in the mountains. She comes across a dog that helps her find her parents. She wants to keep the dog, but she knows her parents do not like animals. She manages to convince them after crying and begging a lot.

Narcissism 5, Question 26: There is more than one possible line of interpretation for this scene. The parents who allow the girl to get lost may be a representation of contempt for the daughter, who is helpless and sad. Losing herself can express a girl's defensive attitude of triumphant contempt towards her parents. The dog finds her parents, not the girl, which may indicate the egoic feeling of hopelessness in relation to the parents or a defensive denial of their value and of her need to reach them. Sadness can also be a manifestation of frustration of her manic expectation of her defensive self-sufficiency.

Narcissism 6, Question 29: The couple having remained together while they lost the girl may represent a rivalry with marital appreciation to the detriment of the appreciation of the daughter. The girl's rivalling superego revenge can manifest itself in two ways: convincing her parents by crying, imposing her will in the argument with them, and fuelling a rivalry between the parents and the dog, which would be the winner of the girl's preference.

Board 16: The story describes a place of peace where the people were good and fair, which is very different from reality. This world was created by the imagination of a depressed girl, who was going through a very difficult phase, without the will to live and believing that no one cared about her.

Narcissism 3, Question 9: The lack of will to live may represent the weakened ego of the girl feeling hopeless being attacked by her cruel superego, which in turn can be massively projected into others as an expectation that no one cares about her.

Narcissism 9, Question 36: The place of peace in which people are good and just may be an omnipotent manifestation of her needs as a demanding ego ideal in relation to which the ego is perceived as a failure.

The analysis of the projective material that was done by the clinician during the assessment indicated that the patient has a fragile and unstable mental state, with internal restlessness and anxiety due to feelings of inferiority, incapacity, and dissatisfaction, using inhibitory defences that suppress the expression of feelings and lead to withdrawal.

The inability to handle interpersonal relationships in a profound way leads to contact avoidance, with coldness and distance from the outside world. The patient has little ability to establish spontaneous social contacts, feels ashamed, and has difficulty to correctly evaluate her own potential, with intense concern for social criticism. This difficulty is also expressed in her sexuality, as she suffers from feelings of maladjustment in relation to her body. The patient tends to be at the mercy of the decisions of others, assuming a passive position.

The patient reported expecting to have her desires satisfied; to be stroked, loved, guided, and comforted; and to seek support and protection. She would like to feel more valued, important and admired by people. She is susceptible to feelings or anxiety of abandonment and insecurity when not satisfied, and she fears being taken over by anger, irritation and hatred. She fears identifying with things that she considers ugly and undesirable and tends to perceive the world as hostile and persecutory.

The patient has demonstrated to be ambitious, with a desire to excel, overcome obstacles and maintain high standards of achievement. However, faced with difficulties performing some tasks, she feels frustrated, angry, and sad.

Final remarks

The narratives that the patients constructed for the TAT boards were analysed on the basis of hypotheses of potential underlying intrapsychic dynamics related to narcissism. The TAT is a projective test in which the examinee's narratives about the boards are interpreted by the examiner according to a set of criteria. We sought to offer a possible interpretation of the material produced by the examinee from the psychoanalytical point of view defined at the beginning of the chapter, considering the clinical experience.

This exploratory analysis is not intended to be conclusive. The psychic aspects of narcissism indicate that the two patients with autism experience significant suffering in which ego fragility and helplessness in the face of idealizations and persecutory anxieties prevail. Primitive psychic mechanisms such as massive projection and introjection, splitting, denial and idealization involving the ego, the ego ideal, and the superego were highlighted.

The integration of this analysis with material that had been previously collected during interviews and obtained through the application of personality assessment instruments indicates that the profile of narcissistic suffering in both cases is based in vulnerability. The patients also exhibit significant difficulties in emotion regulation, decreased self-esteem, and confidence. Impairments in their ability to communicate feelings and emotional needs make it difficult to detect this profile in clinical work.

Although it is not possible to generalize, the vulnerability profile described here is the one most frequently observed in clinical practice, even when its expression is masked by compensatory strategies developed by patients or by their autistic manifestations. Conversely, the grandiose profile, while rare, may also present. However, it is often more challenging to address therapeutically due to the inherent inaccessibility and defensiveness of these patients.

In the clinical care of people with autism, difficulties believed to arise from this diagnosis, such as the occurrence of restricted and repetitive interests, as well as difficulties in social interaction and communication, are addressed more often. These characteristics are expected for people with autism, which leads relatives, patients, and clinicians to not suspect that other psychic aspects which are not pathognomonic of autism may have a role in mental suffering and relationships.

A deeper exploration of emotional dynamics often requires accessing experiences such as those described above, with the aim of benefiting both patients and their families. This exploratory study highlights the importance of continued research, especially in light of the growing emphasis on personality assessments discussed in the introduction. Expanding our understanding of how personality traits or profiles, particularly narcissistic ones, manifest in individuals with ASD is crucial to deepening our insight into the psychological challenges they face. To achieve this, it is necessary to go beyond surface observations and investigate the underlying psychic mechanisms that prevail in such situations.

As a next step, we plan to systematically assess individuals with autism using the *Structured Interview of Personality Organization* (STIPO-R-BR). This approach may contribute to the growing body of knowledge derived from psychoanalytic clinical work with ASD patients, shedding light on the intrapsychic difficulties discussed here and their interpersonal consequences. By integrating systematic assessments with clinical observations, we hope to advance our understanding of these dynamics and their impact on patients with ASD.

References

American Psychiatric Association [APA] (2013). *Diagnostic and Statistical Manual of Mental Disorders*, 5th Edn. Washington, DC: American Psychiatric Association.

Broglia, G., Nisticò, V., Di Paolo, B., Faggioli, R., Bertani, A., Gambini, O., & Demartini, B. (2024). Traits of narcissistic vulnerability in adults with autism spectrum disorders without intellectual disabilities. *Autism Research, 17*(1), 138–147. https://doi.org/10.1002/aur.3065

Clarkin, J. F., Caligor, E., Stern, B., & Kernberg, O. F. (2016). *The Structured Interview for Personality Organization-Revised (STIPO-R)*. Weill Medical College of Cornell University.

Constantino, J., & Gruber, C. (2015). *Escala de Responsividade Social – SRS 2*. Hogrefe.

Fulceri, F., Grossi, E., Contaldo, A., Narzisi, A., Apicella, F., Parrini, I., Tancredi, R., Calderoni, S., & Muratori, F. (2019). Motor skills as moderators of core symptoms in autism spectrum disorders: Preliminary data from an exploratory analysis with artificial neural networks. *Frontiers in Psychology, 9*, 2683.

Garcia Durand, J., Batista Geraldini, S. A. R., Perez Paschoal, L., Cangueiro, L., Tamarozzi Mamede, D., Scandiuzzi de Brito, T., Vaz Marques, M., David, V., &

Lerner, R. (2019). Case-contrast study about parent–infant interaction in a Brazilian sample of siblings of children with autism spectrum disorders. *Infant Mental Health Jouranl, 40,* 289–301. https://doi.org/10.1002/imhj.21772

Kernberg, O. F. (1975). *Borderline Conditions and Pathological Narcissism.* Jason Aronson.

Kernberg, O. F. (1984). *Severe Personality Disorders: Psychotherapeutic Strategies.* Yale University Press.

Leme, I. F. A. S., Rabelo, I. S., & Alves, G. A. S. (2013). *Inventário Fatorial de Personalidade-II (IFP-II) Manual Técnico –* São Paulo: Casa do Psicólogo.

Luiz, L. B. (2020). *Tradução, adaptação cultural e evidências de validade da versão brasileira da "Structure Interview of Personality Organization-Revised".* STIPO-R Brasil.

May, T., Pilkington, P., Younan, R., & Williams, K. (2021). Overlap of autism spectrum disorder and borderline personality disorder: A systematic review and meta-analysis. *Autism Research, 14*(9), 2071–2083. https://doi.org/10.1002/aur.2619

Murray, H. A. (1967). *Teste de apercepção temática.* Mestre Jou.

Nascimento, E. (1997). *Adaptação e padronização de uma amostra brasileira.* São Paulo: Casa do Psicólogo.

Nunes, C. H. S., Hutz, C. S., & Nunes, M. F. O. (2013). *Bateria Fatorial de Personalidade – BFP: questionário auto aplicativo que avalia características do comportamento emocional (Bateria Fatorial de Personalidade (BFP) – Manual técnico.* Itatiba, SP: Casa do Psicólogo.

Rinaldi, C., Attanasio, M., Valenti, M., Mazza, M., & Keller, R. (2021). Autism spectrum disorder and personality disorders: Comorbidity and differential diagnosis. *World Journal of Psychiatry, 11*(12), 1366–1386. https://doi.org/10.5498/wjp.v11.i12.1366

Strunz, S., Westphal, L., Ritter, K., Heuser, I., Dziobek, I., & Roepke, S. (2015). Personality pathology of adults with autism spectrum disorder without accompanying intellectual impairment in comparison to adults with personality disorders. *Journal of Autism and Developmental Disorders, 45,* 4026–4038.

Trentini, C. M., Yates, D. B., Stumpf, & Heck, V. (2014). Adaptação brasileira da Escala Wechsler abreviada de Inteligência (WASI): São Paulo: Casa do Psicólogo.

6 Types of narcissism
A neuropsychoanalytic contribution

Mark Solms

Introduction

It is hard to imagine a satisfactory theory of mental functioning in health and disease that doesn't include the concept of 'narcissism'. Yet, this concept was introduced into psychology and psychiatry barely more than a century ago (Ellis, 1898; Näcke, 1899) and it still has no place in neuroscience (or pitifully little place; see Solms, 1995).

From the start, Freud's (1914) conception of narcissism—which represented a giant leap beyond those of Ellis and Näcke—was intimately bound up with his drive theory. In the first such theory, in which he classified our innate drives dualistically under the headings of 'sexual' and 'self-preservative' (Freud, 1915), he conceptualized narcissism as a libidinal disposition in which the sexual drive selects the ego as its love object (this is 'self-love' versus 'object-love'). Freud (1920) was prompted to revise this drive theory partly by his subsequent observation that self-preservation was motivated, at bottom, by narcissism. That is, Freud observed that we want to continue existing only because we love ourselves. But this is not an *innate* disposition; some people do not love themselves enough to want to continue existing—they take no pleasure in their own being, and they can even hate themselves to the extent of killing themselves. This removed Freud's justification for distinguishing between sexual and self-preservative drives. He therefore combined them under the heading of 'life' drives, which he now contrasted with a 'death' drive: an innate tendency to self-destruction, which secondarily becomes aggression when it is deflected outwards. This radical revision of his drive theory introduced new depth to our understanding of narcissism, which had previously been conceptualized in purely libidinal terms. Freud now recognized that narcissism has a *destructive* aspect; that the deflection outwards of the so-called death drive, too, is attributable to narcissism. This was epitomized by his shocking claim that 'hate, as a relation to objects, is older than love' (Freud, 1915, p. 122). Henceforth, narcissism was associated not only with self-love and the introjection of all that is good but also with object-hatred and the projection of all that is bad (Freud, 1925). The theory of 'destructive narcissism' was developed

DOI: 10.4324/9781003565284-9

further after Freud's death by British psychoanalysts, mainly with reference to the notion of primary envy (e.g., Klein, 1957).

Although the entire Kleinian development was predicated upon Freud's second drive theory, at least initially, most psychoanalysts today do not rely upon this theory anymore (and if they do, they use it in essentially metaphorical terms). This loss of confidence in Freudian drive theory has led to an abandonment of drive theory in general; that is, psychoanalysts today have largely abandoned the concept of 'drive' altogether.

This is a lamentable situation, since it is via the drives that the mind is *embodied*. Freud's definition of 'drive' (as opposed to his classification of the drives) remains as serviceable today as it ever was: 'a measure of the demand made upon the mind for work in consequence of its connection with the body' (1915, p. 107). Who can deny that imperative demands are made upon the mind for work in consequence of bodily needs—such as hunger, thirst, sleepiness, pain and the like—let alone sexuality?

Be that as it may, the aim of the present paper is not to make the point that if we have lost confidence in Freudian drive theory then we are obliged to replace it with another drive theory (on that point, see Solms, 2021). Rather, the aim of this paper is to consider some of the consequences for the concept of narcissism if we replace Freud's final classification of the drives with an alternative one, which was developed in the last decade of the 20th century under the banner of 'affective neuroscience' (Panksepp, 1998).

It is unnecessary to set out the reasons why a *neurobiological* taxonomy of the drives should replace the classical psychoanalytical one (on that, again, see Solms, 2021). This cross-disciplinary borrowing is precisely what Freud predicted would happen, and should happen:

> I am altogether doubtful whether any decisive pointers for the differentiation and classification of the drives can be arrived at on the basis of working over the psychological material. This working over seems rather itself to call for the application to the material of definite assumptions concerning the life of the drives, *and it would be a desirable thing if those assumptions could be taken from some other branch of knowledge* and carried over to psychology.
>
> (Freud, 1915, pp. 109–110, emphasis added)

> It should be made quite clear that the uncertainty of our speculation [about the drives] has been greatly increased by *the necessity for borrowing from the science of biology*. Biology is truly a land of unlimited possibilities. We may expect it to give us the most surprising information, and we cannot guess what answers it will return in a few dozen years to the questions we have put to it. They may be of a kind which will blow away the whole of our artificial structure of hypothesis.
>
> (Freud, 1920, p. 57, emphasis added)

So, given the fact that Freud's conception of narcissism was intimately bound up with his drive theories, and given that his second drive theory underpinned a (if not the) major subsequent development of the concept in psychoanalysis, let us now consider what happens to it if we adopt the currently authoritative neurobiological classification of the drives, according to which there are not two emotional drives but rather *seven*. The consequences, surely, must be far reaching. Freud thought that all pleasure was libidinal (and that the satisfaction of self-preservative drives only became pleasurable through 'anaclisis'); but it turns out that there are many different types of pleasure in the brain.

Before I can delineate the consequences of this for the concept of narcissism, a brief introduction to the current neurobiological drive theory is required.

Homeostasis

Freud's definition of drive ('a measure of the demand made upon the mind for work in consequence of its connection with the body') is understood nowadays as a manifestation of the most fundamental mechanism in biology: namely, homeostasis.

Every living thing must remain within its viable bounds, if it is to stay alive. This applies across a wide range of parameters, such as—in the case of us human beings—core body temperature, blood pressure, oxygen level, water level, sugar level, amount of sleep, etc. The ideal points between these viable bounds are called 'set-points'. Deviations away from set-points are called 'needs', which represent measures of bodily demand for work: the animal must *do something* to reduce this measure (i.e., the quantity of deviation) back towards the set-point. To this end, it deploys 'predictions', most of which are innate and operate automatically (e.g., perspiration and panting are predicted to reduce body temperature; slowed heart rate and vasodilation are predicted to reduce blood pressure). These innate physiological predictions are called 'reflexes'. Their psychological equivalents are 'instincts'.[1]

Reflexes and instincts are stereotyped responses to need, which succeed only in *expected* environments: that is, in the environmental niches for which they were naturally selected. The respiratory reflex, for example, which is automatically deployed to meet our oxygen needs, succeeds only if ambient air contains the expected level of oxygen. If it does not, then the need is *felt* in the form of suffocation alarm—that is, it becomes conscious. It is at this point that the body starts to make demands upon *the mind* for work. Therefore, it is at this point that we begin to speak of 'drive' (as opposed to 'need').

In accordance with what Freud called the 'pleasure principle', increasing drive demand is felt as unpleasure and decreasing demand as pleasure. In addition to this extremely important dimension (called 'valence'), each drive also has a categorical *quality*. Thus, the unpleasant feeling of suffocation differs from the unpleasant feeling of thirst and from that of sleep deprivation, and so on. The quality of the feeling has the value of identifying *which* category of need is being prioritized.

The reason why drives are felt is because the subject, being in an unexpected situation in which its innate prediction has failed, must make behavioural *choices*, and choices must (necessarily) be underwritten by a value system: one which distinguishes between 'good' and 'bad' alternatives. This is what feelings do: they enable us to *feel our way* through uncertain situations. In this way, they underwrite voluntary (as opposed to automatic) behaviour.

Moreover, feeling our way through situations enables us to *learn* from the experiences. This is called the 'law of effect', which states: 'responses that produce a satisfying effect in a particular situation become more likely to occur again in that situation, and responses that produce a discomforting effect become less likely to occur again in that situation'. In other words, feeling our way through life's problems enables us to supplement our innate predictions with more flexible, acquired ones.

Panksepp distinguishes seven 'emotional' drives from the bodily drives that I have mentioned so far. These are the drives which are of greatest interest to psychoanalysts, so I will focus on them for the remainder of this chapter. Before discussing the types of narcissism that are associated with each of these drives, I will briefly enumerate them, identify their set-points and their associated instinctual predictions, and describe the feelings that announce the success or failure of predictions.

The seven emotional drives

1. LUST. The set-point for this drive is: 'a sexual object is freely available to me'. (Please note: the viable bounds of the sexual drive serve the preservation of the species—not the individual.) The individual subject is not motivated by remote evolutionary mechanisms but rather by here-and-now feelings. This is why sexual behaviours—of which there are a great variety—do not by any means typically result in reproduction. (In fact, in the case of *all* drives, we sentient beings are motivated by feelings; knowledge of the biological imperatives that led to the evolution of those feelings is superfluous.) The instinctual predictions associated with LUST include: lordosis, mounting, intromission and thrusting behaviours. These crude and stereotyped actions which are predicted to satisfy the sexual drive do not get you very far. Everything else that you need to know about how to get people to have sex with you—and especially those individuals that you want to have sex with—must therefore be *learned* through experience. Successful prediction in respect of the LUST drive is felt as erotic pleasure, which peaks at orgasm, and failure is felt as pent-up desire.

2. SEEKING. Much of what Freud conceptualized under the heading of 'libido' extends well beyond the confines of the LUST drive, as we understand it in neurobiology today. A substantial portion of what Freud called libido is nowadays called SEEKING (a drive which is mediated not by sex hormones but rather by dopamine).[2] The set-point for this drive is: 'I am actively engaging with something interesting'. In this sense, it may be described as 'epistemophilic': a drive to *know*. Engaging proactively with novelty reduces ignorance about the world—the world in which we must satisfy our needs—therefore, it enhances our chances of survival and reproductive success, in the long run. The instinctual behaviour associated with SEEKING is foraging—that is, exploration—which may be translated into words via the biblical phrase: 'seek and you shall find'. Since this is not strictly true (sometimes we seek and do not find), this prediction must be supplemented by learning. Successful SEEKING predictions are felt as curiosity, intertest, enthusiasm and optimistic expectancy; unsuccessful ones are felt as boredom, emptiness, apathy and pessimistic despair. An important distinction between LUST and SEEKING is that the set-point of the former is *consummatory*, whereas the set-point of the latter is *appetitive*; in other words, the SEEKING drive is never 'satiated'. (For this reason, SEEKING is active even while we sleep; and it is the driving force behind dreaming; see Solms, 2011.)[3]

3. RAGE. This drive is not synonymous with aggression. It involves a particular type of aggression, which we call 'hot' aggression. The aggression associated with SEEKING is 'cold' or 'predatory'. (Think of a prowling lion.) Later, we will learn about a third drive associated with aggression—of the 'territorial' or 'dominance' type—namely, the drive to PLAY. The latter type of aggression involves symbolic 'display' behaviours (thus, we say of a dog defending its territory that 'its bark is worse than its bite'). The set-point for RAGE is: 'there are no impeding objects getting between me and what I need'. The instinctual behaviour that is predicted to rectify things when this imperative is frustrated is called 'affective attack'; that is: lunging, hitting, kicking and biting, until the obstacle is vanquished. The pleasurable and unpleasurable feelings associated with RAGE are obvious: the sweet satisfaction of an opponent relenting versus mounting irritation and anger. Equally obvious is the fact that affective attack cannot be deployed in all (actually, in most) situations in which your needs are impeded. Whose mother never frustrated them, for example? Thus, through learning from experience, the blind rage of a screaming infant gives way through development (notwithstanding the occasional tantrum) to more nuanced, sophisticated and context-sensitive predictions for dealing with life's frustrations.

With these few remarks, we have entered an important theme that will be developed later: the fact that the seven emotional drives and their associated instincts *conflict* with one another and with reality, leading to the necessity for what Freud called 'drive fusion' and 'compromise formation'. We will see later that successful negotiation of this provides the essential foundation for the transition from narcissism to object love (from what Klein called 'part' to 'whole' object relations, and from the 'paranoid schizoid' to 'depressive' positions through integration of good and bad parts of the self and its objects).

4. FEAR. The set-point for this drive is: 'I am not facing danger to life and limb'. The innate prediction as to how to return to these viable bounds is to freeze or flee. The feelings which announce failure versus success in this respect are trepidatious anxiety versus relief upon returning to safety. However, if all that you ever do when you are scared is to freeze or flee, then you are suffering from an anxiety disorder (think of the common phobias and PTSD). Thus, you must learn what else to do to feel safe, in a context-sensitive fashion. RAGE commonly conflicts with FEAR: you dare not attack an object that is bigger than you, no matter how frustrating it might become.

5. PANIC/GRIEF. We mammals cannot fend for ourselves when we are young; so, we must 'attach' to a caregiving object. In the case of human infants, this occurs during the first six months of life, after which separation anxiety and stranger anxiety set in. Attachment occurs again, repeatedly throughout life, with other objects. It is mediated by endogenous opioids, which are highly *addictive*. The set-point for PANIC/GRIEF is 'my attachment object is close at hand'. If s/he is not, panicky feelings akin to opiate withdrawal set in. The instinctual prediction as to how this can be rectified is to emit 'separation distress vocalizations' (i.e., crying, in the case of humans) and search behaviours. If this does not succeed, PANIC shifts to GRIEF. Now the instinctual prediction becomes: give up. This is felt as hopelessness and all the other emotions associated with negative SEEKING (since GRIEF entails a shutting down of SEEKING). If this state persists— that is, if the subject cannot come up with a better prediction than simply giving up—then we speak of depression: dysphoria, anhedonia, abulia, etc. The opposite is the warm fuzzy feeling of reunion; a feeling which, unfortunately, can also be achieved by 'self-medication' with codeine, morphine, heroin, etc. Bowlby (1969) called the PANIC phase of the separation distress response 'protest', and he called the GRIEF phase 'despair'. *Protest* is a particularly felicitous term, since it captures the admixture of RAGE that frequently accompanies abandonment. As Bion said: a good object absent is a bad object present. Hence, RAGE comes into conflict with PANIC/GRIEF, like it does with FEAR. As I said before, whose mother never frustrated them?

6. CARE. Attachment is a bidirectional process. We do not need only to be looked after by a caregiving object; we need also to nurture our offspring (and other dependent or vulnerable objects, such as pets and patients). The set-point for CARE is: 'my dependent object is safe and contented'. If it is not, we suffer feelings of agitated concern, and we can become overwhelmed

by our inability to rectify things. An extreme example is post-partum depression (CARE is mediated by specific hormones and peptides which increase massively during pregnancy and childbirth). The instinctual predictions available to us in this respect include picking up the baby, holding it close to us, rocking it, making soothing noises ('motherese'), etc. As every parent knows, these actions do not always succeed. Hence, a lot more must be learnt through experience. There is an intimate link between PANIC/ GRIEF and CARE; there is strong empirical evidence that those who were not adequately cared for (and therefore suffered PANIC/GRIEF) have particular difficulty in nurturing their offspring.

7. PLAY. Since mammals are social species, we *need* to play. This is how we form viable groups, achieve acceptance by a group, and attain status within it. The set point for PLAY is something like: 'I have friends who want to be with me; who respect me, and, ideally, admire me'. The instinctual behaviour for this drive is 'rough-and-tumble play'. Successful PLAY entails fairness (epitomized by the '60:40 rule', which states that playmates must take turns in calling the shots). So, through PLAY, children learn about cooperation and collaboration, reciprocity, mutuality and empathy. The bully might control all the toys, but nobody wants to play with him. It is through PLAY that we become socialized and civilized. Unsuccessful PLAY is often characterized by cheating, lying and deception (think of character pathology) and by a preoccupation with dominance and submission (think of perversion). PLAY is all about respecting boundaries and obeying rules. Successful PLAY requires compliance with the 'as if' rule, too, which states that play fighting (for example) must not become real fighting. If it does, then PLAY becomes RAGE (and FEAR). In other words, PLAY is fundamentally symbolic. For this reason, as Winnicott (1971) taught us, it underwrites the whole of cultural life. The pleasurable feelings associated with this drive include a sense of fun, social belonging and pride. Its unpleasurable feelings are the opposite: joylessness, isolation and shame.

The ensuing types of narcissism

1. LUST. The narcissism associated with this drive was the first to be recognized, historically. It is literally 'self-love', associated with auto-erotic behaviours. I have little to add to what Ellis, Näcke and Freud taught us in this regard, apart from the following. The transition from self-love to object-love does not, on the neuropsychoanalytic view, involve a 'stage in the development of the libido', but rather a fusion of LUST with PANIC/ GRIEF. To the extent that the sexual object which must be freely available (in accordance with the set-point for LUST) is not the own self and body but rather those of an external object, to that extent the subject must tolerate *dependence* upon an object. That is, the self must learn to tolerate vulnerability in relation to *loss* of its love object. This is the so-called depressive position, which seems to entail (in this respect) an integration of lustful feelings

with loving feelings—a fusion of what Freud called 'erotic' currents and 'affectionate' ones.

2. SEEKING. As stated, Freud conflated this drive, too, with LUST. For that reason, he conceptualized *omnipotence* (i.e., the narcissism associated with overly optimistic mania and megalomania and with delusions of grandeur) as 'self-love' in the libidinal sense. In light of what we know about the SEEKING drive, it now becomes apparent that these mental states—which can be produced artificially by administration of dopamine boosters—have little, if anything, to do with sexuality (once we recognize that not all forms of pleasure are sexual). Since SEEKING is the drive to *know*—i.e., to reduce uncertainty—it becomes reasonable to suggest that all delusions (all pathological 'certainties') are narcissistic phenomena of the SEEKING type. It is surely no accident that antipsychotic drugs—which suppress the positive but not the negative symptoms of psychosis—are dopamine blockers. The depressive position does not require only the tolerance of dependence, as just mentioned, but also tolerance of *not* knowing. Thus, the omnipotent prediction 'seek and you shall find' must be amended to something along the lines of: 'seek and you shall *sometimes* find'. As Mick Jagger put it: 'you can't always get what you want'. Foregoing what you cannot have, once again, entails tolerance of loss. Moreover, mature romantic love does not entail only successful fusion of LUST with PANIC/GRIEF but also with SEEKING, because commitment to one romantic partner requires forgoing the many other enticing potential partners out there. (For more details on SEEKING narcissism, see Solms, 2022.)

At this point, the general trend mentioned in the previous section comes into view: *the transition from narcissism to object love involves drive fusion and compromise formation.*

3. RAGE. As we have seen, Freud introduced the concept of destructive narcissism in 1915 already. On his view, object-hate was the necessary corollary of self-love. It is of the essence of objects that they are independent of the egocentric purview of the subject. For this reason, following Freud, we see destructive narcissism as the expression of an innate destructive drive, but in neuropsychoanalysis, we do not consider this drive to be only *secondarily* deflected outwards: we see RAGE as the *primary* response to frustrating objects. Another thing we can add to our existing understanding is that narcissistic RAGE is the fount of the primitive superego. If the set-point for this drive is 'there are no impeding objects getting between me and what I need', then the superego is bound to be the primary object of affective attack; since what is the superego if not an impeding object?— the internalized parent that says 'no', or 'thou shalt not'. In this sense, the superego is an 'internal object' par excellence; it entails the internalization of objects *as* objects (an other within the self). As I have said already, RAGE conflicts sharply with FEAR and with PANIC/GRIEF; this is a theme that I will develop further under the next two headings. As I do so, it will become apparent that maturation of the superego has everything to do with management of such conflicts through drive fusion and compromise formation.

4. FEAR. The conflict between RAGE and FEAR is rooted in the fact that if you attack someone who is bigger than you (like a parent, perhaps especially a father), then they might well retaliate. The urge to attack such an object is therefore felt not only as RAGE but also as FEAR, by the law of talion: an eye for an eye. However, since the feeling of FEAR in such instances does not emanate from an actual hostile object, but rather within the imagination of the subject, the appropriate term for it is 'paranoia'. Paranoia, then—which is a basic attitude of the ego in relation to the primitive superego—is revealed to be the narcissistic type of FEAR. This is a more satisfying account of the relationship between narcissism and the self-preservative drive of FEAR than the notion that we want to preserve ourselves only because we are in love with ourselves. Tempering RAGE towards the superego (i.e., developing better predictions in relation to it than simple affective attack), then, plays a central role in superego maturation—by which I mean, of course, achieving a more realistic sense of the dangers posed by internalized parents.

5. PANIC/GRIEF. The conflict between RAGE and PANIC/GRIEF is rooted in the fact that if you attack someone upon whose love you depend (like a parent, perhaps especially a mother) then you might well lose their love. The urge to attack is therefore inhibited and directed inward ('I am bad'), yielding the feeling called *guilt*. This is a very common occurrence in depression, as Freud (1916–1917) recognized long ago. Thus, guilt (self-directed RAGE) is revealed to be a second type of narcissistic RAGE, alongside paranoia. Since guilt is another basic attitude of the ego in relation to the primitive superego, it too is reduced to more realistic proportions through the tempering of RAGE towards the superego. If guilt is a narcissistic type of RAGE, the question arises: what is the PANIC/GRIEF type of narcissism? The answer comes from the fact that, unlike the other drives, PANIC/GRIEF is *dependent* upon an object; accordingly, its satisfaction is uniquely contingent upon the disposition of the object towards the subject (or at least upon the subject's experience of that disposition).[4] In consequence, PANIC/GRIEF narcissism involves the degree to which the subject feels loved—and, indeed, lovable. Deficits in this type of narcissism are, sadly, not easily remedied. One narcissistic deployment of the PANIC/GRIEF drive, therefore—a solution which is not uncommon—is the illusion that one can look after (can care for) oneself. You cannot, in reality, satisfactorily attach to yourself.

6. CARE. The principal way in which the CARE type of narcissism manifests itself is the extent to which the caregiver recognizes that the dependent object is not an extension of itself but rather a separate object, with needs and a mind of its own. Failures in this respect take many forms, ranging from living one's life vicariously through one's children, to requiring one's children to validate one's caregiving prowess, to rejection of 'dud' children in favour of 'trophy' ones, etc. Clearly, narcissism of the CARE type entails a fundamental failure to nurture—the caregiving self prioritizes its own needs over those of the object-to-be-cared-for. The transition

from narcissism to object-love in this respect entails nothing more (or less) than becoming a 'good enough' mother.

7. PLAY. This (social) type of narcissism centres on the relationship between the individual and the group. It manifests mainly in preoccupations with status and power. One need only consider the conspicuous display of wealth (or the appearance of it) with designer brands—so commonplace nowadays—to realize how ubiquitous this type of narcissism is. It is easy to recognize it in the personalities of many Presidents of countries and companies. The bully mentioned in my description of PLAY in the previous section is a narcissist—but he is a very different type of narcissist than is a parent who lives vicariously through their children, or a guilt-ridden melancholic, or a compulsive masturbator, etc. The essential attributes of this type of narcissist map directly onto the two 'rules' of PLAY which were mentioned in the previous section: (a) they have an excessive tendency to dominate rather than to collaborate and cooperate—which necessarily entails a failure of empathy—and (b) they are excessively concrete. To put it colloquially, they take everything in life 'too seriously'. They do not have fun. I have mentioned already the roles of RAGE, FEAR and PANIC/GRIEF in the neuropsychoanalytic understanding of superego maturation, which yields paranoia and guilt. *Shame* is the third basic attitude of the ego in relation to the superego. This emotion arises from an unfavourable comparison by the ego of its own attributes relative to those of what Freud called the 'ego ideal'. On the neuropsychoanalytic view, this narcissistic ideal is primarily a social construct; it is a product of the PLAY drive. This aspect of PLAY narcissism involves wanting to be *seen* to be at the top of the hierarchy, rather than enjoying the private satisfactions that come with genuine, everyday achievements attained through fair play.

Conclusion

There is much more that could be said about narcissism from the neuropsychoanalytic perspective. This applies especially to narcissistic *defences* (see Solms, 2024). Unfortunately, word-count limitations don't allow for this. Nevertheless, I hope that I have been able to provide an adequate heads-of-argument outline of the ways in which our understanding of narcissism is deepened by this revision of drive theory—which not only updates psychoanalytic theory in line with recent scientific developments but also has direct clinical applications.

Notes

1 Here the necessity for distinguishing between 'drive' and 'instinct' becomes abundantly apparent. Strachey translated both of the equivalent German terms (*Trieb* and *Instinkt*) with the single English term 'instinct'. This leads to confusion, since an instinct is an innate *response* to a drive—it is not the drive itself—and drives can be responded to in other ways than by instincts, as the next paragraph explains.

2 Freud observed repeatedly that alkaloid toxicity and withdrawal (caused by cocaine use, which boosts dopamine) is akin to actual neurosis; that is, to dammed-up libido. Here is an example: 'The [actual] neuroses, which can be derived only from disturbances of sexual life, show the closest clinical similarity to the phenomena of intoxication and abstinence that arise from the habitual use of toxic, pleasure-producing substances (alkaloids)' (Freud, 1905, p. 191).

3 Freud was always puzzled by the fact that *increasing* sexual desire (e.g., in foreplay, which postpones orgasm) is pleasurable. This is because he conflated appetitive SEEKING with consummatory LUST. Interestingly, the German word *'Lust'*, unlike its English equivalent, denotes both 'desire' and 'pleasure'.

4 It is noteworthy that all the drives, as they are conceptualised in affective neuroscience, are intrinsically object-related. This is significantly different from Freud's conception of the drives as 'objectless'.

References

Bowlby, J. (1969). *Attachment*. London: The Hogarth Press.

Ellis, H. (1898). Auto-Erotism: A Psychological Study. *Alienist and Neurologist*, 19: 260.

Freud, S. (1905). Fragment of an Analysis of a Case of Hysteria. *RSE*, 7: 1–108.

Freud, S. (1914). On Narcissism: An Introduction. *RSE*, 14: 58–89.

Freud, S. (1915). Drives and their Vicissitudes. *RSE*, 14: 97–123.

Freud, S. (1916–17). Mourning and Melancholia. *RSE*, 14: 211–231.

Freud, S. (1920). Beyond the Pleasure Principle. *RSE*, 18: 1–61.

Freud, S. (1925). Negation. *RSE*, 19: 233–241.

Klein, M. (1957). *Envy and Gratitude*. London: The Hogarth Press.

Näcke, P. (1899). Kritisches zum Kapitel der normalen und pathologischen Sexualität. *Archiv für Psychiatrie*, 32, 356.

Panksepp, J. (1998). *Affective Neuroscience*. New York: Oxford University Press.

Solms, M. (1995). Is the Brain More Real than the Mind? *Psychoanalytic Psychotherapy, 9*, 107–120.

Solms, M. (2011). Neurobiology and the Neurological Basis of Dreaming.' In P. Montagna, & S. Chokroverty (eds.), *Handbook of Clinical Neurology*, 98 (3rd series) Sleep Disorders—Part 1. New York: Elsevier, pp. 519–544.

Solms, M. (2021). Revision of Drive Theory. *Journal of the American Psychoanalytic Association, 69*, 1033–1091.

Solms, M. (2022). A Neuropsychoanalytic Note on Omnipotence. In J. Arundale (ed.), *The Omnipotent State of Mind: Psychoanalytic Perspectives*, London: Routledge, pp. 115–121.

Solms, M. (2024). The Mechanism of Change in the 'Talking Cure': A Neuropsychoanalytic Perspective. In S. Gullestad, E. Stänicke, & M. Leuzinger-Bohleber (eds.), *Psychoanalytic Studies of Change: An Integrative Perspective*, London: Routledge, pp. 114–127.

Winnicott, D. W. (1971). *Playing and Reality*. London: Penguin.

7 Diagnosis and evaluation of narcissism

Stephan Doering

The myth of narcissus

Almost everyone will know that narcissism as a term and a concept can be traced back to the myth of Narcissus, the charismatic beauty, who fell in love with himself and couldn't love anyone else. Some of the details of his story might be less well-known; Narcissus was conceived during a rape: "Liriope, a water-lady whom Cephisus raped within a winding brook and nearly drowned her" (Ovid, 1958, p. 74). Cephisus was a river-god, Liriope a water nymph. After she had given birth to a son, whom Liriope called Narcissus, she went to consult the blind seer Tiresias. He presaged that Narcissus would live to old age "only if never he comes to know himself" (p. 75). The boy grew up and at the age of 16, he was of tremendous beauty admired by boys and girls, whom he rejected in a contemptuous way. His most pertinacious admirer, the nymph Echo, he rejected fiercly: "No, you must not touch—go, take your hands away, may I be dead before you throw your fearful charms around me" (p. 76).

Narcissus fell in love with his own reflection on the surface of a spring, he admires his own beauty until he recognizes:

> Look! I am he; I've loved within the shadow of what I am, and in that love I burn [...] Am I the lover or beloved? Then why make love? [...] O may I fall away from my own body—and this is odd from any lover's lips—I would my love would go away from me.
>
> (p. 78 f.)

Soon after this, Narcissus dies—after his dead body had disappeared, narcissus flowers grew from this very place.

Ovid's "character study" coincides in a surprising way with contemporary descriptions of narcissistic personality pathology. We see grandiosity and self-admiration as well as a lack of empathy and contemptuous rejection and devaluation of others. Most interesting is the seer's prediction that Narcissus will not tolerate self-awareness, which turns out to be true.

DOI: 10.4324/9781003565284-10

A narcissistic person is by all means trying to maintain a grandiose self that is threatened by recognition of the real self. A narcissistic person avoids inferiority and dependency, which mounts into severe difficulties in object relations. Another person cannot be loved as distinct individual completely separated from the self. A self-object, that is "like me", under my control, and continuously "mirroring me" is the only compromise. Thus, falling in love with the own reflection is a beautiful metaphor for being in need of a self-object and for the intolerance of mature object love.

In the 1st century, Plinius (1999, p. 99) pointed out that it was not Narcissus, who gave his name to the flower, but the other way around: The flower received the name due to its narcotizing smell; the Greek ναρκη (narke) translates into "sleep, numbness". Hartmann (2018, p. 14) points out that "Narcissus deadened or narcotized his own unbearable feelings about the lack of attention and mirroring by his primary objects" (translation S. D.).

The term "narcissism" was used for the first time by the British poet Samuel Taylor Coleridge in 1822 when he complained about the society's—obviously self-centered—"time-murder" at social events (Coleridge, 1971, p. 196). Oscar Wilde called his seminal hero Dorian Gray a Narcissus when he kissed the lips of his own portrait—"Morning after morning he had sat before his portrait wondering at its beauty" (1891/1961, p. 109).

Early concepts of narcissism

The first one, who referred to Narcissus in a psychopathological context, was the French psychologist Alfred Binet: "La fable du beau Narcisse est une image poétique de ces tristes perversions" (1887, p. 267). He regarded Narcissus as suffering from a specific kind of fetishism, in which the self takes on the function of the object. Most of the time, Havelock Ellis, the British sexologist, is quoted as the first one, who described narcissism as a perversion of auto-erotism of mainly women, who are "absorbed, and often entirely lost in self-admiration" with an "exclusion of any attraction for other persons" (Ellis, 1898, p. 280). Paul Näcke, the German psychiatrist, referred to Ellis when was talking of "real narcissism" (*echtem Narcismus*) as a very rare condition and the most severe manifestation of auto-erotism as a perversion (1899, p. 496).

It was Sigmund Freud in his seminal paper "On narcissism: An introduction" (1914), who redeemed narcissism when he stated: "Narcissism in this sense would not be a perversion, but the libidinal complement of the egoism of the instinct of self-preservation, a measure of which may justifiably be attributed to every living creature" (p. 73 f.). Following Freud's view, a modern formulation of narcissism could be: Healthy self-love goes along with the satisfaction of succeeding, the joy of being accepted and acknowledged, as well as self-confidence in taking responsibility and exercise power in a socially responsible manner.

Psychiatric classification

In line with the previous statement, modern classifications would not regard narcissism per se a mental disorder. It is only pathological narcissism that justifies a diagnosis. In case of the psychiatric classification, the label would be *narcissistic personality disorder*.

The Diagnostic and Statistical Manual of Mental Disorders (DSM-5; American Psychiatric Association, 2013) follows the "classical" categorical line of diagnosing personality disorders. General criteria have to be fulfilled (Table 7.1) before one out of ten specific personality disorders can be diagnosed (Table 7.2). The general criteria define a pathological pattern of "experience and behavior that deviates" from cultural norms and expectations is "inflexible and pervasive" in different social situations, causes "distress" and can be "traced back at least to adolescence" (p. 646 f.).

For the diagnosis of narcissistic personality disorder, in addition five out of nine specific diagnostic criteria have to be fulfilled (see Table 7.2).

The above-mentioned categorical system is currently being replaced by a new dimensional system. DSM-5 contains an "Alternative Model" in its annex called "Section III" (p. 761–781). The core general diagnostic criterion of this model is an "impairment in personality (self/interpersonal) functioning" (Table 7.3).

Criterion A is operationalized as the "level of personality functioning" (Table 7.4), i.e., the person's way to get along with oneself and others.

Extensive operationalizations of five levels of personality functioning are given for each of the four domains given in Table 7.3 (little or no, some,

Table 7.1 General criteria for the diagnosis of a personality disorder in DSM-5 (American Psychiatric Association, p. 646 f.)

A   An enduring pattern of inner experience and behavior that deviates markedly from the expectations of the individual's culture. This pattern is manifested in two (or more) of the following areas:

  1 Cognition (i.e., ways of perceiving and interpreting self, other people, and events).
  2 Affectivity (i.e., the range, intensity, lability, and appropriateness of emotional response).
  3 Interpersonal functioning.
  4 Impulse control.

B   The enduring pattern is inflexible and pervasive across a broad range of personal and social situations.
C   The enduring pattern leads to clinically significant distress or impairment in social, occupational, or other important areas of functioning.
D   The pattern is stable and of long duration, and its onset can be traced back at least to adolescence or early adulthood.
E   The enduring pattern is not better explained as a manifestation or consequence of another mental disorder.
F   The enduring pattern is not attributable to the physiological effects of a substance (e.g., a drug of abuse, a medication) or another medical condition (e.g., head trauma).

Table 7.2 Specific diagnostic criteria for narcissistic personality disorder according to DSM-5 (American Psychiatric Association, p. 669 f.)

A pervasive pattern of grandiosity (in fantasy or behavior), need for admiration, and lack of empathy, beginning by early adulthood and present in a variety of contexts, as indicated by five (or more) of the following:

1 Has a graniose sense of self-importance (e.g., exaggerates achievements and talents, expects to be recognized as superior without commensurate achievements).
2 Is preoccupied with fantasies of unlimited success, power, brilliance, beauty, or ideal love.
3 Believes that he or she is "special" and unique and can only be understood by, or should associate with, other special or high-status people (or institutions).
4 Requires excessive admiration.
5 Has a sense of entitlement (i.e., unreasonable expectations of especially favorable treatment or automatic compliance with his or her expectations).
6 Is interpersonally exploitative (i.e., takes advantage of others to achieve his or her own ends).
7 Lacks empathy: is unwilling to recognize or identify with the feelings and needs of others.
8 Is often envious of others or believes that others are envious of him or her.
9 Shows arrogant, haughty behaviors or attitudes.

Table 7.3 General diagnostic criteria of the Alternative DSM-5 Model for personality disorders (American Psychiatric Association, p. 761)

The essential features of a personality disorder are

A Moderate or greater impairment in personality (self/interpersonal) functioning.
B One or more pathological personality traits.
C The impairments in personality functioning and the individual's personality trait expression are relatively inflexible and pervasive across a broad range of personal and social situations.
D The impairments in personality functioning and the individual's personality trait expression are relatively stable across time, with onsets that can be traced back to at least adolescence or early adulthood.
E The impairments in personality functioning and the individual's personality trait expression are not better explained by another mental disorder.
F The impairments in personality functioning and the individual's personality trait expression are not solely attributable to the physiological affects of a substance or another medical condition (e.g., severe head trauma).
G The impairments in personality functioning and the individual's personality trait expression are not better understood as normal for an individual's developmental stage or sociocultural environment.

moderate, severe, and extreme impairment) and an overall level of personality functioning is determined.

Criterion B, the pathological personality traits are the second part of the diagnostic description; the alternative model contains 5 trait domains (negative affectivity, detachment, antagonism, disinhibition, psychoticism) and 25 specific trait facets. Every diagnosis is individually composed from

Table 7.4 The elements of personality functioning of the Alternative DSM-5 Model for personality disorders (American Psychiatric Association, p. 762)

Self:

1 **Identity:** Experience of oneself as unique, with clear boundaries between self and others; stability of self-esteem and accuracy of self-appraisal; capacity for, and ability to regulate, a range of emotional experience.

2 **Self-direction:** Pursuit of coherent and meaningful short-term and life goals; utilization of constructive and prosocial internal standards of behavior; ability to self-reflect productively.

Interpersonal:

1 **Empathy:** Comprehension and appreciation of others' experiences and motivations; tolerance of differing perspectives; understanding the effects of one's own behavior on others.

2 **Intimacy:** Depth and duration of connection with others; desire and capacity for closeness; mutuality of regard reflected in interpersonal behavior.

Table 7.5 Prototypical description of narcissistic personality disorder according to the Alternative DSM-5 Model for personality disorders (American Psychiatric Association, p. 767 f.)

A Moderate or greater impairment in personality functioning, manifested by characteristic difficulties in two or more of the following areas:

1 **Identity:** Excessive reference to others for self-definition and self-esteem regulation; exaggerated self-appraisal inflated or deflated, or vacillating between extremes; emotional regulation mirrors fluctuations in self-esteem.

2 **Self-direction:** Goal setting based on gaining approval from others; personal standards unreasonably high in order to see oneself as exceptional, or too low based on a sense of entitlement; often unaware of own motivations.

3 **Empathy:** Impaired ability to recognize or identify with the feelings and needs of others; excessively attuned to reactions of others, but only if perceived as relevant to self; over- or underestimate of own effect on others.

4 **Intimacy:** Relationships largely superficial and exist to serve self-esteem regulation; mutuality constrained by little genuine interest in others' experiences and predominance of a need for personal gain.

B Both of the following pathological personality traits:

1 **Grandiosity** (an aspect of **Antagonism**): Feelings of entitlement, either overt or covert; self-centeredness; firmly holding to the belief that one is better than others; condescension toward others.

2 **Attention seeking** (an aspect of **Antagonism**): Excessive attempts to attract and the focus of the attention of others; admiration seeking.

the trait domains and trait facets; however, prototypical descriptions of the "classical" personality disorders are given by the alternative model (Table 7.5).

Since the "classical" categorical DSM-5 description of narcissistic personality disorder depicted a merely grandiose narcissism, the alternative model mentions that narcissism can be covert, the self can be deflated, or the effect on others can be underestimated; a hint to another kind of narcissistic pathology that can be less obvious and of a rather self-devaluating nature. The paragraph "associated features supporting diagnosis" of the "classical" classification (p. 671) points toward a similar direction pointing out that people with narcissistic personality disorder can be "sensitive" to "injury" from criticism or defeat, "feeling humiliated, degraded, hollow, and empty"; show "social withdrawal or an appearance of humility"; and suffer from "sustained feelings of shame or humiliation and the attendant self-criticism".

The new International Classification of Diseases, 11th revision (ICD-11; World Health Organization, 2024) adopted the DSM-5 alternative model as the one and only diagnostic classification into its main body.

Grandiose and vulnerable narcissism

Many authors suggested a dichotomy of two different types of pathological narcissism. Pincus and Lukowitsky (2010) summarize beginning with Kohut's (1971) horizontal and vertical split via Rosenfeld's (1987) distinction of tick-skinned and thin-skinned narcissists to their own description of grandiose and vulnerable types of narcissism. Pincus and Lukowitsky suggest that both types can occur overtly as well as covertly. The latter types do not exhibit their narcissistic traits, but hide them so that only after thorough examination they can be uncovered. Moreover, in every narcissistic patient, both grandiosity and vulnerability are present.

Otto Kernberg's classification

From his very early writings on, narcissism was one the Kernberg's main foci. In his 1975 book *Borderline Conditions and Pathological Narcissism*, he defined normal narcissism as "libidinal investment of the self" (p. 315) whereas a pathological narcissistic self is "infiltrated by aggression" (1984, p. 290) to a higher degree than by libidinal forces. As soon as the aggression exceeds a certain degree malignant narcissism might result that manifests in a specific way in the transference relationship:

> (1) paranoid regressions in the transference, including "paranoid micropsychotic episodes"; (2) chronic self-destructiveness or suicide as a triumph over the analyst; (3) major and minor dishonesty in the transference; and (4) overt sadistic triumph over the analyst, or malignant grandiosity.
>
> (1984, p. 290)

According to the level of personality organization, Kernberg would distinguish narcissistic personality disorder on a higher borderline level from malignant narcissism on a lower borderline level and antisocial personality disorder on the lowest level of personality organization. On this continuum, impulse control decreases, whereas antisocial behaviors increase.

Later, Kernberg extended his model by describing nine different types of narcissistic pathology on different levels of personality organization (2014).

1 High-level narcissistic personality disorder as described in *DSM-5*, a grandiose type with higher level of personality organization.

2 The thick-skinned narcissist according to Rosenfeld (1987), a grandiose type with "brief dissociated, devastating experiences of self-devaluation, depression, and suicidal tendency" (Kernberg, 2014, p. 869).

3 The thin-skinned narcissist according to Rosenfeld (1987), a more fragile type on a lower organizational level with ego-syntonic sadistic features and often severely traumatized in childhood (Kernberg, 2014, p. 872).

4 The syndrome of arrogance as described by Bion (1957), an extremely arrogant behavior toward the therapist in combination with an incapacity for cognitive reflection and inordinate curiosity toward the life of the therapist (Kernberg, 2014, p. 873).

5 The intolerance of triangulation (Britton, 2004), this type shows an omnipotent control of the analyst, severe regression, and a characteristic incapacity to tolerate any thoughts that are different from his/her own (Kernberg, 2014, p. 876).

6 The severely suicidal narcissist shows a non-impulsive slowly developing suicidality in combination with seemingly "normal" behavior, massive devaluation of external reality, and a sense of superiority derived from overcoming all feelings of fear or pain and death (Kernberg, 2014, p. 877).

7 The dead mother syndrome as described by Green (1993) characterized by rejection of any significant relationship out of identification with an internalized imago of a dead mother, frequently derived from the early experiences with a severely depressed, unavailable mother (Kernberg, 2014, p. 879)

8 The sado-masochistic narcissist with the most severe negative therapeutic reactions and an unconscious attempt to transform all relationships into hostile interactions and severely sadomasochistic involvements (Kernberg, 2014, p. 880)

9 Malignant narcissism and antisocial personality disorder with an increasing loss of protective superego functions and a rise in antisocial features (Kernberg, 2014, p. 882).

I would add the high-functioning vulnerable personality disorder, which corresponds to the avoidant personality disorder of DSM-5 (American Psychiatric Association, 2013, p. 672).

Figure 7.1 shows the different types of narcissistic personality pathology according to Kernberg's model.

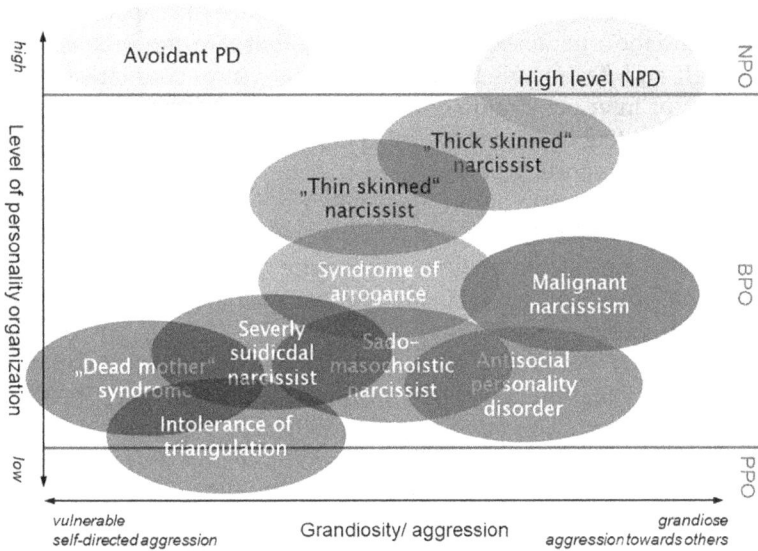

Figure 7.1 Narcissistic personality pathology according to Kernberg (2014). BPO, borderline personality organization, NPO, neurotic personality organization, PPO, psychotic personality organization.

Table 7.6 Basic transference patterns in narcissistic patients

Patient	*Therapist*	
	Grandiose	Devalued
	Grandiose	Grandiose
	Grandiose	Devalued
	Devalued	Devalued

Transference patterns

Two core motives seem to drive the narcissistic way of relating: (1) the fear of inferiority and (2) the fear of dependency. The major manifestations of narcissistic pathology can be understood as a strategy of avoidance or a defensive formation, respectively: A person's dependency and inferiority must not become visible for the self as well as for the object.

The major defensive actions are idealization and devaluation. In a dyadic relational constellation, both, self and object, can either be idealized or devaluated. This results in four basic transference patterns (see Table 7.6).

There are two complementary patterns with one—therapist or patient—idealized and the other one devaluated. In the first case, the patient idealizes his/her self and devaluates the therapist. The typical countertransference is a feeling of inferiority and contamination. In an ego-syntonic way, the therapist might feel he/she is too inexperienced and not sufficiently competent for this demanding patient.

In the opposite constellation, the patient devaluates him-/herself and idealizes the therapist. The therapist might feel that this patient is untreatable and lacks motivation and/or intelligence ("It is beneath me to waste my time with this P. It is not surprising that everybody rejects him, he is such a disagreeable person!").

The two other patterns are concordant ones; either both patient and therapist are devaluated or both are idealized. In the first case, the therapist might feel incompetent while the patient feels like a failure. In the countertransference, the therapist might be convinced that this patient is too difficult, that the he/she (the therapist) is too inexperienced and will never succeed with this patient.

The idealized dyad consists of an ideal team. The perfect patient finds the best therapist of the world. Healing is guaranteed, both will celebrate a tremendous success with their treatment.

These four transference constellations correspond to a "Glossary of the most Prominent Prototypical Transference-Patterns-List" (Caligor et al., 2019) that was created as a didactic tool for Transference-Focused Psychotherapy (TFP).

The dyad devaluated therapist/grandiose patient corresponds to the "narcissistic detached" pattern:

> Total denial of any relationship; patient is detached and unavailable, and therapist feels sealed off from patient. Emptiness, doubts in the therapist's own qualification and ability to help, feeling of the absence of any transference. Loss of hope for any change and doubt in the necessity of the treatment. The treatment might become intellectualized aiming at merely cognitive learning.

The dyad of a devaluated patient /idealized therapist can be found in the "narcissistic paranoid" transference:

> A split, implicitly aggressive relation between a grandiose, dismissive or devaluing ideal self and a devalued therapist. A power struggle might result with the countertransference of either defeating the patient or submitting to his/her grandiosity and attacks. Many role reversals might occur.

The concordant patterns are described as "narcissistic masochistic" in the case of the devaluated participants:

A split relationship between a manifestly submissive but ultimately grandiose, covertly hostile and controlling self in relation to a controlled and devalued therapist. Might go along with an omnipotent control of the therapist by severe physical or social self-harming behavior.

(negative therapeutic reaction)

Two idealized protagonists would be mirrored by the "narcissistic grandiose" transference:

Either a dyad of an idealized and a devalued aspect of the self, each assigned to the therapist and the patient, respectively; or a collusive grandiosity with a joint conviction of the ability to accomplish great things, achieve tremendous success in the treatment. Therapist might be caught by a countertransference of grandiose self-idealization, being the best and only therapist with the fantasy of creating a "new and unique treatment strategy custom made for this patient only"; alternatively, the therapist may be caught in unwarranted self-devaluation, with the patient in the position of the superior self.

Diagnostic instruments

In unclear cases, for training purposes, for court expert reports, or for research, structured diagnostic instruments can be employed—these are either structured interviews or questionnaires.

Regarding diagnoses according to DSM-5, the "Structured Clinical Interview for DSM-5 (SCID-5)" represents the official instrument that is used for reliable diagnosis. There are two different interviews when it comes to personality disorders: (1) SCID-5-PD assesses the classical categorical diagnoses for personality disorders (First, et al. 2016; see Tables 7.1 and 7.2). The SCID-5-AMPD (First et al., 2018; see Tables 7.3 and 7.4) covers the Alternative Model for DSM-5 Personality Disorders including the levels of personality functioning as well as the trait diagnoses. A well-established and freely available alternative to part 1 of the SCID-5-AMPD is the "Structured Interview for Personality organization" (STIPO-R; Clarkin et al., 2016)[1]. This interview provides dimensional scores for six domains of personality functioning/organization and an additional narcissism score. The Operationalized Psychodynamic Diagnosis (OPD-3; Arbeitskreis OPD, 2023) serves the same purpose. Gunderson and Ronningstam published the "Diagnostic Interview for Narcissism" (1990) that covers five dimensions of narcissism with 134 items.

A number of questionnaires are available for the assessment of personality functioning, e.g., the "Inventory of Personality Organization" (IPO, Clarkin et al., 2001) and the Structure Questionnaire of the Operationalized Psychodynamic Diagnosis (Ehrenthal et al., 2012). Finally, the Levels of Personality Functioning Scale—Self Rating Questionnaire (LPFS-SR; Morey, 2017). For self-report of the personality traits (part II of the DSM-5 AMPD), the "Personality Inventory for DSM-5" (PiD-5; Krueger et al., 2013) has been developed.

Finally, narcissistic traits can be assessed with either the "Narcissistic Personality Inventory" (NPI; Raskin & Hall, 1979) or the "Pathological Narcissism Inventory" (PNI; Pincus et al., 2009).

Note

1 Free download at https://istfp.org/publications/diagnostic-instruments/.

References

American Psychiatric Association. (2013). *Diagnostic and Statistical Manual of Mental Disorders*, Fifth Edition, DSM-5. Washington, DC: American Psychiatric Press.

Arbeitskreis OPD. (2023). *OPD-3 – Operationalisierte Psychodynamische Diagnostik. Das Manual für Diagnostik und Therapieplanung.* Göttingen: Hogrefe.

Binet, A. (1887). Le fétichisme dans l'amour. *Revue Philosophique de la France et de L'Étranger XXIV*, 143–167, 252–274.

Bion, W. R. (1957). On arrogance. In: *Second Thoughts: Selected Papers on Psychoanalysis*. New York: Basic Books, pp. 86–92.

Britton, R. (2004). Subjectivity, objectivity, and triangular space. *Psychoanal Q, 73*, 47–61.

Caligor, E., Doering, S., & Kernberg, O. F. (2019). *A Glossary of the most Prominent Prototypical Transference Patterns.* New York: International Society of Transference-focused Psychotherapy (unpublished manuscript).

Clarkin, J. F., Caligor, E., Stern, B. L., & Kernberg, O. F. (2016). *Structured Interview of Personality Organization–Revised (STIPO-R).* New York: Weill Medical College of Cornell University.

Clarkin, J. F., Foelsch, P. A., & Kernberg, O. F. (2001). *The Inventory of Personality Organization.* New York: Weill Medical College of Cornell University.

Coleridge, S. T. (1971). *Collected Letters of Samuel Taylor Coleridge.* Volume V – 1820–1825. edited by Karl Leslie Griggs. Oxford: Clarendon Press.

Ehrenthal, J. C., Dinger, U., Horsch, L., Komo-Lang, M., Klinkerfuss, M., Grande, T., & Schauenburg, H. (2012). *The OPD structure questionnaire (OPD-SQ): First results on reliability and validity. Psychotherapie, Psychosomatik, Medizinische Psychologie, 62*(1), 25–32.

Ellis, H. (1898). Auto-erotism: A psychological study. *Alienist and Neurologist, XIX*, 260–299.

First, M. B., Skodol, A. E., Bender, D. S., & Oldham, J. M. (2018). *Structured Clinical Interview for the DSM-5 Alternative Model for Personality Disorders (SCID-5-AMPD).* Arlington, VA: American Psychiatric Publishing.

First, M. B., Williams, J. B. W., Smith Benjamin, L., & Spitzer, R. L. (2016). *Structured Clinical Interview for DSM-5 Personality Disorders (SCID-5-PD).* Arlington, VA: American Psychiatric Publishing.

Freud, S. (1914/1957). *On Narcissism: An Introduction.* Standard Edition XIV. London: Hogarth Press, 73–102.

Green, A. (1993). *On Private Madness*. Madison, CT: International Universities Press.

Gunderson, J. G., Ronningstam, E., & Bodkin, A. (1990). The diagnostic interview for narcissistic patients. *Archives of General Psychiatry, 47*(7), 676–680. https://doi.org/10.1001/archpsyc.1990.01810190076011

Hartmann, H. P. (2018). *Narzissmus und narzisstische Persönlichkeitsstörungen*. Göttingen: Vandenhoeck & Ruprecht.

Kernberg, O. F. (1975). *Borderline Conditions and Pathological Narcissism*. Oxford: Jason Aronson.

Kernberg, O. F. (1984). *Severe Personality Disorders: Psychotherapeutic Strategies*. New Haven, CT: Yale University Press.

Kernberg, O. F. (2014). An overview of the treatment of severe narcissistic Pathology. *International Journal of Psychoanal, 95*, 865–888.

Kohut, H. (1971). *The Analysis of the Self. A Systematic Approach to the Psychoanalytic Treatment of Narcissistic Personality Disorders*. Chicago: University of Chicago Press.

Krueger, R. F., Derringer, J., Markon, K. E., Watson, D., & Skodol, A. E. (2013). *Personality Inventory for DSM-5 (PID-5)*. Washington, DC: American Psychiatric Association.

Morey, L. C. (2017). Development and initial evaluation of a self-report form of the DSM-5 level of personality functioning scale. *Psychological Assessment, 29*, 1302–1308.

Näcke, P. (1899). Die sexuellen Perversitäten in der Irrenanstalt. *Wiener Klinische Rundschau XIII(27-28)*, 435–438, 458–460, 478–481, 496–497.

Ovid. (1958). *The Metamorphoses. A Complete New Version by Horace Gregory*. New York: The Viking Pass.

Pincus, A. L., Ansell, E. B., Pimentel, C. A., Cain, N. M., Wright, A. G. C., & Levy, K. N. (2009). Initial construction and validation of the pathological narcissism inventory. *Psychol Assess, 21*(3), 365–379.

Pincus, A. L., & Lukowitsky, M. R. (2010). Pathological narcissism and narcissistic personality disorder. *Annu Rev Clin Psychol, 6*, 421–446.

Plinius. (1999). *Naturkunde*. Bücher XXI/XXII. Zürich: Artemis & Winkler.

Raskin, R. N., & Hall, C. S. (1979). A narcissistic personality inventory. *Psychol Rep, 45*, 590.

Rosenfeld, H. (1987). *Impasse and Interpretation: Therapeutic and Anti-Therapeutic Factors in the Psychoanalytic Treatment of Psychotic, Borderline, and Neurotic Patients*. London: Tavistock.

Wilde, O. (1891/1961). *The Picture of Dorian Gray*. New York: Airmont Publishing.

World Health Organization. (2024). *Clinical Descriptions and Diagnostic Requirements for ICD-11 Mental, Behavioural and Neurodevelopmental Disorders*. Geneva: World Health Organization.

8   Therapeutic approaches to narcissism in transference-focused psychotherapy

John F. Clarkin, Nicole Cain, Eve Caligor, and Julia Sowislo

Introduction

Transference-focused psychotherapy (TFP) is a psychoanalytic object relations approach that was initially developed for the treatment of patients with borderline personality disorder (BPD) (Clarkin, Yeomans, & Kernberg, 1999; Clarkin, Yeomans, & Kernberg, 2006; Yeomans, Clarkin, & Kernberg, 2015). TFP has been empirically investigated and supported for patients with BPD by members of the Personality Disorders Institute at the Weill Medical College of Cornell University in New York (Clarkin, Levy, Lenzenweger, & Kernberg, 2007) and colleagues in Vienna and Munich (Doering, Horz, Rentrop, et al., 2010). With the shift from focus on categorical diagnoses of personality pathology to assessment of the functional severity of personality pathology in both DSM-5 alternative model (American Psychiatric Association, 2013) and ICD-11 (World Health Organization, 2021), the principles of TFP are being applied to the range of personality dysfunction (Caligor, Kernberg, Clarkin, & Yeomans, 2018) including narcissism (Diamond, Yeomans, Stern, & Kernberg, 2021). In this chapter, we discuss the assessment and treatment of narcissistic pathology at two different levels of severity in patients functioning at a borderline level.

Co-occurrence of BPD and narcissism

The co-occurrence of BPD with narcissistic personality disorder (NPD) has been found in major studies to range from 53.1% to 46% (see Horz-Sagstetter, Diamond, Clarkin, et al., 2018 for a review). Within a group of female patients diagnosed with borderline personality disorder, the differences between patients with and without co-occurring NPD were examined. The BPD/NPD patients presented with significantly fewer symptom disorders than the BPD only group. However, the BPD/NPD group met criteria for more personality disorder diagnoses than the BPD only group. The limitation of this study is the reliance upon DSM criteria for NPD which are too narrowly focused on grandiose narcissism. As reported in this chapter,

DOI: 10.4324/9781003565284-11

the detection of different presentations of narcissism, including grandiose, vulnerable and malignant narcissism, is revealed more clearly with trait measures.

Multiple faces of narcissism

Based upon his clinical observations, Kernberg (1984) was one of the first to describe the dimensional nature of narcissism ranging from normal and pathological narcissism in increasing levels of severity and disruptions in daily functioning. He described pathological narcissism as involving a grandiose self with excessive self-reference and a need to be loved and admired. This exaggerated self-reference is accompanied by a relative absence of capacity for an integrated concept of others with lack of empathy for others while maintaining some degree of normal functioning. These characteristics can lead to boredom in intimate relations, lack of an ability to love another, and relationship infidelity. The most severe level of pathological narcissism involves the lack of impulse control, and a disposition to explosive and chronic rage reactions and/or paranoid distortions. A most important characteristic is the extent that aggression has been integrated into the pathological grandiose self. Malignant narcissism refers most specifically to the infiltration of aggression into the pathological grandiose self. The resulting picture of malignant narcissism may include paranoia, psychopathic features, and sadism. The internal aggression in the representation of self and others is often manifested in the patient's interpersonal interactions with others. For example, these patients often have a suspicious, distorted view of other's actions and intentions, which may result in acting out (or fantasizing) narcissistic rage and/or sadistic cruelty. They often exhibit a willingness to socially dominate others, without self-awareness or remorse.

There has been a recent upsurge of interest in the trait description of narcissism in the psychological literature. Using trait instruments on both community (often college students) and clinical samples, the focus has been on two prototypes of narcissism, namely grandiose and vulnerable narcissism. The core of narcissism is seen as antagonism by some, and entitlement by others, with the expression of the core dependent upon other traits that result in either grandiose or vulnerable presentations or some variation of the two depending upon the environmental circumstances. Using the Pathological Narcissism Index (PNI) (Pincus, Ansell, Pimentel, et al., 2009) in a network approach with a large community sample, Di Pierro and colleagues (2019) found grandiose fantasies, contingent self-esteem, and entitlement rage constituted a core of narcissism. The relationship of narcissism to antisocial traits has been pursued under the title of the dark triad (Paulhus & Williams, 2002), described as the conjunction of narcissism with psychopathic traits. In addition to the dark triad, Miller and colleagues (Miller, Dir, Gentile, et al., 2010) have posited that there is a vulnerable triad composed of vulnerable narcissism, psychopathy, and BPD.

Wright and Woods (2020) have emphasized the necessity to understand narcissism and other personality deficits not only with between individuals' differences (such as with traits) but also within person variation. Within person variation refers to the specifics of the behavior pattern for the individual, e.g., when, with whom, and under what conditions a particular behavior is exhibited. The goal is to not only identify the pathology, but also to understand when and under what conditions to personality deficit/pathology arises for a particular individual. This within person variance is most relevant to clinical intervention and approaches an understanding of the functional usefulness of pathological behavior such as narcissism. Individuals with narcissism react poorly to others who take a dominant position in an interaction. In those situations, such as what might arise between therapist and patient, the patient with narcissism is likely to react with negativity and irritation to any behavior that is perceived as dominance on the part of the therapist. In this chapter, we provide information on two patients utilizing both between individual data (traits) and within person data from the use of electronic diary material.

Measurement of malignant narcissism

Contemporary research on pathological narcissism emphasizes the importance of assessing both grandiosity and vulnerability (Cain, Pincus, & Ansell, 2008; Miller, Lynam, Hyatt, & Campbell, 2017; Pincus & Lukowitsky, 2010). This conceptualization demands that one go beyond the DSM diagnostic criteria for narcissistic personality disorder as they place almost exclusive emphasis on grandiose narcissism. In addition, the trait literature is approaching what Kernberg has termed malignant narcissism with the research on traits that constitute the dark triad.

To develop an index of malignant narcissism congruent with the Kernberg theoretical conception, we (Cain, Sowislo, Caligor, & Clarkin, 2024) utilized the existing database from a larger TFP treatment study. Items from two self-report questionnaires, the Psychopathic Personality Inventory-Revised (PPI-R; Lilienfeld & Widows, 2005) and PNI (Pincus, Ansell, Pimentel, et al., 2009) were reviewed to ensure comprehensive coverage of Kernberg's construct of malignant narcissism. Scores on all three factors of the PPI-R were used to create the index: Fearless Dominance (FD; social potency, stress immunity, and fearlessness), Self-Centered Impulsivity (SCI; carefree non-planfulness, impulsive non-conformity, Machiavellian egocentricity, and blame externalization), and Coldheartedness (sadistic aggression and meanness). The PNI is a self-report measure that assesses seven characteristics spanning narcissistic grandiosity (grandiose fantasy, exploitativeness, self-sacrificing self-enhancement) and narcissistic vulnerability (contingent self-esteem, entitlement rage, devaluing, hiding the self). Both the narcissistic grandiosity and narcissistic vulnerability subscales of the PNI were used to ensure adequate coverage of the grandiosity, exploitativeness, entitlement rage, and devaluation relevant to malignant narcissism (Diamond et al., 2021; Kernberg, 1984). Scores on these two measures were standardized to ensure a commensurable metric across both measures. The summed *z*-scores for each of these two measures created a value for each subject on what we termed the malignant narcissism index.

Individual cases selected from an empirical trial

Empirical psychotherapy research has focused on analysis of large groups of patients with the same official diagnosis treated by two or more carefully described treatments with a goal of identifying the superior treatment for the average patient identified by means scores in the two or more groups. However, as every clinician is keenly aware, no two patients with the same psychiatric diagnosis are exactly alike, and individual patients with their own unique personality organization respond to treatment with very different levels of engagement and motivation for change. In our empirical investigations of patients with reliable diagnoses of BPD, we have found that a number of these patients present with varying degrees of narcissism, ranging from vulnerable narcissism and/or grandiose narcissism to malignant narcissism. This addition of a narcissistic orientation may present the possibility of significant impact on treatment process and outcome.

An alternative approach to the RCT alone is to study intensely individual cases embedded within empirical psychotherapy trials (Fishman, Messer, Edwards, & Dattilio, 2017). In a series of articles reporting on single cases enhanced with data, we have asked a few specific questions about the process and impact of TFP for BPD. One single case study utilized electronic diary material to examine the patient's change in relationship to the therapist (i.e., transference) as related to changes in relations with significant others across 18 months of treatment (Meehan, Cain, Roche, et al., 2023). Another study compared the patient pathology and treatment process of a patient who significantly improved compared to a patient who did not improve in TFP (Levy, Meehan, Clouthier, et al., 2017). Another single case study examined the positive change in not only borderline symptoms but also depression during a year of TFP (Clarkin, Petrini, & Diamond, 2019).

TFP approach to the treatment of narcissism

TFP provides a framework for the treatment of personality pathology at different levels of personality organization severity (see Table 8.1). In general, TFP focuses on the examination of the patient's dominant object relations, i.e., frequent self-perceptions and perceptions of the other with associated affects. The treatment of narcissism focuses on perceptions of self and other characteristic of NPD. These perceptions organize the disruptions in self-functioning and functioning associated with the disorder and are expressed in the relationship with the therapist.

The object relations model posits a central relationship between narcissism and aggression, with the quality and centrality of aggression increasing

Table 8.1 Levels of personality organization and impact on TFP treatment planning and process

	Neurotic organization	High borderline organization	Mid-borderline organization	Low borderline organization
Objectives of treatment	Increase flexible functioning in areas of conflict	Increase in depth and stability in experience of self and others	Resolution of destructive behavior and greater depth in experience of self and others	Behavior control with modulation of aggression
Structuring of Treatment via a Verbal Contract	Little need for structured contract	Need for an explicitly agreed upon treatment contract	Carefully constructed treatment contract is essential	Contracting must be extensive; focus on secondary gain and safety of patient and therapist
Treatment Alliance	Available for a working alliance	Ambivalence about seeking help; early alliance unstable or superficial	Suspicion, with fear of critical attack or exploitation by therapist; alliance may improve with time	Therapist seen as corrupt, arrogant, exploitative; limits capacity to form an alliance
Transference Developments	Affectively well-modulated; realistic and stable perception over time	Early idealized transferences can keep paranoid object relations contained	Rapid, affectively charged and extreme. Confusing with role reversals and abrupt shifts.	Affectively charged; predominantly paranoid
Countertransference Developments	Therapists affected in subtle and socially appropriate ways	Subtler than in mid/low BPO Therapist feels less controlled and has more inner space to reflect	Therapist feels uncomfortable, controlled and driven to action	Therapist feels uncomfortable, controlled and driven to action

with level of severity of pathology (Kernberg, 2018). A pathological, gran-diose sense of self (referred to as the "pathological grandiose self") defines NPD and can stabilize functioning in less severe presentations. For individuals in this group, direct expressions of aggression may be defended against. In contrast, in more severe presentations, the grandiose self is infiltrated with aggression, which expressed in relationships with others characterized by overt hostility and depreciation and at more extreme levels, ego syntonic sadism and cruelty.

The presence of narcissism in the personality pathology picture presents specific challenges to the treatment. For example, in the beginning phase of treatment, the patient's need to maintain superiority will often lead to rejections of the therapist's help or acknowledgement of the therapist's expertise. In this context, the rate of drop-out is high. A transference dyad of a knowing patient and a devalued therapist can quickly emerge (Caligor et al., 2018). The initial dominant transference paradigm is often one in which there is a relationship between a grandiose, entitled, superior self (patient) in relationship with an impotent, devalued, inferior other (therapist). This general transference paradigm can take on variations depending upon the "thick skinned" versus the "thin skinned" narcissistic individual (Kernberg, 2018). Patients with more "thin skinned" presentations may initially experience themselves in the devalued position in relation to a therapist experienced as superior and entitled. These variations have been indicated in the trait literature as the grandiose and vulnerable forms of narcissism, and we discuss their assessment later in the chapter.

Two cases involving varying degrees of narcissism

One of the limitations of the RCT approach is its focus on patients with a specific diagnosis such as BPD, even though many of the patients in such a group have different comorbid difficulties, other symptoms, strengths, etc. A common comorbid condition with BPD patients is the occurrence of various degrees of narcissism, including malignant narcissism. In prior research, we have found that the presence of malignant narcissism retards the process of positive change in psychotherapy for BPD patients (Lenzenweger, Clarkin, Caligor, et al., 2018). However, this general finding leads to the further question of what process events might be related to this retarded change process. The case study has the potential to provide some information concerning this question. We report here on two patients who completed 18 months of TFP. Some details of the cases are changed to protect their identity. We refer to "Sally" (for severe borderline organization) and to "Martha" (for moderate borderline organization) and their treatment.

Sources of information

There are multiple sources of information about each patient in the empirical trial reported on here. A research assistant obtained information from the patient using semi-structured interviews, self-report questionnaires, and rating scales. The therapist provided periodic ratings on the process of the psychotherapy, including reports on transference and countertransference.

The peer consultants to the therapists made periodic evaluations of the therapeutic process by watching video recordings of sessions and providing feedback.

Patient demographics and reason for seeking treatment

Sally is a 30-year-old single heterosexual female of Asian descent. Sally applied for treatment following the painful breakup of relationship with a live-in male companion of nine months duration. She was very dependent and submissive to the male companion who was dominant, controlling, and aggressive, at times physically abusive. Her treatment goal was to find a new mate. She was employed full-time in computer programming.

Martha is a 27-year-old single heterosexual white female. Martha applied for treatment with a goal of improving her relationships with men. She was in an exclusive relationship with a male companion, but the relationship was tumultuous with frequent verbal fights. She resented any attempt by her partner to be her equal. She was employed in free-lance publishing.

Diagnosis and related pathology

Diagnoses were made with the use of semi-structured interviews. Sally met criteria for BPD and NPD. She also met criteria for symptom disorders of persistent depressive disorder, social anxiety disorder, generalized anxiety disorder, and ADHD. Her structural diagnosis as revealed on the Structured Interview for Personality Organization—Revised (STIPO-R, Clarkin, Caligor, Stern, & Kernberg, 2016) indicated low level (severe) personality organization with severely disturbed scores for the domains of identity, quality of object relations, and aggression, with a score of moderately severe for moral values (see Table 8.1).

She had above average scores on the PNI scales of grandiose and vulnerable narcissism. Her score on our malignant narcissism index was one standard deviation above the mean for the patients (N=60) in the entire study. Her responses on a questionnaire for interpersonal problems indicated problems being over controlling and hostile in relationships. Her relationship style was rigid. She expressed high degrees of distress about her ways of relating to others, which is usually a positive prognostic sign.

Martha met criteria for BPD, paranoid, avoidant, and obsessive-compulsive personality disorder. She also met criteria for major depressive disorder in partial remission, generalized anxiety disorder, and ADHD. Her STIPO-R scores for identity, quality of object relations, aggression, and moral values were in the moderately severe range of personality organization (see Table 8.1). She obtained above average scores on the PNI for both grandiose and vulnerable narcissism. Her malignant narcissism index was at the mean for the entire sample. She reported that she was overcontrolling in relationships and tended to dominate in a rigid way. She was distressed about this pattern and wanted to change.

Sally manifested more symptom disorders than Martha, but that did not fully document Sally's malignant narcissism and Martha's less serious indications of narcissism. Both had indications of depression and anxiety. Both reported being controlling in relationships. The major difference between the two patients was the very high score on malignant narcissism as obtained by Sally in contrast to the mean level of this condition as exhibited by Martha.

Relational functioning: start and course of treatment

As indicated in Table 8.1, TFP is a structured treatment that begins with a verbal contract between therapist and patient specifying the responsibilities of both participants for treatment to be effective. As the severity of patient pathology increases, there is an increasing need for the clear statement and negotiation of the treatment contract. Both Sally and Martha agreed to the treatment contract. Both patients started treatment with adherence to the contract with regular, on-time attendance; however, the early emerging transference differed sharply between the two patients.

Sally developed an intense connection to the therapist from the very beginning of treatment, more like a need to fuse rather than a relationship. Sessions were dominated by her report of fantasies involving sexual and aggressive content between her and the therapist. The dominant object relationship theme was one in which the therapist was domineering and the patient was left out and discarded. The dominant transference themes were rated by therapist as paranoid.

In her free associations, the patient revealed minute details about the therapist, his professional work, and his family. Upon some questioning from the therapist around the 12 months of treatment, the patient revealed that she was stalking the therapist on the internet, seeking to discover minute details about his professional standing and personal history. She also began following him, without his knowledge, as he left his office after work hours. The therapist experienced these intrusions into his life as aggressive and frightening. With direction from his peer consultation group, the therapist informed the patient that she was breaking the therapeutic contract by her stalking, and the behavior must stop for the treatment to continue. The patient was able to comply with this boundary setting and transformed the behavior into an exploration of her desire for intimacy, albeit dominated by aggression. Subsequently, the patient was able to reflect on the possibility of friendships in her life filled with affection without the dominance of aggression. During the second half of the treatment, Sally developed a platonic relationship with a gay man. The transference with the therapist became slightly erotic without significant aggression.

Martha entered treatment with her male TFP therapist by keeping her distance, gradually gaining more trust and slowly revealing more of the fabric of her life. Her relationship with her male companion was fraught with conflict. Without her companion's knowledge, she was sexually unfaithful. She dominated him and resented any attempt on his part to be a co-equal partner with her. She expressed a fear of closeness as it might leave her vulnerable to humiliation. This intense fear invaded not only her intimate relationship with male companion, but also her transference with her TFP therapist who rated the transference at three months as a paranoid one.

Gradually, Martha became more open with the therapist. Her transference pattern remained a paranoid one at 12 months, but by 15 months, it shifted to a narcissistic transference. She made advances in her work in publishing. At the same time, she ended the relationship with the male companion, and subsequently initiated a new exclusive relationship with a male companion with whom she began to develop a more equal relationship with much less conflict.

Treatment outcome: symptoms and love/work

The research data obtained over the duration of the treatment provides another view of treatment impact. Sally made important gains as symptoms of anger and depression decreased, and moral functioning improved. Her narcissistic symptoms became less severe. During the 18 months of TFP, Sally's relationship with the therapist was intense, and at the same time, she abstained from any extra-therapy intimate relations. She did develop some satisfying platonic relationships, and fantasies of intimate relations without sadomasochistic elements emerged.

As part of the research procedure, we asked patients to rate themselves and others in their daily life using smartphone technology (i.e., ecological momentary assessment or EMA) at three timepoints in the 18-month treatment. This enables us to track important shifts in self-other representations, shifts that the patient may not be aware of. At the beginning of treatment, Sally's perceptions of others in her daily life were rigid, extreme, and mostly negative. During the 18 months of TFP, her perceptions became much more nuanced. Her capacity to view others as warm, friendly, and more benign, particularly around themes of dominance and control, emerged over the course of treatment. She also began to view herself as more capable of warmth and affiliation as treatment progressed.

Martha's presenting symptoms of aggression and conflict in intimate relations decreased over time. Her part-time free-lance work became more successful and rewarding. Her conflicted relationship with her male companion was terminated. She began a new intimate relationship during the second half of the treatment and this relationship was more compatible and less conflicted and without dominant aggression.

On the electronic diary, Martha showed a trajectory of change that was expressed first with her therapist (at nine months) and later with extra-therapy relationships. At the beginning of treatment, she perceived dominance in her relationships, both her own and that of others, as cold, reflecting her assumption that agency and assertion were corrupted by control and being controlled. By nine months there was a perception that the therapist's agency was warm, but no change in the perception of agency in others. By the end of treatment, she perceived agency of others as potentially warm. She was by this time seeing her own agency with the therapist as warm.

Discussion

We have posited that between the rich, clinical-near experience of a psycho-analytic case study and the average results of a randomized clinical trial of psychotherapy there is another possibility to obtain valuable information. A single case drawn from a larger empirical trial can provide both rich clinical information combined with data obtained in reliable ways. In this chapter, we have utilized two such cases with both clinical and empirical data to examine the impact of malignant narcissism in the context of diagnosed BPD on treatment process and outcome.

The typical BPD patient has co-occurring personality disorders, and narcissism is a frequent co-occurring condition. In this combination of borderline pathology and varying degrees of narcissism, the patient experiences a very negative view of self with at the same time a superior and grandiose view of self in relation to others including the therapist. Trait research suggests (Miller et al., 2010) suggests that vulnerable narcissism is an essential aspect of BPD and this was present in both cases presented in this chapter. As observed by Kernberg (1984), the extent of aggression invading the individual's orientation to self and others can lead to a condition he termed malignant narcissism. The two cases presented here were similar in many ways, but a salient difference was the greater degree of aggression manifested by Sally which indicated the presence of malignant narcissism.

Criterion A of the DSM-5 alternative model is helpful in distinguishing the two patients reported here, with ratings in the pathology range on empathy, for example. However, domains such as aggression and moral values are covered more directly in the STIPO-R than the DSM-5 alternative model. Criterion B is based on traits, and we found traits measured on the PNI and PPI-R to be essential in indicating differences in malignant narcissism in these two patients. It is not clear if the traits in DSM-5 alternative model would have provided such a precise result.

The patient with malignant narcissism (Sally) expressed affectively charged aggression in free associations and transference material for 15 months of the TFP treatment episode. The therapist felt the impact of the aggression in the transference and reacted with counter transference feelings of impotence, fear, and doubt about treatment effectiveness. The therapist was grateful for the support of the peer consultation group and considered the consultation was essential to treatment continuation. In contrast, the treatment of Martha was relatively benign if not somewhat distant in the relationship between patient and therapist. Only with time did the patient begin to expand her communication with the therapist and simultaneously develop a relatively conflict-free relationship with a male companion.

We suggest that clinicians be alert to the possible presence of malignant narcissism in their initial evaluations of borderline patients. In our research, malignant narcissism stands out as an important confounding issue in the treatment of these patients. The treatment of BPD patients with malignant narcissism requires a highly structured treatment with the goal of interpreting the aggression and impaired moral functioning in relations with the therapist and significant others.

Using individual cases within a sample of patients treated in an empirical study stimulates a more in-depth view of what might be unique to one patient and what aspect might generalize to similar patients. With the emphasis on the uniqueness of each individual patient (despite having the same PD diagnosis), we are interested in what is unique and what aspects do seem to generalize to other patients. For example, the intense attachment if not fusion with the therapist that characterized the treatment of Sally from the beginning of TFP with subsequent stalking behavior toward the therapist is rare in our clinical and experimental work. What does, in our view, generalize from this case is the malignant narcissism index that is one standard deviation above the mean indicating the potential for aggression manifesting during the treatment, aggression that will challenge the limitations of the therapist.

Another issue raised by these two cases is the timing of the intervention during the course of the patients' illness. Both patients were in their late 1920s and early 1930s, beyond the intense acting out period for BPD individuals in their teens and early 1920s. Sally had 11 previous suicide attempts, but that phase seemed to be over by the time of this treatment episode. Both were in relationships, showing some desire and capacity for intimacy; however, both marred by narcissism infiltrated with a degree of aggression.

References

American Psychiatric Association. (2013). *Diagnostic and statistical manual of mental disorders* (5th ed.). American Psychiatric Association Press.

Cain, N. M., Pincus, A. L., & Ansell, E. B. (2008). Narcissism at the crossroads: Phenotypic description of pathological narcissism across clinical theory, social/personality pathology, and psychiatric diagnosis. *Clinical Psychology Review, 28*, 638–656.

Cain, N. M., Sowislo, J., Caligor, E., & Clarkin, J. F. (2024). Developing an index to assess malignant narcissism in patients diagnosed with borderline personality disorder using measures of pathological narcissism and psychopathy. *Psychoanalytic Psychology, 41*, 129–136.

Caligor, E., Kernberg, O. F., Clarkin, J. F., & Yeomans, F. E. (2018). *Psychodynamic therapy for personality pathology: Treating self and interpersonal functioning*. Washington, DC: American Psychiatric Association Publishing.

Clarkin, J. F., Cain, N., & Caligor, E. (2024). Trajectory of change in the individual and the diagnostic group: Transference-focused psychotherapy (TFP) and the treatment of personality pathology. In S. E. Gullestad, E. Staenicke, & M. Leuzinger-Bohleber (eds.), *Psychoanalytic studies of change: An integrative perspective.* London and New York: Routledge, pp. 9–23.

Clarkin, J. F., Caligor, E., Stern, B. L., & Kernberg, O. F. (2016). *The structured interview of personality organization-revised (STIPO-R).* Unpublished manuscript.

Clarkin, J. F., Levy, K. N., Lenzenweger, M. F., & Kernberg, O. F. (2007). Evaluating three treatments for borderline personality disorder: A multiwave study. *American Journal of Psychiatry, 164*(6), 922–928.

Clarkin, J. F., Petrini, M., & Diamond, D. (2019). Complex depression: The treatment of major depression and severe personality pathology. *Journal of Clinical Psychology, 75,* 824–833.

Clarkin, J. F., Yeomans, F. E., & Kernberg, O. F. (1999). *Psychotherapy for borderline personality.* New York: Wiley and Sons.

Clarkin, J. F., Yeomans, F. E., & Kernberg, O. F. (2006). *Psychotherapy for borderline personality: Focusing on object relations.* Washington, DC: American Psychiatric Association Publishing.

Diamond, D., Yeomans, F. E., Stern, B. L., & Kernberg, O. F. (2021). *Treating pathological narcissism with transference-focused psychotherapy.* New York: Guilford.

Di Pierro, R., Costantini, G., Benzi, I., Madeddu, F., & Preti, E. (2019). Grandiose and entitled, but still fragile: A network analysis of pathological narcissistic traits. *Personality and Individual Differences, 140,* 15–20.

Doering, S., Horz, S., Rentrop, M., Fischer-Kern, M., Schuster, P., Benecke, C., Buchheim, A., Martius, P., & Buchheim, P. (2010). Transference-focused psychotherapy versus treatment by community psychotherapists for borderline personality disorder: Randomised controlled trial. *British Journal of Psychiatry, 196*(5), 389–395.

Fishman, D. B., Messer, S. B., Edwards, D. J. A., & Dattilio, F. M. (Eds.) (2017). *Case studies within psychotherapy trials: Integrating qualitative and quantitative methods.* New York: Oxford University Press.

Horz-Sagstetter, S., Diamond, D., Clarkin, J. F., Levy, K. N., Rentrop, M., Fischer-Kern, M., Cain, N. M., & Doering, S. (2018). Clinical characteristics of comorbid narcissistic personality disorder in patients with borderline personality disorder. *Journal of Personality Disorders, 32*(4), 562–575.

Kernberg, O. F. (1984). *Severe personality disorders: Psychotherapeutic strategies.* New Haven: Yale University Press.

Kernberg, O. F. (2018). *Treatment of severe personality disorders: Resolution of aggression and recovery of eroticism.* Washington, DC: American Psychiatric Association Publishing.

Lenzenweger, M. F., Clarkin, J. F., Caligor, E., Cain, N. M., & Kernberg, O. F. (2018). Malignant narcissism in relation to clinical change in borderline personality disorder: An exploratory study. *Psychopathology, 51*(5), 318–325.

Levy, K. N., Meehan, K. B., Clouthier, T. L., Yeomans, F. E., Lenzenweger, M. F., Clarkin, J. F., & Kernberg, O. F. (2017). Transference-focused psychotherapy for adult borderline personality disorder. In D. B. Fishman, S. B. Mosser, D. J. A. Edwards, & F. M. Dattilio (eds.), *Case studies within psychotherapy trials: Integrating qualitative and quantitative methods.* New York: Oxford University Press, pp. 190–245.

Lilienfeld, S. O., & Widows, M. R. (2005). *Psychopathic Personality Inventory—Revised (PPI-R) professional manual.* Odessa, FL: Psychological Assessment Resources.

Meehan, K. B., Cain, N. M., Roche, M. J., Fertuck, E. A., Sowislo, J. F., & Clarkin, J. F. (2023). Evaluating change in transference, interpersonal functioning, and trust processes in the treatment of borderline personality disorder: A single-case study using ecological momentary assessment. *Journal of Personality Disorders, 37*(4), 386–403.

Miller, J. D., Dir, A., Gentile, B., Wilson, L., Pryor, L. R., & Campbell, W. K. (2010). Searching for a vulnerable dark triad: Comparing factor 2 psychopathy, vulnerable narcissism, and borderline personality disorder. *Journal of Personality, 78,* 1529–1564.

Miller, J. D., Lynam, D. R., Hyatt, C. S., & Campbell, W. K. (2017). Controversies in narcissism. *Annual Review of Clinical Psychology, 13,* 291–315.

Paulhus, D. L., & Williams, K. M. (2002). The dark triad of personality: Narcissism, Machiavellianism and psychopathy. *Journal of Research in Personality, 36,* 556–563.

Pincus, A. L., Ansell, E. B., Pimentel, C. A., Cain, N. M., Wright, A. G., & Levy, K. N. (2009). Initial construction and validation of the Pathological Narcissism Inventory. *Psychological Assessment, 21*(3), 365.

Pincus, A. L., & Lukowitsky, M. R. (2010). Pathological narcissism and narcissistic personality disorder. *Annual Review of Clinical Psychology, 6,* 421–446.

World Health Organization. (2021). *International classification of diseases, 1th Revision (ICD-11).* Author.

Wright, G. C., & Woods, W. C. (2020). Personalized models of psychopathology. *Annual Review of Clinical Psychology, 16*(15), 1–15.

Yeomans, F. E., Clarkin, J. F., & Kernberg, O. F. (2015). *Transference-Focused psychotherapy for borderline personality disorder: A clinical guide.* Washington, DC: American Psychiatric Association Publishing.

9 Are personality disorders disease variants or (extreme) normal variants?—fragments of an ongoing debate

Stephan Hau

Introduction

The diagnosis of personality disorders in diagnostic manuals has consistently sparked fundamental discussions, likely due to the inherent challenge of fitting personality disorders into the biological-medical disease model upon which the DSM and ICD are based. This chapter briefly outlines the historical evolution of personality disorder diagnosis before addressing whether mental disorders can be adequately described using a medical disease model. It also explores the potential advantages of function-oriented diagnostics.

Mental health—mental illness

To help individuals who are mentally ill, we not only need effective psychotherapies but also need a reliable system of diagnosis and assessment to identify the appropriate treatment method for each patient. In other words, we must be able to reliably distinguish between health and ill-health. The WHO defines mental health as a state in which individuals can realize their potential, work productively, and contribute to society. However, defining mental illness is far more challenging. A distinction can be made between "mental problems" and "psychiatric conditions." Only "psychiatric conditions," which are further categorized into "mental diseases and syndromes" and "developmental mental dysfunctions," require psychotherapeutic treatment. These conditions are associated with a psychiatric diagnosis and corresponding diagnostic codes.

Attempts to develop a psychiatric diagnostic system

In the early 20th century, a debate emerged about how to classify psychological and psychiatric disorders. A significant contribution came from German psychiatrist Emil Kraepelin (1856–1928), who made a pioneering effort to systematize all psychiatric diagnoses. Kraepelin is considered the

DOI: 10.4324/9781003565284-12

founder of modern scientific psychiatry, psychopharmacology and psychiatric genetics.

His fundamental idea was to classify psychiatric diseases using the same systematology applied to other medical conditions: the premise that psychiatric diseases are rooted in pathological biological processes. This approach extended even to deviations in personality—what we now define as personality disorders. Kraepelin believed that, like physiological diseases, psychiatric disorders could be classified based on symptomatology. From his perspective, personality disorders were viewed as milder forms of severe mental illnesses and could be categorized within the same framework as other diseases. This foundational assumption proved highly influential and remained a guiding principle in the development of diagnostic classification systems, such as the ICD-10 and DSM-IV, until very recently.

Kraepelin's view, however, did not go unchallenged. The question of whether personality disorders are disease variants or extreme forms of normal personality traits was debated by other prominent German psychiatrists, such as Karl Jaspers and Kurt Schneider. Both disagreed with Kraepelin's unifying approach that classified all personality disorders as variants of diseases. In 1923, Schneider introduced an additional category he referred to as "abnormal variants of mental being," which he distinguished from mental abnormalities caused by illnesses. This new category encompassed personality disorders, separating them conceptually from disease-related conditions.

In 1946, Jaspers made an effort to define the boundaries of the psychopathological method. He identified "psychiatric prejudices," such as the tendency to associate all mental illnesses with brain pathologies and the assumption that mentally ill individuals must be suffering from brain diseases. According to Jaspers, mental processes can only be accessed indirectly through patients' reports of their experiences. As a result, no definitive parameters for psychological disorders can be established independently of patients' reports and psychopathological analyses. He argued that diagnostic approaches in psychiatry fundamentally differ from analytic procedures in the natural sciences.

Both Jaspers and Schneider emphasized a distinction between disease processes and personality processes. Unlike the rapid and unpredictable onset of diseases—such as those caused by infections or trauma—personality traits are better understood through a historical perspective. Personality disorders often develop gradually over a person's lifetime and are closely tied to the life circumstances they have experienced. As a result, disease classification should be distinguished from the description of personality variants. The latter should be described as "ideal types," rooted in societal norms—what a society considers tolerable as normal variations versus what it deems excessively deviant and, therefore, pathological.

Within psychiatry, Kraepelin's approach prevailed, and his concept of differentiating between various psychiatric diagnoses within a classification system remains a core pillar of the DSM and ICD frameworks today.

DSM and ICD

About half a century after Kraepelin's approach, the World Health Organization (WHO) initiated its own classification system: the *International Classification of Diseases* (ICD). Currently in its 11th edition, the ICD includes psychiatric diagnoses under Chapter F.

A similar approach was adopted in the United States with the development of the DSM system (*Diagnostic and Statistical Manual of Mental Disorders*), first published in 1952. After World War II, the US Department of Defense sought to investigate the effects of war on soldiers' mental health, leading to the creation of the first American diagnostic system. Today, the DSM is published by the American Psychiatric Association (APA) and is currently in its fifth edition.

While DSM-II, published in the 1960s, had a strong psychosocial foundation, DSM-III and DSM-IV shifted toward a medical disease model. The focus became distinguishing psychiatric disorders based solely on objectively assessable criteria for various symptoms—criteria-based categories with clear definitions and boundaries. Diagnoses were made using polythetic criteria groups, and a separate axis was introduced specifically for personality pathology.

This design of the DSM can be interpreted as a capitulation to the medical disease model. Many categorizations were criticized as hypothetical or lacking sufficient research. Above all, diagnoses of personality disorders highlighted that the longstanding question of whether mental disorders are milder forms of more serious illnesses (as Kraepelin had suggested) or deviations from a norm defined by society had still not been resolved.

Narcissistic personality disorders

The criteria for narcissistic personality disorder (NPD) have evolved over the years. NPD was not included in the first edition of the *Diagnostic and Statistical Manual of Mental Disorders* (DSM-I). It wasn't until the late 1960s, when the second edition of the DSM (DSM-II) was developed, that Heinz Kohut introduced narcissism as an independent clinical concept. NPD was then included as a Cluster B personality disorder in the DSM.

The DSM differentiated three clusters of personality disorders: Cluster A, Cluster B, and Cluster C, with each cluster having its own distinct characteristics. Cluster A includes personality disorders with odd or eccentric traits, such as paranoid personality disorder, schizoid personality disorder, and schizotypal personality disorder. Cluster B consists of personality disorders characterized by dramatic, emotional, or erratic features, including antisocial personality disorder, borderline personality disorder, histrionic personality disorder, and NPD. Finally, Cluster C lists personality disorders marked by anxious and fearful traits, such as avoidant personality disorder, dependent personality disorder, and obsessive-compulsive personality disorder.

The cluster system has been used for diagnosing personality disorders for many years; however, there are limitations when approaching personality disorders in this manner. For example, the cluster classification is not consistently validated in the literature (see, e.g., Tackett et al., 2008). Additionally, there are very few studies that help to understand the etiology of NPD. Some behavioral genetic studies have shown that NPD, along with other Cluster B personality disorders, is highly heritable (Torgersen et al., 2012; Torgersen et al., 2000).

Other medical conditions have also been discussed, often in relation to personality disorders or personality changes. The focus here has been on pathologies that may damage neurons, including head trauma, cerebrovascular diseases, cerebral tumors, epilepsy, and a range of other diagnoses, such as Huntington's disease, multiple sclerosis, and endocrine disorders (see Leppla et al., 2021).

Criticism

The DSM and ICD diagnostic systems have been repeatedly criticized for their descriptive diagnoses. In particular, diagnoses related to personality disorders have been criticized as overly complex, with many categories that partially overlap. Not all categories are based on a coherent model or theory; instead, descriptions seem to have evolved from historical precedent, clinical experience, and committee consensus. Furthermore, the classification has been criticized as inconsistent with available data, with most evidence suggesting that personality disorders are distributed along a single dimension (cf. Kessler et al., 2005, 2011).

Since the 1990s, there have also been discussions regarding a dimensional model of personality disorders.

Short description of the criteria for PND

NPD has been attempted to be diagnosed as a clearly defined mental illness for many years, using the diagnostic criteria provided by the two major diagnostic systems: DSM and ICD. After some general remarks, the following criteria for NPD are outlined in the DSM-5-TR: A pervasive pattern of grandiosity, a need for admiration, and a lack of empathy are evident in interpersonal settings. These behavioral patterns have their origin in early adulthood and are seen as persistent across various contexts. Five of the following clinical features must be present:

- Having a grandiose sense of self-importance, such as exaggerating achievements and talents, expecting to be recognized as superior even without commensurate achievements.
- Preoccupation with fantasies of success, power, beauty, and idealization.

- Belief in being "special" and that they can only be understood by or associated with other high-status people (or institutions).
- Demanding excessive admiration.
- Sense of entitlement.
- Exploitation behaviors.
- Lack of empathy.
- Envy toward others or belief that others are envious of them.
- Arrogant, haughty behaviors and attitudes.

One of the problems with these criteria is that narcissistic traits are not inherently pathological. On the contrary, narcissistic qualities are a normal part of human development. There is also a described developmental process in which narcissism emerges around age eight, peaks during adolescence, and decreases in adulthood (cf. Thomaes et al., 2009).

It becomes evident that diagnosing NPD is challenging without considering the social context and individual life circumstances. This highlights a key issue with a symptom-oriented diagnostic approach. The fact that personality disorders, despite not being fundamentally different in origin from other psychiatric disorders, remained difficult to fit into the categorization systems is reflected in their placement on a separate axis. This demonstrates that they did not truly align with the existing diagnostic frameworks. The questions raised by Jaspers and Schneider have still not been satisfactorily answered.

Other diagnostic approaches

The dissatisfaction with the diagnostic approaches offered by DSM and ICD has led to the development of alternative methods that are fundamentally development-oriented and/or person-centered, as opposed to symptom-based diagnoses. These approaches focus on developmental pathways from infancy to adulthood and on disorders related to developmental tasks. It is assumed that complex interactions between biological and psychosocial factors are expressed throughout the lifespan (Lingiardi & McWilliams, 2017; Luyten & Blatt, 2011; Luyten et al., 2012; McWilliams, 2011).

The two basic assumptions are:

1 A person-centered, development-focused psychopathological approach must be central to psychiatric classification.
2 Functionality: Psychopathology is often seen as an attempt at adaptation.

Adopting a developmental psychopathology perspective means grounding psychiatric classification in longitudinal developmental research (Caspi et al., 2014). It is more effective to conceptualize mental disorders not as static end-states but as complex, dynamic conflict-defense constellations.

Psychopathology is viewed here as a dynamic process striving for functionality. It should be seen as failed adaptation attempts, reflecting variations in personality development.

Individuals are constantly negotiating different developmental tasks, and problems in negotiating these tasks can manifest in various ways throughout the lifespan. Therefore, it is important to provide a "taxonomy of people" (rather than a "taxonomy of diseases") and to aim to describe "what one *is* rather than what one *has*" (Lingiardi & McWilliams, 2017, p. 17).

Psychological "disorders" are thus not static end-states but functional attempts at adaptation. These adaptation attempts may be highly inappropriate for the individual or their environment, yet they can still be considered the best possible balance between the person's psychological endowment, biological predispositions, and environment.

Another approach takes a transdiagnostic perspective. With the increasing recognition that mental disorders often share common mechanisms, there has been renewed interest in transdiagnostic interventions (Barlow et al., 2014; Weisz et al., 2012). Transdiagnostic research challenges the notion that psychiatric diagnoses are well-defined entities. The primary argument is that the current diagnostic manual, with its hundreds of diagnoses that a person must either have 100% or not at all, poorly captures reality. It is more likely that psychiatric problems are normally distributed in the population, meaning everyone is at some risk for every disorder.

Another example of an alternative diagnostic approach is the concept of "symptom networks," which assumes that psychiatric symptoms influence each other more than any underlying hypothetical disease. Symptom networks are constructed by the patient themselves. A specific set of problems is identified, along with the severity and emotional impact these problems have for the patient. Additionally, the patient is asked to describe the causal relationships between the various problems (cf. Koernigs & Lönnroos, 2022).

New diagnostic approach in DSM-5 Appendix 3 and ICD-11: the focus on structure and functioning

A significant change in the diagnosis of personality disorders, including NPD, occurred with the publication of DSM-5 and ICD-11. These new diagnostic approaches represent a clear effort to return to a diagnostic process that takes into account the structure and functional level of an individual.

While DSM-5 has not fully embraced this shift and continues with the old approach (defining various personality disorders using polythetic criteria), it introduces the new model as an "alternative" diagnostic model in Appendix 3. Upon closer inspection, one can see that the focus is now on "psychic functioning," particularly how the Self operates and how interpersonal relationships are structured.

In contrast, ICD-11 fully adopts this change, abandoning the previous system of distinct personality disorder diagnoses. Instead, it introduces three levels of functioning for personality disorders, which focus on different aspects of functioning, including identity, self-esteem, the ability to form intimate relationships, impulse control, and adaptation of interpersonal behavior.

ICD-11 distinguishes between three levels of personality disorder: mild, moderate, and severe.

On a general level, personality disorders in ICD-11 are described as follows:

> Personality disorder is characterized by problems in functioning of aspects of the self (e.g., identity, self-worth, accuracy of self-view, self-direction), and/or interpersonal dysfunction (e.g., ability to develop and maintain close and mutually satisfying relationships, ability to understand others' perspectives and to manage conflict in relationships) that have persisted over an extended period of time (e.g., 2 years or more). The disturbance is manifest in patterns of cognition, emotional experience, emotional expression, and behavior that are maladaptive (e.g., inflexible or poorly regulated) and is manifest across a range of personal and social situations (i.e., is not limited to specific relationships or social roles). The patterns of behavior characterizing the disturbance are not developmentally appropriate and cannot be explained primarily by social or cultural factors, including socio-political conflict. The disturbance is associated with substantial distress or significant impairment in personal, family, social, educational, occupational or other important areas of functioning.

Three different levels of severity are distinguished. In its milder form, a personality disorder is described as:

> All general diagnostic requirements for Personality Disorder are met. Disturbances affect some areas of personality functioning but not others (e.g., problems with self-direction in the absence of problems with stability and coherence of identity or self-worth), and may not be apparent in some contexts. There are problems in many interpersonal relationships and/or in performance of expected occupational and social roles, but some relationships are maintained and/or some roles carried out. Specific manifestations of personality disturbances are generally of mild severity. Mild Personality Disorder is typically not associated with substantial harm to self or others, but may be associated with substantial distress or with impairment in personal, family, social, educational, occupational or other important areas of functioning that is either limited to circumscribed areas (e.g., romantic relationships; employment) or present in more areas but milder.

A moderate-level personality disorder is described as follows:

> All general diagnostic requirements for Personality Disorder are met. Disturbances affect multiple areas of personality functioning (e.g., identity or sense of self, ability to form intimate relationships, ability to control impulses and modulate behavior). However, some areas of personality functioning may be relatively less affected. There are marked problems in most interpersonal relationships and the performance of most expected social and occupational roles are compromised to some degree. Relationships are likely to be characterized by conflict, avoidance, withdrawal, or extreme dependency (e.g., few friendships maintained, persistent conflict in work relationships and consequent occupational problems, romantic relationships characterized by serious disruption or inappropriate submissiveness). Specific manifestations of personality disturbance are generally of moderate severity. Moderate Personality Disorder is sometimes associated with harm to self or others, and is associated with marked impairment in personal, family, social, educational, occupational or other important areas of functioning, although functioning in circumscribed areas may be maintained.

Finally, a severe level of personality disorder is described:

> All general diagnostic requirements for Personality Disorder are met. There are severe disturbances in functioning of the self (e.g., sense of self may be so unstable that individuals report not having a sense of who they are or so rigid that they refuse to participate in any but an extremely narrow range of situations; self-view may be characterized by self-contempt or be grandiose or highly eccentric). Problems in interpersonal functioning seriously affect virtually all relationships and the ability and willingness to perform expected social and occupational roles is absent or severely compromised. Specific manifestations of personality disturbance are severe and affect most, if not all, areas of personality functioning. Severe Personality Disorder is often associated with harm to self or others, and is associated with severe impairment in all or nearly all areas of life, including personal, family, social, educational, occupational, and other important areas of function.

Parallels to psychoanalytic approaches

The method of diagnosing personality disorders described here represents a complete departure from the symptom-oriented, descriptive diagnosis of distinct personality disorder types. Instead, it focuses on general patterns of functioning and experiences of self and relational contexts, described across different organizational levels.

Although not explicitly stated by the authors of the latest versions of the DSM or ICD systems, the emphasis on functional aspects of personality disorders, self-experiences, and relational dynamics, as well as the division into three levels of functioning, clearly parallels Otto Kernberg's (see Kernberg & Caligor, 2005) diagnostic framework. Kernberg's model divides personality organization into three levels—neurotic, borderline, and psychotic—offering similar descriptions of varying levels of functioning.

Another well-established psychodynamically based framework for describing different levels of psychic structure can be found in the *Operationalized Psychodynamic Diagnostic* (OPD) system, recently published in its third edition (Arbeitskreis OPD, 2023).

The way personality disorders are defined in the ICD-11 and the alternative diagnostic approach of the DSM-5 strongly resembles concepts introduced over 30 years ago in the definitions of different categories for levels of psychological structure, as outlined by the OPD System (OPD-Taskforce, 2008). Developed in Germany by psychoanalysts dissatisfied with the unreliable subjectivity of psychiatric diagnoses on the one hand, and the limited scope of existing diagnostic systems on the other, the OPD seeks to complement the descriptive, symptom-oriented diagnoses of the DSM and ICD with a comprehensive, operationalized framework. This framework includes the assessment of repetitive relational patterns, the identification of unconscious conflicts, and the description of four levels of psychic structure (high, moderate, low, and disorganized). The axis addressing the psychological structure of a patient further defines varying levels of self-integration across four distinct areas, each analyzed from both a self- and object-related perspective.

Self-perception is defined as the ability for self-reflection, the development of a self-image, and the maintenance of a coherent self-image over time, including psychosexual and social identity. It also encompasses the ability to distinguish between various internal processes, particularly the differentiation of affects. *Object perception*, on the other hand, refers to the capacity to distinguish between internal and external reality and to perceive others as whole individuals with their own goals, rights, contradictions, and the ability to empathize with them.

Another aspect of assessing the level of psychic structure focuses on the abilities of self-regulation and the regulation of object relationships. *Self-regulation* is defined as the capacity for initiating competent action, guiding and integrating needs and emotions, enduring stress, and restoring balance. A particularly important aspect is the ability to maintain realistic self-esteem and regulate its fluctuations. The *regulation of object relationships* is defined as the ability to preserve and nurture relationships, such as balancing differing interests. Additionally, two dimensions assess the emotional capacity to *communicate* both *internally* and *externally*. This includes the ability to emotionally engage with and address others, interact with them, and interpret their affective signals.

Finally, the assessment also examines the presence of *attachments to internal or external objects*.

The OPD construction of the axis for personality structure was heavily inspired by and relies significantly on Otto Kernberg's earlier definition of different levels of personality organization (see Kernberg, 2004). The recent changes in diagnosing personality disorders in the DSM and ICD have created opportunities for psychoanalytic approaches to gain visibility and connect with mainstream psychiatric research on personality disorders. While the psychoanalytic roots of the current diagnostic concepts in the DSM and ICD are not explicitly acknowledged, it is nonetheless gratifying to see psychodynamic concepts and perspectives reintroduced into these systems. However, these connections are not made clear to the reader or user. At the same time, this shift in diagnostic approaches for personality disorders may also serve as a reminder that the fundamental question—whether personality disorders are milder forms of severe mental illness or normative variations of socially accepted behavior—remains unresolved.

Discussion of different perspectives on mental processes

The challenges in identifying an adequate approach for diagnosing personality disorders, such as NPD or Borderline Personality Disorder, reflect a broader conceptual issue regarding how mental processes are diagnosed. This question will be explored further at the end of this chapter.

Many researchers operate on the assumption that there are neurophysiological correlates for mental disorders. This perspective underpins the hypothesis that distinct, brain-based pathological types of mental disorders can be defined. The approach assumes that, in investigating, diagnosing, treating, and reporting cases of mental illness, we are dealing with discrete pathological types. Paradoxically, despite decades of intensive research, this hypothesis has not been validated. No reliable biological markers have been identified that covary with operationally defined clinical syndromes to support a valid, brain-based classification of mental disorders. One common explanation for this failure is that the self-organized and context-sensitive dynamics of brain function are not yet sufficiently understood. Advocates for this view argue that more effort should be directed toward exploring non-linear, computational models of mental disorders (see Thagard, 2008). This line of reasoning seems to echo a weakened version of the medical model for understanding mental disorders.

However, one could propose the opposite hypothesis: that there are no distinct, brain-based types of mental disorders. The connections between mind, brain, and behavior may simply not align with the framework of the medical model. The complexities of mental processes cannot be adequately represented by a model that conceptualizes the brain as a gland "secreting" behavior, similar to how hormones are produced, or as a computer generating output in the form of behavior. Instead, one might view the brain as a tool for cultural practice, with its internal structure being highly individualized, intricately interconnected, and psycho-economically shaped by cultural influences. From this "culturalist" perspective, it seems unlikely that mental disorders would correspond neatly to specific, damaged brain states.

Mark Solms (2021) is clear when he states: We cannot directly observe psychological processes (mind), only indirect and incomplete conclusions can be drawn about how the psyche works, e.g., we can only observe representations of the psychic apparatus and how it works. "Mind" is never directly observable; we only have indirect representations available.

The conclusion is that one can distinguish between two different kinds of observation of mental functioning: One can either observe mental functioning via an external perception surface (the brain) or via an internal perception surface (introspection). In the natural sciences, the first option has mostly been chosen, when looking for neural correlates of conscious processes. This is what Chalmers (1995) described as "the simple problem" and this is exactly what one tries to do when looking for specific neural correlates that exist in contexts of mental disorders.

Mark Solms (2021) makes a compelling point when he states: We cannot directly observe psychological processes (the mind); only indirect and incomplete conclusions can be drawn about how the psyche operates. For instance, we can only observe representations of the psychic apparatus and its functioning. The "mind" is never directly observable; we have access only to indirect representations. The conclusion is that there are two distinct ways to observe mental functioning: either through an external perception surface (the brain) or an internal perception surface (introspection). In the natural sciences, the first approach has predominantly been chosen, focusing on neural correlates of conscious processes. This corresponds to what Chalmers (1995) referred to as "the simple problem." Specifically, this is the method employed when researchers aim to identify neural correlates associated with mental disorders. According to Chalmers, there is a far more challenging question to address: Why and how does the quality of subjective experience arise from objective neurophysiological events? To explore this, Solms and Friston (2018) use memory processes as an example. A memory, they argue, is both the subjective re-experience of an event and the objective activity of neural networks that encode that event. This leads to the conclusion that memory is neither purely subjective (mental) nor purely objective (physically measurable). Instead, memory—and by extension, mental processes—encompasses both dimensions (cf. Solms & Friston, 2018; see also contribution of Solms in this volume).

But there is a third aspect to consider: we cannot exist outside of relationships. We are constantly engaged in interactions and embedded in affective psychosocial contexts with others. This means that explanatory models for mental processes are insufficient if they focus solely on the individual. We must also account for the psycho-social interactional context in which a person lives. From birth, we exist in relation to others—we are received by others, engaged in constant dialogue, and in ongoing exchanges. Knowledge about the external world and about ourselves can only be generated through the relational detour via the minds of others, i.e., through interaction. This idea resonates with the research approach of Embodied Cognitive Science, which reflects similar foundational assumptions (cf. Pfeifer & Scheier, 2001; Leuzinger-Bohleber, 2015). In this framework, the psyche is not described as a simple input-output system but rather as a dynamic field of interaction between mind, body, and environment, characterized by ongoing feedback processes during these interactions.

Building on what we have developed so far, we can engage in a thought experiment described by Markus Pawelzik (2018). Imagine that we could fully separate the objective, biological "body" from the intersubjective, social dimension of being human. In this scenario, we could conceptualize a patient as having two distinct and distinguishable sides. When diagnosing, we might approach the patient as an organism whose malfunctions need to be identified and addressed. This perspective would focus on the biological mechanisms that constitute the organism, particularly the neural processes responsible for generating problematic behaviors. However, if we were to examine this individual purely from a biological standpoint, gaining complete control over all neural processes—what, then, could we infer about this person's psychological state? Could we truly understand his/her inner world by examining neurons alone?

As clinicians, we may adopt an interpersonal perspective and begin by engaging with the patient about their problems and the symptoms he/she is experiencing. We would explore the patient's development and form hypotheses about possible connections between internal and external conditions. When we interact with the patient, we bring our own cultural background and interpersonal skills to the conversation. Through this process, we may come to understand where the "problem" lies and, perhaps, why it has arisen. This approach allows us to draw conclusions about the patient's life history and contextualize their experiences. During the conversation, we process not only explicit information but also implicit cues, which can offer deeper insights. From this perspective, we can conclude that without considering the specific situation the patient is in—and without understanding the patient's meaningful social and cultural context, as well as their life-world perspective—the patterns of activity observed in the patient's nervous system would remain devoid of meaning.

This dialogical approach to the patient enables the development of an individualized case conception in which symptoms and problems are articulated in a way that the patient can understand. The relational approach also fosters the establishment of a "therapeutic relationship," which ideally encourages the patient to open up, engage in self-reflection, and embrace the possibility of learning and change. I fully agree with Pawelzik's assertion that only this interpersonal perspective allows clinicians to meet the patient where they are psychologically.

This approach aligns with the current frontier of psychological research. Increasingly, it is recognized that an individual perspective is insufficient to fully explain mental states, as it fails to account for the social context in which a person exists. Consequently, there is growing interest in adopting a dyadic perspective. For example, Wheatley et al. (2024) refer to this as "the emerging science of interacting minds." It is within this framework that the future of effective psychological diagnostics lies.

References

American Psychiatric Association. (2022). *Diagnostic and Satistical Manual of Mental Disorders* (5th ed., text rev.). https://doi.org/10.1176/appi.books.9780890425787

Arbeitskreis OPD (Hrsg.) (2023). *Operationalisierte Psychodynamische Diagnostik.* Göttingen: Hogrefe.

Barlow, D. H., Sauer-Zavala, S., Carl, J. R., Bullis, J. R., & Ellard, K. K. (2014). The nature, diagnosis, and treatment of neuroticism. *Clinical Psychological Science, 2,* 344–365. https://doi.org/10.1177/2167702613505532

Caspi, A., et al. (2014). Caspi, A., Houts, R. M., Belsky, D. W., et al. (2014). The p factor: One general psychopathology factor in the structure of psychiatric disorders? *Clinical Psychological Science, 2,* 119–137. https://doi.org/10.1177/2167702613497473

Chalmers, D. J. (1995). Facing up to the problem of consciousness. *Journal of Consciousness Studies, 2*(3), 200–219.

Jaspers, C. (1946). *Allgemeine Psychopathologie. Ein Leitfaden für Studierende, Ärzte und Psychologen.* 4., völlig neu bearbeitete Auflage: Berlin/Heidelberg 1946.

Kernberg, O. F. (2004). Borderline personality disorder and borderline personality organization: psychopathology and psychotherapy. In J. J. Magnavita (Ed.), *Handbook of Personality Disorders: Theory and Practice* (pp. 92–119). Hoboken, NJ: John Wiley & Sons Inc.

Kernberg O. F., & Caligor E. (2005). A psychoanalytic theory of personality disorders. In M. F. Lenzenweger, & J. F. Clarkin (Eds.), *Major Theories of Personality Disorder.* (pp. 114–156). New York: The Guilford Press

Kessler, R. C., Chiu, W. T., Demler, O., Merikangas, K. R., & Walters, E. E. (2005). Prevalence, severity, and comorbidity of 12-month DSM-IV disorders in the National Comorbidity Survey Replication. *Archives of General Psychiatry, 62,* 617–627. https://doi.org/10.1001/archp syc.62.6.617

Kessler, R. C., Ormel, J., Petukhova, et al. (2011). Development of lifetime comorbidity in the World Health Organization world mental health surveys. *Archives General Psychiatry, 68,* 90–100. https://doi.org/10.1001/archgenpsychiatry.2010.180

Koernigs, F., & Lönnroos, A. (2022). *Självskattade symtomnätverk.* Stockholm, SU: Examensuppsats.

Leppla, I., Fishman, D., Kalra, I., & Oldham, M. A. (2021). Clinical approach to personality change due to another medical condition. *Journal of the Academy of Consultation-Liaison Psychiatry, 62*(1), 14–21. [PubMed]

Leuzinger-Bohleber, M. (2015). *Finding the Body in the Mind.* London: Routledge.

Lingiardi, V., & McWilliams, N. (2017). *Psychodynamic diagnostic manual: PDM-2.* Guilford Press, p. 17. New York, NY.

Luyten, P., & Blatt, S. J. (2011). Integrating theory-driven and empirically-derived models of personality development and psychopathology: A proposal for DSM-V. *Clinical Psychology Review, 31,* 52–68. https://doi.org/10.1016/j.cpr.2010.09.003

Luyten, P., Mayes, L. C., Target, M., & Fonagy, P. (2012). Developmental research. In G. O. Gabbard, B. Litowitz, & P. Williams (Eds.), *Textbook of Psychoanalysis* (2nd ed., pp. 423–442). American Psychiatric Press. Washington DC.

McWilliams, N. (2011). *Psychoanalytic Diagnosis: Understanding Personality Structure in the Clinical Process,* 2nd ed. Guilford Press, p. 17. New York, NY.

OPD Taskforce (2008). *Operationalized Psychodynamic Diagnosis OPD-2.* Göttingen: Hogrefe.

Pawelzik, M. (2018). Gibt es psychische Störungen? *Journal für Philosophie & Psychiatrie,* 1–28, https://www.jfpp.org/119.98.html

Pfeifer, R., & Scheier, C., (2001). *Understanding Intelligence Cambridge, MS.* MIT Press.

Schneider, K. (1923): *Die psychopathischen Persönlichkeiten.* In Gustav Aschaffenburg (Hrsg.): *Handbuch der Psychiatrie.* Spezieller Teil, 7. Abt., 1. Teil. Deuticke, Leipzig; 2. wes. veränd. Aufl. 1928 und weit., zuletzt 9. Aufl. 1950

Solms, M. (2021): *The Hidden Spring: A Journey to the Source of Consciousness.* London: Profile Books.

Solms, M., & Friston, K. (2018). How and why consciousness arises. *Journal of Consciousness Studies, 25*(5–6), 202–238.

Tackett, J. L., Silberschmidt, A. L., Krueger, R. F., & Sponheim, S. R. (2008). A dimensional model of personality disorder: Incorporating DSM cluster A characteristics. *Journal of Abnormal Psychology, 117*(2), 454–459. [PubMed]

Thagard, P. (2008). Explanatory coherence. In J. E. Adler, & L. J. Rips (Eds.), *Reasoning: Studies of Human Inference and its Foundations* (pp. 471–513). Cambridge University Press, Cambridge, UK. https://doi.org/10.1017/CBO9780511814273.026

Thomaes, S., Bushman, B. J., Orobio de Castro, B., & Stegge, H. (2009). What makes narcissists bloom? A framework for research on the etiology and development of narcissism. *Dev Psychopathol, 21*(4), 1233–1247. [PubMed]

Torgersen, S., Lygren, S., Øien, P. A., Skre, I., Onstad, S., Edvardsen, J., Tambs, K., & Kringlen, E. (2000). A twin study of personality disorders. *Comprehensive Psychiatry, 41*(6), 416–425. [PubMed]

Torgersen, S., Myers, J., Reichborn-Kjennerud, T., Røysamb, E., Kubarych, T. S., & Kendler, K. S. (2012). The heritability of cluster B personality disorders assessed both by personal interview and questionnaire. *Journal of Personality Disorders, 26*(6), 848–866. [PMC free article] [PubMed]

Weisz, J. R et al. (2012). Testing standard and modular designs for psychotherapy treating depression, anxiety, and conduct problems in youth: A randomized effectiveness trial. *Archives of General Psychiatry, 69,* 274–282. https://doi.org/10.1001/archgenpsychiatry.2011.147

Wheatley, T., Thornton, M., Stolk, A., & Chang, L. (2024). The emerging science of interacting minds. *Perspectives on Psychological Science, 19*(2), 355–373. https://doi.org/10.1177/17456916231200177

World Health Organization (WHO). (2019/2021): *International Classification of Diseases, Eleventh Revision (ICD-11),* https://icd.who.int/browse11.

Part III

Confronting contemporary cultural challenges

10 Confronting modern zeitgeist

Visions of psychoanalysis in life and mental health care

Erik Stänicke and Helene Amundsen Nissen-Lie

In the Western world, we are used to taking for granted a postmodern position. There is no singular way to believe, live, or consume. Likewise, psychological treatments are not singular either, besides striving toward the ideal of being evidence-based. Moreover, there is little consensus about what it means to be a therapist. Due to this, and given a zeitgeist that stresses efficiency and quick relief from suffering, it is understandable that psychoanalysis is not the first choice of treatment when a person needs mental health care, no more than it is an obvious vocation for someone who wants to become a skilled therapist.

Within a neoliberal worldview, with its defense of free markets, deregulation, individualized responsibility, promotion of competition in every area of life, as well as an evidence-based policy, psychoanalysis is expected to fare poorly in modern societies. Does psychoanalysis propose values and viewpoints that collide with today's general worldview? In order to answer this, we must first state what is meant by a worldview to think more clearly about the position of psychoanalysis today. Indeed, does psychoanalysis contend a "Weltanschauung"?

As many will know, Freud (1933) argued against the possibility of psychoanalysis providing humankind with a Weltanschauung, a worldview. He began his last lecture in *New Introductory Lectures on Psychoanalysis* by saying that he was "constantly being asked in other quarters: does psychoanalysis lead to a particular Weltanschauung and, if so, to which?" (p. 158). He strongly argued against the idea that psychoanalysis leads to a specific worldview. In his thinking, theories that promise a worldview present an "overriding hypothesis, which, accordingly, leaves no question unanswered and in which everything that interests us finds its fixed place" (p. 158). A worldview has the aim of making each of us "feel secure in life" (p. 158).

Thus, according to Freud, a worldview can only be an illusion, an idealization, a defense against reality. Even if he admitted that science is a kind of worldview, one that is on par with psychoanalysis, he insists that science is a worldview that does not provide us with fixed solutions and feelings of security. On the contrary, science is always about raising questions, being willing to change one's opinion in the face of new observations, and

DOI: 10.4324/9781003565284-14

disclosing our lack of knowledge when we find out that we do not know. Freud's (1933) typical examples of worldviews are religion, some types of art, and especially typical perspectives of time, such as Marxism. However, if we understand Weltanschauung more as concerning value-anchored ideas that resonate with us on a deeper level, can psychoanalysis be seen to represent a Weltanschauung, i.e., an overarching worldview that may help us in understanding what it is to be human? Indeed, it is our contention that psychoanalysis be conceptualized as a broader vision or a worldview that can make us feel validated and understood, and which can help us in the great task of trying to make sense of ourselves and the world. As such, psychoanalysis can represent a specific *vision of the human condition*. If this is true, the question for this chapter is whether a *psychoanalytic vision* confronts or even collides with our time.

Contemporary society and its discontent

Since the work of Nietzsche, Marx, and the Frankfurter school—and, of course, Freud (1916, 1933)—we have had critical, diagnostic views on society. In more contemporary times, there are too many scholars to mention, but Christopher Lasch (1979) is a strong candidate. He criticized the Western culture in the 1970s, especially the American, for fostering beliefs that idolize individualism, self-centeredness, and shallowness. Lasch described a whole generation that developed virtues out of vices like self-realization at the expense of the community and social responsibility. This *narcissistic culture* is made possible by changes in society with consumerism, mass media, and a "therapeutic culture" that aim at individual satisfaction. The symptom is emptiness and alienation. Over 20 years later, Hartmut Rosa (2013) published in 2005 his social diagnostics, and in his view, society fared no better. On the contrary, he describes an acceleration in several major areas of problematic social living. Firstly, he describes a technological acceleration that aims not only for production efficiency but also efficient human communication. When Rosa points to human communication as accelerating, he did not even have a chance to take the effects from social media into account. Secondly, he was concerned about an acceleration in changes in social norms and roles that demand us to constantly adapt. Thirdly, we see an acceleration in daily activities. We want to do more, travel more, eat more, meet new people, and try out new careers. Later, Byung-Chui Han (2015) writes about our achievement society, where we are constantly expected to optimize ourselves to be competitive and effective. The symptoms are burnout, fatigue, and depression.

Mental health care and its discontent

Thus, since Lasch (1979), the human condition in contemporary society is even more concerning. With this as a background, we want to look at the state of modern health care. Here too we seem to live in a time where efficiency is highly valued and often used as a standard of care. Treatment shall be efficient. In some ways, this is, of course, an imperative; a patient should not need to suffer more than necessary. It goes without saying in somatic medicine and, to a degree, in psychotherapy. However, as psychoanalysts, we know that efficient treatment makes compromises. Short-term treatment often has guidelines that are carved out before the single meeting between therapist and patient, and thus, it must define the problem and solution to it, which is the treatment, before even meeting the patient. In intensive short-term dynamic therapy, the therapist is trained to listen for specific defense mechanisms, specific dynamic conflicts, and pathways for development, such as defense against aggression, which avoids an inner conflict of anger toward people the patient cares for, such as parents, and where the solution is to help the patient getting in touch with his anger, rage, and even murderous fantasies of killing one's parents, and then helping the patient to tolerate guilt feelings and then wishes to repair the relationship (e.g., Abbass, 2021). However, the problem is that this pathway in therapy is already decided before even meeting the specific patient! It is theory-driven, a top-down kind of therapy. And maybe it must be since it also aims at being efficient. Thus, it seems that acceleration has become a virtue also in health care, even in psychotherapy.

The question we want to raise is if this efficient short-term therapy is based on specific visions of the human being and his potential for suffering. Furthermore, if these specific visions are on a collision with psychoanalysis, and if so, how it is on a collision? Could it be that efficient short-term psychotherapies have ideologies and visions of reality that are anchored deeply within the large political zeitgeist? Discussing these questions seems to be of uttermost importance since we analysts have a challenge in communicating with health politicians and patients about why treatment is sometimes efficient if it is done three to five times a week over several years.

Visions of reality

Roy Schafer's (1970) seminal paper—*Visions of Reality*—may aid us in understanding what kind of worldview psychoanalysis offers and what our Zeitgeist promotes. Schafer claims four visions of reality that constitute the patient, his pathology, and his cure differently. Schafer argues that all four visions of reality—that we also may understand as four different views of the human condition—must be heralded by each analyst. He writes that one or two visions may dominate one's thinking but that a good clinician should be able to use all four. However, we think, in today's situation, it is more recognizable to see the four visions as representing substantially different perspectives on health care and psychotherapy. Schafer was inspired broadly by theories in humanities when he proposed to divide psychoanalysis into four visions, named the *comical*, the *romantic*, the *tragic*, and the *ironic*. Others have later discussed these visions further (Messer & Winokur, 1984; Strenger, 1997), but we will stick to Schafer (1970):

Firstly, we have a *comical vision of reality*. Schafer writes that it focuses selectively on external, controllable, and predictable aspects of a situation and persons. It is a vision that values the power of positive thinking and social agreement and, thus, shies away from conflicts. You may ask why this vision is called comical, but it is a good definition of what happens in slap-stick humor. Think of how all ages laugh at clowns who make the same mistake time after time and try to amend their problems by manipulating external objects. In many ways, we think that our time, with its belief in science and technology to ever produce more efficient ways of treatment, is comical in this specific sense of Schafer's definition.

Secondly, we have a *romantic vision of reality*. This is a vision that sees life as a journey, an adventure. The journey is considered potentially dangerous, heroic, and an immense individual challenge. The life journey aims to experience the sublime, holiness, the beautiful, and the good. This is a vision that we may find in psychoanalysis, such as in part of self-psychology or Winnicott's thinking. Just think of great psychoanalytic books with titles such as "On Learning from the Patient" (Casement, 1985), it is the message of psychoanalysis as a journey where the analyst is educated by the patient. We think we also find this vision in existential psychotherapy with its focus on authenticity, confronting the finality that each of us must face death on our own and that therapeutic change follows from the truth itself.

Thirdly, we have a *tragic vision* which may be seen as the quintessential Weltanschauung of psychoanalysis. The tragic vision shows a strong interest in dilemmas, paradoxes, ambiguities, and fragility of the human being and our dependency. This vision makes one sensitive to dangers, mysteries, and absurdities in life. With this attitude toward life, one will feel that every victory consists of loss, that satisfaction produces pain, that justified actions also imply guilt, that passion and duty never can be reconciled, and that every life choice consists of the loss of other opportunities.

Finally, according to Roy Schafer (1970), we have an *ironic attitude toward reality*. It has affinities to the tragic vision with its focus on conflicts, ambiguities, and paradoxes. However, it looks at these from a distance, and it takes nothing for granted. The ironic viewpoint aims at limiting human engagement at the same time as it makes strong claims about life being difficult. It is a vision of reality that aims to make subjective experience trivial and insignificant. Even if this vision seems negative, Schafer argues that it, at its best, stands for sobriety, and creates a needed balance for the other visions.

Schafer (1970) makes the point that, as psychoanalysts, we need all four visions. He argues that we analysts usually have a bias toward the tragic and, to a degree, the romantic vision. Yet, we also need the comic and ironic vision—we need flexibility in understanding the patient and the treatment from different viewpoints. However, we will point out that, as analysts, we not only have a bias toward the tragic vision, correctly stated by Schafer, but that we live in a time where the tragic vision is more under pressure than ever before. In contemporary political discussions or health care systems, we do not see it being based on tragic values and visions. On the contrary, we seem to live in a time where comical and sometimes ironic visions dictate the discourse. Just think of the demand the health care system makes use of evidence-based treatments even if these, such as CBT, DBT, or EMDR, only help a portion of patients. In every field of society—school system, prisons, and police force—we see the comical aim of getting everything under control and describe every move as a procedure. In today's society, this has reached an extreme to warrant the old critical theory of "the total administrated society" (Marcuse, 1964). There is not much room for paradoxes and dilemmas, not to say room for unconscious communication, all problems shall only be solved and fixed.

Hence, we seem to live in a time where psychoanalysis is an oddball. We invite patients to meet us several times a week over many years without guarantees for a cure and a clearly defined procedure or manual. Many of us have met non-psychoanalytic colleagues who seem to think that psychoanalysis is dangerous and shocked that it is not illegal. Thus, maybe it is time to discuss the prospect of psychoanalysis in our time. One may respond by saying that psychoanalysis has always been controversial, and that this situation is not new. That is true, yet every generation must rediscover psychoanalysis (Freud, 1916; Ogden, 2009) and accordingly find ways of conveying its radical message to the public.

Freud (1933) states that psychoanalysis does not need to be a worldview, but even more strongly, he states that it is incapable of being one. In today's climate, it is, in our opinion, a surprising statement, but Freud underlines that the worldview in psychoanalysis is embedded in a scientific one. Possibly, this scientific and secular worldview of his, where he holds it as a significant virtue to live in line with reality principle and thus, tolerate life's hard facts, such as loss and mourning (Whitebook, 2017), may have been radical enough for Freud. But today, the climate is another, secularism and even scientism are common attitudes. Thus, in our contemporary context, psychoanalysis proposes a tragic view of man that seems not only odd for its time but, for many, downright provoking. We are, of course, aware of Freud's lamenting that psychoanalysis was unpopular and provoking in his Victorian time, but we contend that is for different reasons. In Freud's time, psychoanalysis was, for many, impossible to accept because of its statements of infantile sexuality. Today, psychoanalysis is infuriating because it focuses on our vulnerability and dependency. Not so much sexuality but more on our infantile relational needs as pervasive throughout life.

In our opinion, psychoanalysis is a worldview with a specific understanding of the human condition that in no way "solves all problems"— that is Freud's (1933) definition of Weltanschauung. It is a worldview that underlines life as endless rounds of suffering, consisting of loss, grief, and shortcomings in our capacity to protect us from unbearable stimuli from not only the world but also from within.

The omnipotent therapist as an answer to a modern zeitgeist

In our view, and in line with the reasoning above, a predefined, symptom-based, time-efficient solution to therapy is grounded in a specific vision of the human being—a vision that is deeply anchored in a larger narcis-sistic zeitgeist (e.g., Lasch, 1979; Rosa, 2013), and which collides funda-mentally with a psychoanalytic (especially a tragic) vision of reality in Schafer's terms. The implications of this for the practicing psychotherapist are enormous; we can be lured into an omnipotent position, a savior that is expected to cure complex psychological and social problems "in less than ten sessions." To reconcile these expectations with our professional iden-tity, we must opt for an attitude of *hubris*.

In Greek mythology, hubris was considered a dangerous human limita-tion: When man looked upon himself with qualities reserved for the Gods, he displayed an arrogance that evoked the indignation and punishment of the Gods. In the myths, the healer Asclepius, son of the god Apollo and the woman Coronis, provoked Zeus when attempting to bring the dead back to life—something only the Gods could do. As a response, Zeus punished Asclepius' omnipotence with a deadly, lightning strike. Asclepius' father, Apollo, was outraged by his son's murder and had him sent as immortal to Olympus, where the injuries from the lightning strike enabled Asclepius to heal others. Thus, from the myth of Asclepius, we get two essential mes-sages: the danger of hubris and the notion of "the wounded healer" (Jung, 1951) who can heal, not *despite*, but *because of* one's own wounds. We will come back to the latter point.

In line with the central argument of this chapter, as we see it, there are different forces driving the therapist into omnipotence, and they are inter-linked. The pressures from society, including those embedded in clinical guidelines provided by health authorities committed to narrow cost-benefit calculations, and based on findings brought to us by academics who rarely see a patient, are one potent force. The patient's wish for a "quick fix" may add considerable weight to that. Finally, the pressures can also come from within, from our own emotional vulnerability.

Sometimes, on one level, patients want an omnipotent expert who can quickly relieve them of their pain and who knows better than them. The therapist becomes an idealized parental figure who can ease them of the heavy burden of personal responsibility, which it takes maturity to embrace (Maroda, 2022). This demand or "pull" is particularly promi-nent at the beginning of therapy, where the need for a steady, confident person who knows the direction in a time of overwhelming chaos over-rides the need for autonomy, which will appear later, after some work.

As therapists, it is tempting to enact our role in these encounters and play the part of an omnipotent parental figure. Some of us will be more prone to this enactment, which we will discuss below. For now, we recognize the fact that this pressure from the patient may force us into becoming more of an expert than there is reason to be; because we cannot stand the patient's disappointment—or because it fits with our own inner demands.

In addition to the pull that comes from the patient, we have managers at mental health clinics and policymakers who will further exacerbate this demand for quick and cost-effective "administration" of the patients entering their clinics. Whether positive and meaningful change takes place is of less importance to them. In the public mental health services, today we are introduced to new routines and procedures, which, in order to be competent employees, mean that we need to transform ourselves into superhumans who can quickly solve complex mental, societal, and existential life challenges. The rapidly increasing status of mental health professionals only adds to the pressure, and we seem to have created a therapist role that is elevated to a God-like creature rather than a "fellow human being" with professional knowledge of mental health problems and treatment (e.g., Madsen, 2014).

What motivates a person to seek the profession of psychotherapy in this climate? Along with increased status for psychotherapists, young people may enter the profession for other reasons than curiosity and interest in the human condition and a wish to help (see Farber et al., 2005); the idea of being a high status (omnipotent) healer of mental health problems may become a driving force. In our view, therapists must all possess what might be called a "sound narcissism." That is, the idea that one can make a difference in someone's life, despite the complexity of the problems presented (an idea that might to some seem absurd). However, a darker, more vulnerable form of narcissism is when we *need* the affirmation (or even "love") from the patient or therapeutic progress to keep us going (see Maroda, 2022; Jørgensen, 2025).

To complicate matters, we know that while therapists who have struggled with their own problems can be more sensitive and compassionate toward clients—a notion captured in "the wounded healer," our wounds may also create "blind spots," which can make the therapist unconsciously take control of situations where he previously felt powerless (Miller, 1997; Nissen-Lie, 2014). Therapists who have grown up in emotionally demanding or disturbed families, thus, can develop a sensitivity that may represent an important resource in their work. However, in Klein's thinking, on a more unconscious level, such an upbringing may have also left the person with a fundamental feeling of inadequacy, which can contribute to shame or guilt. The feeling of inadequacy can exist alongside an experience of having been useful as a helper and "negotiator" in the family, a dynamic that can form part of the motivational basis for becoming a psychotherapist

(Nissen-Lie, 2014). It is precisely in the therapeutic work that one is given the opportunity to be affirmed as "a good person."

Hubris on the part of the therapist can thus act as compensation but will particularly affect the more narcissistic among us. Such narcissistic vulnerability, in turn, makes it difficult to meet the opposition or criticism from the patient in a constructive manner (Maroda, 2022; Jørgensen, 2025). We talk about a match between the pull from the patient, from the system, and from within for a therapist who must hide his humanity and vulnerability to manage.

Despite the lure of omnipotence fostered by these forces, recent advances in psychotherapy research have demonstrated, much to the surprise of several researchers, that the virtue of humility, stressed by the existential philosopher Søren Kierkegaard some 150 years ago, is actually a beneficial attitude in the art of helping (see Kierkegaard, 1859). We will end on that note.

The power of professional humility

Recent research has established that the person of the therapist is likely more important for the outcome of therapy than the method he or she uses (Heinonen & Nissen-Lie, 2020). This does not mean that being informed by theory or using a particular therapeutic method does not play a role. Of course, it does, but the result for the patient will depend on *how* the method is used by a given therapist, and the quality of the relationship with the patient.

What are the therapists' characteristics that matter in this work? In direct contrast to a zeitgeist underlining self-confidence and omnipotence, as we have discussed in this chapter, several recent findings converge toward suggesting the power of professional humility and that "an expert therapist is first and foremost a humble therapist" (Hook et al., 2015).

In a line of research, we found that therapists' self-reported scores on a scale called *Professional Self-Doubt* (*PSD*) were positively linked to the patient-rated working alliance (as well as change in patient-rated interpersonal problems measured (e.g., Nissen-Lie et al., 2017). In line with the values inherent in our "comic" zeitgeist, one could argue that psychotherapists should possess professional self-*confidence*, not professional self-*doubt* (which entails a more tragic vision). Recent findings from Germany and the US on the role of under- and over-estimation of one's own effectiveness as a therapist relative to the patient's scores corroborate this finding. For example, when Ziem and Hoyer (2020) compared therapists' assessments of their clients' progress with clients' measurements of their actual improvement, they found that more modest or conservative therapist estimations (relative to their clients' actual improvement) predicted *larger* reductions of clients' symptoms and greater improvements in quality of life as assessed by the therapists themselves. Similarly, in a recent American study, Constantino et al. (2023) found that therapists who consistently overestimated their (problem-specific) effectiveness had patients who reported worse global outcomes than patients whose therapist more accurately estimated their effectiveness. Even more strikingly, the therapists who *under*estimated their problem-specific effectiveness (i.e., assessed their effectiveness to be lower than it was) had patients who reported *better* outcomes than patients whose therapist over or accurately estimated their effectiveness. These findings indicate that a more modest attitude, or professional humility, paves the way for behaviors that foster client change.

It is plausible that a therapist who is willing to accept that they may not be optimally knowledgeable or effective, or indeed is not a superhuman, will be motivated to continuously learn and truly be open to listening to the other person (i.e., the patient). In short, humility paves the way for the therapists' reflective practice (Bennett-Levy, 2019) and appropriate responsiveness toward a changing situation that is unique to each dyad taking place in it (Stiles, 2009).

Studies of Cultural Humility in the United States are another strand of research which put humility on the map as a virtue in mental health care—despite forces from the authorities to administer the work with efficiency. Patients from different minority backgrounds who went to therapists they perceived as more culturally humble, experienced greater improvement in psychotherapy (Owen et al., 2014). Being culturally humble involves adopting a curious, non-judgmental, and sensitive attitude about what the client's cultural affiliation (sexual, ethnic, religious, and other) means to them.

In our view, there is no reason to think that this is limited to cultural phenomena (i.e., religious or ethnic issues and so on), but is relevant in meeting all kinds of experiences (emotions, thoughts, dreams, reactions to us, political ideas) the client shares with us. In essence, an attitude of humility is a prerequisite for learning, the willingness to correct oneself, and a sign of the notion of *negative capability* (Bion, 1962; Strømme, 2012).

From the old Greek myths, we learn that above the entrance to the Oracle of Delphi—who made predictions about the future for people who sought her out—were the following words in Greek: Γνώθι Σεαυτόν (or: "Gnothi seauton"). The words have most often been translated into the famous dictum, "Know thyself" and are referred to by many thinkers in psychotherapy to underline the importance of self-knowledge (Castonguay et al., 2017).

A more precise translation of what is in this statement, however, should be: "Remember that you are human, not God" (Zachrisson, 2021).

Some concluding reflections

Psychoanalysis may be unpopular for the same reason it is an important corrective of our time. It proposes a tragic vision in Schafer's (1970) meaning of the word. Contrary to the current prevailing vision in society of technological optimism, individualism, and expectancy of efficiency in health care, psychoanalysis proposes a radical understanding of the human condition in at least five areas. Firstly, with its theory of the unconscious and psychodynamics of conflictual motivations and needs, psychoanalysis reminds us that we, as subjects, are not in full control of our impulses, feelings, and actions. Even if we strive toward realistic and disciplined self-control, there will be parts of ourselves that will always elude transparency. Secondly, we live in a time with a high expectancy of individual success and an assumed close link between success and well-being. Yet, we all experience that life consists also of loss and pain. With secularism, many expect health care to relieve us of our pain, but we all know professionally and even, more painfully, personally that this falls short. Thirdly, psychoanalysis corrects the contemporary illusion of perfectionism. A deep psychoanalytic experience is that humans—even if they put all their efforts into it—will never reach harmony or existence without shortcomings and faults. Fourthly, psychoanalysis proposes a deeper understanding of human relations. With its theories of splitting, projection, and projective identification, to mention but a few, psychoanalytic thinking sheds light on conflicts in family life, organizations, and even between nations. It is a worldview that has realistic claims and expectancies and not "excessive positivity," to borrow a term used by Han (2015). Finally, psychoanalysis, with its focus on vulnerability, relational fragility, and dependency, comes with a reminder of our mortality. Thus, psychoanalysis reminds us of the significance of not being locked into society's expectancy of hubris and omnipotence, but rather to be humble. It is first and foremost with a negative capability that we can really listen to another person, it is not primarily with self-confidence and skills. Of course, psychoanalysis is not alone in reminding us of this. Maybe one can claim that existentialism has marked this turf even harder, but we will contend that psychoanalysis has its own take on it: Since humans never get rid of our vulnerability and dependency, even when we are at our strongest and most autonomous, our mortality is always present. Death is not only something we can be reminded of in the future. It is ever-present.

References

Abbas, A. (2021). Intensive short-term dynamic psychotherapy: Methods, evidence, indications and limitations. *Tidsskrift for Norsk psykologforening, 58*(10), 874–879.

Bennett-Levy, J. (2019). Why therapists should walk the talk: The theoretical and empirical case for personal practice in therapist training and professional development. *Journal of Behavior Therapy and Experimental Psychiatry, 62*, 133–145. https://doi. org/10.1016/j.jbtep.2018.08.004

Bion, W. R. (1962). *Learning from experience*. Abingdon: Heinemann.

Casement, P. J. (1985). *Learning from the patient*. London: The Guilford Press.

Castonguay, L. G., & Hill, C. E. (eds.) (2017). *How and why are some therapists better than others? Understanding therapist effects.* American Psychological Association. https://doi.org/10.1037/ 0000034–000

Constantino, M. J., Boswell, J. F., Coyne, A. E., Muir, H. J., Gaines, A. N., & Kraus, D. R. (2023). Therapist perceptions of their own measurement-based, problem-specific effectiveness. *Journal of Consulting and Clinical Psychology, 91*(8), 474–484. https://doi.org/10.1037/ccp0000813

Farber, B. A., Manevich, I., Metzger, J., & Saypol, E. (2005). Choosing psychotherapy as a career: Why did we cross that road? *Journal of Clinical Psychology, 61*(8), 1009–1031. https://doi.org/10.1002/jclp.20174

Freud, S. (1916). Introductory lectures on psychoanalysis. *Standard Edition, 15*, 1–240.

Freud, S. (1933). New introductory lectures on psychoanalysis. *Standard Edition, 22*, 1–182.

Han, B.-C. (2015). *The burnout society.* Stanford: Stanford University Press.

Heinonen, E., & Nissen-Lie, H. A. (2020). What are the characteristics of effective psychotherapists? A systematic literature review. *Psychotherapy Research, 30*(4), 417–432. DOI: 10.1080/10503307.2019.1620366

Hook, J. N., Watkins, Jr., C. E., Davis, D. E., & Owen, J. (2015). Humility: The paradoxical foundation for psychotherapy expertise. *Psychotherapy Bulletin, 50*(2), 11–13.

Jørgensen (2025). Narsissisme. Hans Reitzels forlag. København. In press.

Jung, C. (1951). *Fundamental questions of psychotherapy.* Princeton: Princeton University Press.

Kirkegaard, S. (1859). *Fra synspunkter fra min forfattervirksomhet: En ligefrem meddelelse. Rapport til historien* [*Viewpoints from my authorship: An honest disclosure. Report to history*]. Copenhagen, Denmark: A. E. Reitzel Publishing.

Lasch, C. (1979). *The culture of narcissism: American life in an age of diminishing expectations.* New York: W. W. Norton & Company.

Madsen, O. J. (2014). *The therapeutic turn: How psychology altered Western culture.* Ole Jacob Madsen New York: Routledge.

Marcuse, H. (1964). *The one-dimensional man: Studies in the ideology of advanced industrial society.* Boston: Beacon.

Maroda, K. J. (2022). *The analyst's vulnerability: Impact on theory and practice.* Abingdon and New York: Routledge.

Messer, S. B., & Winokur, M. (1984). Ways of knowing and visions of reality in psychoanalytic therapy and behavior therapy. In H. Arkowitz, & S. B. Messer (ed.), *Psychoanalytic therapy and behavior therapy: Is integration possible?* (pp. 63–100). New York: Plenum Press.

Miller, A. (1997). *The drama of the gifted child. The search for the true self.* Basic Books: New York.

Nissen-Lie, H. A. (2014). Hvorfor velger noen å bli psykoterapeut? Bokkapittel i A. L. von der Lippe, H. A. Nissen-Lie, & H. W. Oddli (Red.), Psykoterapeuten. En antologi om terapeutens rolle i psykoterapi. Oslo: Gyldendal Akademisk.

Nissen-Lie, H. A., Rønnestad, M. H., Høglend. P. A., Havik, O. E., Stiles, T. C., Solbakken, O. A., & Monsen, J. T. (2017). Love yourself as a person, doubt yourself as a therapist? *Clinical Psychology & Psychotherapy, 24*(1), 48–60. DOI: 10.1002/cpp.1977

Ogden, T. H. (2009). Rediscovering psychoanalysis. *Psychoanalytic Perspectives, 6*, 22–31.

Owen, J., Jordan, T. A., Turner, D., Davis, D. E., Hook, J. N., & Leach, M. M. (2014). Therapists' multicultural orientation: Client perceptions of cultural humility, spiritual/religious commitment, and therapy outcomes. *Journal of Psychology and Theology, 42*(1), 91–98. https://doi.org/10.1177/009164711404200110

Rosa, H. (2013). *Social acceleration: A new theory of modernity*. New York: Columbia University Press.

Schafer, R. (1970). The psychoanalytic vision of reality. *International Journal of Psychoanalysis 51*, 279–297.

Stiles, W. B. (2009). Responsiveness as an obstacle for psychotherapy outcome research: It's worse than you think. *Clinical Psychology: Science and Practice, 16*(1), 86–91. https://doi.org/10.1111/j.1468-2850.2009.01148.x

Strenger, C. (1997). Further remarks on the classic and the romantic visions in psychoanalysis: Klein, Winnicott, and ethics. *Psychoanalysis and Contemporary thought, 20*, 207–243.

Strømme, H. (2012). Confronting helplessness: A study of the acquisition of dynamic psychotherapeutic competence by psychology students. *Nordic Psychology, 64*(3), 203–217. https://doi.org/10.1080/19012276.2012.731314

Whitebook, J. (2017). *Freud: An intellectual biography*. New York: Cambridge University Press.

Zachrisson, A. (2021). *Psychoanalysis my way*. Oslo: Kolofon Forlag.

Ziem, M., & Hoyer, J. (2020). Modest, yet progressive: Effective therapists tend to rate therapeutic change less positively than their patients. *Psychotherapy Research, 30*(4), 433–446. https://doi.org/10.1080/ 10503307.2019.1631502

11 Transgender—a challenge for psychoanalysis?[1]

Siri Erika Gullestad

Introduction

Today, psychoanalysis struggles to integrate rapidly developing ideas of gender identity, sex, and sexuality without falling back on normative models. Clinicians are faced with the challenge of encountering transgender people seeking treatment in a quickly changing and multi-polarized cultural environment. In this chapter, I present some of the theoretical and epistemological questions implied in the often-polarized debate about how to understand and help transgender people requesting our help. My concern is the risk of holding on to a biological binary model of sex and a dogmatic understanding of the oedipal complex as well as the danger of pathologizing transgender patients. The chapter underscores that facing the clinical and theoretical challenge of gender diversity and—fluidity has the potential to be creative for our field and for those we try to help.

From a research perspective, different kinds of studies may highlight our theme of transgender identities, e.g. clinical, conceptual, and neurobiological studies. To begin with the latter, neurobiology: In the Sandler conference 2023, also addressing sexual and gender diversity, Mark Solms gave a paper on the *Biological Foundations of Gender* (Solms, 2023) discussing male-female differences. In short, the take home message is that from a biological perspective there is a great deal more that we share than what distinguishes us. As concerns our *therapeutic* approach to transgender identities, clinical studies come forward as essential. In this paper, I will start by highlighting a third line of research, namely historic-conceptual studies, bordering on epistemological questions.

A historical perspective

In our present-day societies, and within psychoanalysis, the debate about sex and gender has become hot and polarized. Problems that previously belonged to the clinic have now moved to courts and politics. However, as historians have argued, attempts to define sex and gender has been a recurrent theme in medical history, a basic question being whether sex

DOI: 10.4324/9781003565284-15

and gender are dichotomies or spectrums. Medicine has always been preoccupied with bodies and identities it has categorized as "abnormal", from homosexuality to trans identity (Slagstad, 2021). In the late 19th century, however, psychiatrists developed a diagnostic framework for so-called abnormal sexuality that previously had been a moral and religious concern. The German psychiatrist Richard von Krafft-Ebing created a taxonomy for what he saw as sexual "perversions", published in *Psychopathia sexualis* in 1896. Krafft-Ebing saw homosexuality as a *degenerative disorder* and spoke about the *delusional* idea of sex transformation, or the feeling of belonging to the "other" sex. On the other hand, however, there were sexual reformists psychiatrists, like Magnus Hirschfeld, who established *Institut für Sexualwissenschaft* in Berlin in 1919. This institute became a place where sexual minorities could come together. Hirschfeld placed sex and sexuality on a spectrum, homosexuality was *part of human variation*: "the human being is not man or woman but man *and* woman" (quoted from Slagstad, 2021, p. 2). Under the supervision of Hirschfeld, doctors performed the first sex-reassignment surgeries on trans people. The institute and its enormous library were burnt by Hitler's gangs in the early 1930s. Certainly, a demonstration of "the political nature of sex" (Slagstad, 2021, p. 1).

Transgender within psychoanalysis

What about psychoanalysis? In *Three Essays* (1905), Freud spoke about our "originally bisexual physical disposition" (p. 141), and again, in 1937, he stated that "every human being is bisexual" (p. 244). "It is important to understand clearly that the concepts of 'masculine' and 'feminine,' whose meaning seems so unambiguous to ordinary people, are amongst the most confused in science", Freud says (1905, p. 219n). There is no pure masculinity or feminity, either *in* a psychological or a biological sense, he continues: "Every individual on the contrary displays a mixture of the character-traits belonging to his own and to the opposite sex" (1905, p. 220n). Thus, Freud opposes seeing masculinity-feminity as a duality or a binary dichotomy, rather emphasizing that these traditional definitions of gender as a dialectic dimension. Addressing the question of homosexuality, Freud opposes all attempts at separating off homosexuals from the rest of mankind as a group of special character (Freud, 1905, p. 145n). Indeed, Freud comes forward as a voice pleading for a broad view on normal variation—a spectrum view on sex.

However, the attitude of open inquiry toward human sexuality that we find in Freud's work has not been dominating neither in psychiatry nor psychoanalysis after Freud. When during the seventies the American Psychiatric Association removed homosexuality as a diagnosis, psychoanalysts protested and tried to reverse the decision (Fonagy & Allison, 2015). The American psychoanalyst Ralph Rougthon has documented how standard psychoanalytic practice for long implied efforts to change gay people's sexual orientation (Roughton, 2000, 2001; Isay, 1985)—a successful analytic outcome was synonymous with attaining a heterosexual orientation.

I had a personal experience with such attitudes. Just before I became president of the Norwegian Psychoanalytic Association, in 2006, our association was "awarded" by the gay community with a cactus, given to persons or associations that represented discriminatory attitudes. It was known in the gay milieu that one of our leading psychiatrists—a very knowledgeable gay man who was a friend of mine—had not been admitted as a candidate for training at our psychoanalytic institute. One reason for refusing him was that he was gay. I remember well talking to one senior colleague maintaining that being gay meant that one had not "resolved" the dynamics of the Oedipal phase!

The current controversial discussion about transgender reminds us of the pathologizing discourse of homosexuality in the past. For example, psychoanalytic authors have regarded transgender as indices of underlying *narcissistic disturbance* (Chiland, 2000; Oppenheimer, 1991, 1992; Quinodoz, 1998; Stein, 1995), as *perversion* (Argentieri, 2009; Limentani, 1979; Socarides, 1970), and as *difficulties in separating* (Coates, 1990, 2006; Coates & Moore, 1998) or *disidentifying from the mother* (Stoller, 1985) (all quoted from Saketopoulou, 2014). Or trans identity is seen as a *defense against castration* and as a refusal of the *classical distinction between man and woman* (Geldhof & Verhaeghe, 2017). Many analysts traditionally approach the body as a bedrock, one regards gender as a factual truth anchored in anatomical differences, implying that a good therapeutic outcome presupposes that patients accept their assigned sex. Today, however, several analytic voices, like Saketopoulou's (2014), maintain that we will understand transpersons better if we treat their gender not as a symptom but as a viable subjective reality.

Of course, this is not easy. To be sure, the way we think about sex and gender has radically changed in the past few decades. A main reason is that young people have been challenging norms that offer only two options: male and female, straight or gay. Increasingly, students have sex with someone of their own gender; and more individuals are identifying as other than gay, bisexual, or straight. Many are identifying as *queer* or *pansexual,* queer being an umbrella term for diverse non-heterosexual identities (Knafo & Lo Bosco, 2020). No wonder that we analysts, as other people, can feel perplexed by this growing profusion of sexual and gender identities. My concern is that we shall manage to meet the challenge presented by gender diversity, without clinging to traditional, normative understanding of development. In short, my worry is the risk of pathologizing transgender.

What is promising, as I see it, is that the different positions within psychoanalysis, e.g., concerning how to define sex and gender, are now being openly debated. An example: The *Psychoanalytic Controversy* section in *IJP* recently reported a long discussion between David Bell and Avgi Saketopoulou. Here the moderator maintains that "however much someone feels he's a girl, the *fact* is that he's a boy" (Blass, 2021, p. 975, my italics). This implies a binary definition,[2] contrasting major medical institutions' broader, more complex spectrum definitions of gender. On the other hand, in 2019, the American Psychoanalytic Association issued a formal apology to the LGBTQ+ community for its previous views and discriminatory actions (Knafo & Lo Bosco, 2020). And in 2022, the psychoanalyst Jack Drescher received the prestigious Sigourney Award for his pioneering work and critical psychoanalytic re-thinking of gender and sexuality on a scientific basis (Drescher, 2020). Most importantly, Drescher contributed to the recent revision of ICD-11 that helped end decades of diagnostic pathologizing of sexual and gender identities.

From a research point of view, I would like to emphasize the importance of systematic studies, e.g., of how non-binary identities develop. In a recent paper titled *Gender identities and identifications in a changing world*, Vittorio Lingiardi (2025) presents a qualitative study of interviews inviting young adults identified as non-binary to narrate the history of their development. The study makes us listen to the young people's voices, to their own subjective experiences, and allows us to become sensitized to their exploration, uncertainty, deconstruction, and need for mirroring. Gender incongruence calls us to the deepest respect for subjectivities, says Lingiardi, which in the current age are sometimes sacrificed in the name of identity politics, with easy media traction. For sure, transgender identity may be binary, often from a very early age, resulting in a need for gender-affirmattive treatment. Non-binary adolescents, however, may understand themselves as subjectivities "beyond the genders". Whereas psychoanalysts traditionally have often looked for the individual's core gender identity, careful listening to the new subjectivities invites new metaphors for describing gender, like "soft assembly" (Harris, 2005), "self-theorization" (Saketopoulou & Pellegrini, 2023), or an "autopoietic dimension" (Bastianini, 2025).

New observations may imply critically revising existing theoretical concepts. For example, Lingiardi (2025) creatively suggests that we revisit the Oedipal "complex" as Oedipal "complexity", arguing that the latter, emphasizing "the third" within the parental couple as well as the "position within generations", may apply irrespective of parents' anatomical characteristics. Such revision allows us to meet the new family constellations of our present Western societies, like growing up with same-gender parents, with an attitude of open inquiry rather than prejudice.

As psychoanalysts, we should attend empathically also to voices expressing gender transformations through literature and photography. Lingiardi calls our attention to Paul Preciado's texts. Strongly critical of a psychoanalysis that, according to Preciado, often represents a medical gaze, Preciado articulates the need for questioning the binary epistemology and the naturalization of genders by affirming that there is an irreducible multiplicity of sexes, genders, and sexualities: "Sexuality is a political theater in which desire—not anatomy—writes the script" (Preciado, 2019).

Certainly, psychoanalysis needs to be in dialogue with our current culture! However, the conceptual opening of identity as subjectively perceived, no longer imposed by biology, but affirmed by desire, is in no way an easy process on the concrete, lived level. To be sure, processes of identification and change may also contain pain, anxiety, and mourning.

Different positions in the field

In what follows, I will try to summarize some of the main issues in today's debate under the points (1) essentialism vs constructivism; (2) the concept of gender; (3) feminist theory; (4) the question of why, and (5) the question of regret.

Essentialism vs constructivism

In a certain perspective, the concepts of essentialism and constructivism, used within epistemology, are new terms, however referring to the age-old debate: Are we "born this way", or do we "become this way", i.e., are heredity or environment crucial factors. A related question is whether one understands gender as primarily given or primarily created. Transgender is an umbrella term that includes both transgender people who transition, and people with gender incongruence or gender dysphoria who do *not* transition. Not all transgender people identify with the term *trans* (etymological *on the other side*) they rather use masculine/ feminine binary distinctions, "I am a girl and has been so from the beginning". On this basis, they may feel that they are, e.g., a woman trapped in a man's body. They have a more "essentialist" definition of themselves, one might say. Such self-definitions must be respected. Others define themselves more "fluidly".

The same contradiction is expressed in psychoanalysts' attitude to identity development and treatment. Winnicott comes forward as a significant author, but who is used in radically different ways. Based on Winnicott's idea of mirroring, Diane Ehrensaft (2015) has created what she calls a "gender affirmative model". She speaks about the "true gender self", i.e., a true self that can be excavated and mirrored, so to speak—what can be called an essentialist model. On the other hand, Oren Gozlan (2018), a Canadian psychoanalyst, himself transgender, uses Winnicott's (1971) idea of "contiguity", i.e., something that touches each other: "In psychoanalytic thinking, continuity must give way to contiguity" (Winnicott, 1971, p. 136). There is no continuity with a true self from the beginning, rather one *becomes* a gendered being. Gender is both inherited and "made", found and "created". One easily forgets, says Gozlan, that biology itself constitutes a changing, unstable basis, "nature" is plastic. Gozlan's project is not to take a position in the dispute, but to explore unspoken assumptions in the debate, including the assumption that the child's development is "natural". Much recent psychoanalytic thinking about transgenderism is inspired by Lacan, who rejects any biological determinism, that is, the idea that there is something natural and inevitable about gender and sexuality. When it comes to the two positions, there seems to be a difference between the USA and Europe. Newer American literature is often in dialogue both with Lacan and with feminism, more concerned with linking to progressive social movements.

To be sure, from a philosophical perspective, the opposition between essentialism and constructivism is theoretically complex, the positions are, in my opinion, mutually dependent, so to speak—there would be no constructivism without essentialism. I cannot discuss this further in this context, but let me shortly say that here, I use the terms as analytical categories aiming at extracting principal positions in the ongoing debate about transgender.

The term "gender"

The term gender was introduced in the 1950s by psychologists and doctors at John Hopkins hospital, among them the psychologist John Money, to distinguish 'gender' from 'sex' (Slagstad, 2021; Eder, 2022) (the Norwegian language does not have this distinction, there is only one term "kjønn"). Inspired by cultural-relativistic trends and ideas about femininity and masculinity as socially determined, the terms "gender" and "gender roles" made it possible to separate sex and gender. Gender roles are not biologically determined. As stated by the sexologist Harry Benjamin: "sex is below the belt, gender is above the belt", meaning that gender is psychosocially constructed, while sex is linked to anatomy and biology. The team at John Hopkins, treating intersex children, claimed that gender is determined by nurture/environment, not nature/biology, i.e., gender is plastic, and can be shaped in the first 18 months of the child's life: If one succeeded in changing the body in a clear masculine or feminine direction, the child would develop a stable identity as man or woman. This was what the clinicians meant by *gender*. What was important was which gender the parents and others attributed to the child—a radical environmental hypothesis that could, however, not be substantiated. In a famous case, treated by Money, a male child was reassigned to be a girl because his penis was damaged due to botched circumcision. As a teenager the girl protested the treatment and changed her gender to become a boy—but Money did not document this part of the child's development. The sex reassignment became a tragedy for the whole family. Money's publications, based on the plastic gender-hypothesis, became a research scandal (Diamond & Sigmundson, 1997).

Influenced by the idea of malleable gender, psychoanalyst Robert Stoller launched the concepts of "gender identity" and "core gender identity". In Stoller's view, a good life presupposes a *match* between biological sex and gender role—again a binary conceptualization of sex and gender. In the clinic Stoller established in Los Angeles, parents sought help for children expressing what parents saw as unwelcome "transgender" behavior. The treatment of, e.g., boys exhibiting so-called feminine behavior consisted in reinforcing "masculine" gender roles—plasticity meant that gender could be bent in conformity with sex assigned at birth. Paradoxically, a kind of behavior therapy, in a clinic led by a psychoanalyst. Indeed, it is ironic that the concept of *gender* which became so important to my generation of feminists—we opposed the idea that sex implied a biological destiny, our sex should not determine specific gender roles—was used to defend traditional notions of masculinity and femininity.

Feminist theory

The debate about "born this way" or "become this way" is not new. Already in 1949 Simone de Beauvoir wrote: "One is not born a woman, rather one becomes a woman" (Beauvoir, 1949). It is society that produces this creature between man and eunuch, which is designated as woman, Beauvoir claimed. She found support in Freud: "Psychoanalysis does not try to describe what a woman is—that would be a task it could scarcely perform—but sets about inquiring how she comes into being" Freud (1933, p. 116). The body is not what the biologists describe, to live in a body is to live in a body in a culture. Radically continuing this point of view, Judith Butler, in *Gender trouble* (2006), develops the idea that gender is *performative* (i.e., something you do). Butler's project was a "subversive confusion" against the categories that keep gender in place. But in their latest book *Who's afraid of gender?* (2024) Butler claims that they may have taken the argument about performatives too far: Some trans people are essentialists and must be respected as such.

However, feminism is not one thing. Radical feminism today includes TERF (trans exclusive radical feminism). Claiming that *trans women are not women* and that they pose a *threat* to women and the feminist movement, the TERFs are clear essentialists. Maintaining, e.g., that trans women come forward as "women with penises in the wardrobe" they form a core of the anti-trans movement—a position shared by influential women like J. K. Rowling, the author of *Harry Potter*. The term "woman born woman" was created by TERF to exclude trans women from particular places, says Kate Bornstein (1994), transgender theorist and activist. Indeed, this demonstrates how difficult it is to answer the question "what is a woman". In a debate on Norwegian television a TERF-feminist raged against a transwoman: "You are a man!"

The question of "why"

When I listen to my patients, it is often with an implicit "why": Why is A afraid of open spaces; why does B have to wash his hands continuously to avoid panicking? Together with the patients, I explore their history to find answers, and the patient is my ally in this exploration. Psychoanalytic theory sheds light on our irrational driving forces, that's why I became a psychoanalyst myself, and that's probably also why psychoanalysis had such a strong position in clinical psychology and psychiatry throughout much of the 20th century. The theory gave an answer to "why". The "why" of psychoanalysis also makes it a critical social theory, allowing for exploration of, e.g., why people become attracted to extreme ideologies. A benign, exploring why is, of course, legitimate and necessary in encounters with trans people, to explore what individuals struggle with, in relation to their experience of gender, and their ways of living and expressing gender.

But why is not a neutral question, claims Avgi Saketopoulou (2021)! The question of etiology is only raised when gender identity does not match the biological body. This means that patients' "normative gender" is accepted at face value, while "non normative gender" must prove its legitimacy. And why should we only question sexual embodiments and identities that differ from the so-called normal, after all erotic desire is complex and potentially disruptive and disorganizing for all of us (Gullestad, 2020; see also Stryker, 2017). As I see it, this is at the heart of the debate—seeing trans identity as deviant and as something to be explained, or as part of human variation that we should recognize and welcome.

On a principal level, the question of "why" concerns whether to treat the patient as a *subject* that should be respected as such, or as an *object*, that is understood by reducing them to underlying explanatory variables (Skjervheim, 1964). We should not forget that analysts with their explanations are in a *power* position. Surely, this is a question of *ethics*. Coming from philosophy, I have always been keenly troubled by reductionism, a tendency also to be found within psychoanalysis.

The question of regret

Treatment (puberty blockers, hormone treatment, surgery) raises questions about regret—a recurring theme in the debate. For some, the fact that someone changes their mind has become the crowning argument against gender-affirming treatment. Therefore, many claim, an investigation must include how likely it is that the young person's self-experience will last, before offering treatment. No one disagrees that a therapist, in dialogue with patients, must assess how confident they are about their wish for example for puberty blockers or hormone treatment. But, as the Norwegian psychologist Reidar Jessen who has researched gender dysphoria maintains, the demand to predict the future is "hubris on behalf of psychologists". The time for omniscient psychologists is over (Jessen, 2023). We are not fortune tellers.

When it comes to the treatment of children with puberty blockers, David Bell has had great impact with his position "First of all, do no harm" (Bell, 2020). Bell argues that "watchful waiting" should be the psychoanalyst's attitude when faced with a prepubertal trans-child's wish for puberty blockers. One argument is the claim that they can *regret* such a decision. However, the argument about regret is not necessarily a valid one. Again Saketopoulou takes the floor: "watchful waiting" is not a neutral position. It involves letting children "experience the development of secondary, sexual characteristics, which is not at all about waiting" (Saketopoulou, 2021, p. 976). Waiting may be experienced as harmful, a harm that one specifically intended to avoid. Doing nothing has effects—we don't know what the harm is ahead of time.

The question of regret also raises a deep philosophical question—we humans regret so much! But the fact that someone regrets medical treatment does not necessarily mean that they would have been better off without treatment, we simply cannot know that. Self-determination is an ethical matter. We have self-determined abortion, even if someone regrets it later in life.

Understanding threat and hatred

The present polarized political debate about transgender seems to bear witness to what has been called a kind of binary terror—panic unleashed when people are faced with the blurring of boundaries (male/female; active/passive) that have been integral to a culture's social fabric. One telling example: The billionaire Elon Musk recently announced that he would move the headquarters of two of his businesses (including the social media platform X) from California to Texas because of a new law intended to protect transgender children. *New York Times* comments that Musk has a personal background for his anti-trans engagement: In 2022, one of his children officially applied for changing her name and gender. Musk was furious and claimed that his child, a transwoman (born a boy), was dead, "killed by the woke mind virus". The daughter refuses to be defined by him: "I no longer live with or wish to be related to my biological father in any way, shape or form". So here we have one of the world's richest men declaring war on his home state for supporting the rights of his children! Indeed, witnessing about a father's need to control his children, but also about the anxiety, threat and panic that transgender may pose.

With our concept of countertransference, psychoanalysts are in a unique position of understanding such anxieties. Why this feeling of threat? My thoughts go to one of Freud's last essays, *Analysis terminable and interminable* (1937). "Masculine protest", Freud says, comes forward as an especially challenging theme in psychoanalytic treatment. It is about a fear of becoming passive and helpless which may represent an almost untreatable resistance in analysis. Patients—and Freud here speaks especially about men—do not want to feel passive in relation to other men, that means being castrated. The passive position is linked to being feminine, Freud also speaks about "repudiation of femininity" (Freud, 1937, p. 250)—meaning that the feminine mode is denied, rejected, disowned. To be sure, it seems that the feminine is here associated with being weak and vulnerable, so often despised in our culture of today. Is contempt for weakness an underlying theme in the masculine protest?

A question comes to my mind: Is misogyny—fear and contempt of the feminine and for weakness—an element in homophobia, and do we find the same element in transphobia? Hatred and prohibition of homosexuality, so dominant in culturally conservative countries, seems to be specifically directed toward *male* homosexuality. Why? The award-winning movie *All of us strangers*, directed by Andrew Haigh, characterized as "the best movie of the year" in Norway 2024, tells the story of a gay man, Adam, and his imaginary encounters with his parents, who died when Adam was a boy. Adam wants to tell them that he is gay. "I always thought you were a bit tutti frutti" the father replies—the term connotes a mélange of different fruit. "You never learnt to play ball as a real boy, there was something girlish about you". As a child, Adam was bullied at school for being « effeminate», now he asks his father why the father did not approach him when he was crying in his room, which he regularly did coming home from school—and the father heard him crying. "I did not want you to be the one who was bullied", the father responds, "if I had been in that schoolyard I might have been among the mob".

"The war on effeminate boys" is the title of an essay by Eve Kosofsky Sedgwick (1993), American founder of queer theory. The point of departure for her essay is a report about adolescent suicide documenting a much higher suicide rate among homosexuals than among other youths. The report highlights condemnation, hostility, and abuse of homosexual adolescents—there is something about feminine boys, "gay" is a word of abuse. While homosexuality was removed as a diagnosis in the seventies, another diagnosis appeared, Sedwick points out: "Gender Identity Disorder in Childhood", a diagnosis given almost exclusively to boys showing "abnormal" interest in "girl stuff". And while the homosexuality diagnosis was removed after forceful protests from activists, the new diagnosis was accepted without further ado, also within psychoanalysis.

To be sure, a discussion of "masculine protest", "repudiation of femininity", and "war on effeminate feminine boys" must take history, culture, and socioeconomic conditions into consideration. Elon Musk's war on transgender takes place in a specific societal context, as do Putin's warfare against liberal Western values and defense of a patriarchal order. Also, as historian Jules Gill-Peterson (2024) explores, modern trans misogyny emerged in particular colonial context. As psychoanalysts, we are in a position of specifically contributing to exploring the *psychological* dynamics of threat and hatred.

What now?

In the past two years, I have had the chance of getting to know some of the work-in-progress on transgender issues by European colleagues, particularly the work of the *IPA Sexual and Gender Diversity Studies Committee*, aiming at discussing how to integrate rapidly developing ideas of gender identity, sex, and sexuality without falling back on normative models. Critical rethinkning of our psychoanalytic theories implies investigating the whole spectrum of subjectivities that have no place in orthodox masculine-feminine duality, i.e., deconstructing the binary masculine/feminine dichotomy, replacing it by a more flexible and open gender concept, thus confronting the clinical and theoretical challenge of gender diversity and fluidity (Thomson-Salo et al., 2025). We must, in my opinion, question the idea of a stable, fixed gender *identity*—we should rather conceptualize gender as dynamically changing over time (Saketopoulou & Pellegrini, 2023). Listening to new ways of expressing and of living gender we must be willing to correct ourselves and, in line with Bion's (1962) *negative capability*, contain the uncertainty of not knowing. In short, we must abandon illusions of understanding in favor of a humble, inquiring attitude.

Notes

1 This chapter is previously published in *Scandinavian Psychoanalytic Review,* 2024.
2 The *American Medical Association* speaks about the "medical spectrum of gender", recognizing that "gender may differ from sex assigned at birth" (Slagstad, 2021).

References

Bastianini, T. (2025 in press). Body, Sexuality, Gender: Between Identifying Project and Desire. In F. Thomson-Salo, L. Bruno, & E. Reichelt (eds.), *Gender, identifications, and identities: Dialogues at the edges.* London: Routledge.

Bell, D. (2020). First Do no Harm. *International Journal of Psychoanalysis, 101*(5), 1031–1038.

Bion, W. ((1962). *Learning from experience.* London & New York: Routledge, 2014.

Blass, R., Bell, D., & Saketopoulou, A. (2021). Can we Think Psychoanalytically about Transgenderism? An Expanded Live Zoom Debate with Avgi Saketopoulou, Moderated by Rachel Blass. *International Journal of Psychoanalysis, 102*(5), 968–1000.

Bornstein, K. (1994). *Gender outlaw. On men, women, and the rest of Us.* New York & London: Routledge.

Butler, J. (2006). *Gender trouble – feminism and the subversion of identity.* London & New York: Routledge.

Butler, J. (2024). *Who's Afraid of gender?* London: Allan Lane.

De Beauvoir, S. (1949). *Le deuxième sexe.* Paris: Gallimard.

Diamond, M., & Sigmundson, H. K. (1997). "Sex Reassignment at Birth. Long-Term Review and Clinical Implications". *Archives of Pediatrics and Adolescent Medicine, 151*(3), 298–304.

Drescher, J. (2020). From Bisexuality to Intersexuality: Rethinking Gender Categories. In L. Hertzmann, & J. Newbigin (eds.), *Sexuality and gender now. Moving beyond heteronormativity.* New York: Routledge, 167–188.

Eder, S. (2022). *How the clinic made gender: The medical history of a transformative idea.* Chicago: University of Chicago Press.

Ehrensaft, D. (2015). Listening and Learning from Gender Non-Conforming Children. *Psychoanal. Study of the Child, 68,* 28–56.

Fonagy, P., & Allison, E. (2015). A Scientific Theory of Homosexuality. In A. Lemma, & P. Lynch, P. (eds.), *Sexualities. Contemporary psychoanalytic perspectives.* London: Routledge.

Freud, S. (1905). *Three essays on the theory of sexuality.* SE, 7, 123–245.

Freud, S. (1933). *Femininity. New introductory lectures.* SE, 22, 112–135.

Freud, S. (1937). *Analysis terminable and interminable.* SE, 23, 209–253.

Geldhof, A., & Verhaeghe, P. (2017). Queer as a New Shelter from Castration. In N. Giffney & E. Watson (eds.), *Clinical encounters in sexuality. Psychoanalytic practice & queer theory.* Punctum books, Earth, Milky Way.

Gill-Peterson, J. (2024). *A short history of trans misogyni.* New York: Verso Books.

Gozlan, O. (2018). From Continuity to Contiguity. A Response to the Fraught Temporality of Gender. *Psychoanalytic Review, 105*(1).

Gullestad, S. E. (2020). The Otherness of Sexuality: Exploring the Conflicted Nature of Drive, Desire and Object Choice. *International Journal of Psychoanalysis, 101*(1), 64–83.

Harris, A. (2005). *Gender as soft assembly.* Hillsdale, NJ: The Analytic Press.

Isay, R. A. (1985). On the Analytic Therapy of Homosexual Men. *Psychoanalytic Study of the Child, 40,* 235–254.

Jessen, R. S. (2023). Feilskritt å avvise kjønnsopplevelse. *Tidsskrift for Norsk Psykologforening, 60*(6), 387. psykologtidsskriftet.no/debatt/2023/05/feilskritt-avvise-kjonnsopplevelse

Knafo, D., & Lo Bosco, R. (2020). *The new sexual landscape and contemporary psychoanalysis.* London: Confer Books.

Lingiardi, V. (2025 in press). Gender Identities and Identifications in a Changing World. In F. Thomson-Salo, L. Bruno, & E. Reichelt (eds.), *Gender, identifications, and identities: Dialogues at the edges.* London: Routledge.

Preciado, P. B. (2019). *An apartment on Uranus: Chronicles of the Crossing.* Semiotext(e): MIT Press.

Roughton, R. (2000). Sometimes a Desire is Just a Desire: Gay Men and Their Analysts. *Gender and Psychoanalysis, 5,* 259–273.

Roughton, R. E. (2001). Four Men in Treatment: An Evolving Perspective on Homosexuality and Bisexuality, 1965 to 2000. *Journal of the American Psychoanalytic Association, 49,* 1187–1217.

Saketopoulou, A. (2014). Mourning the Body as Bedrock: DevelopMental Considerations in Treating Transsexual Patients Analytically. *Journal of the American Psychoanalytic Association, 62*(5), 773–806.

Saketopoulou, A. (2021). Can we think psychoanalytically about transgenderism? An expanded live zoom debate with David Bell and Avgi Saketopoulou, moderated by Rachel Blass. *International Journal of Psychoanalysis, 102*(5), 968–1000.

Saketopoulou, A., & Pellegrini, A. (2023). *Gender without identity.* New York: Uit Books.

Sedgwick, E. K. (1993). How to Bring Your Kids Up Gay: The War on Effeminate Boys. In M. A. Barale, J. Godberg, M. Moon, & E. K. Sedgwick (eds.), *Tendencies.* Durham, NC: Duke University Press, 154–164.

Slagstad, K. (2021). The Political Nature of Sex – Transgender in the History of Medicine. *New England Journal of Medicine, 384,* 1070–1074.

Skjervheim, H. (1964). *Vitskapen om mennesket og den filosofiske refleksjon.* Oslo: Tanum Forlag.

Solms, M. (2023). *The biological foundation of gender. A delicate balance.* Paper presented at the IPA Joseph Sandler Research Conference, Vienna, 2023. The paper was based on

Solms, M., & Turnbull, O. (2002). *The brain and the inner world. An introduction to the neuroscience of subjective experience.* New York: Other Press.

Stryker, S. (2017). Transgender, Queer Theory, and Psychoanalysis. In N. Giffney, & E. Watson (eds.), *Clinical encounters in sexuality. Psychoanalytic practice and queer theory.* Punctum books, 419–426.

Thomson-Salo, F., Bruno, L., & Reichelt, E. (eds.) (2025 in press). *Gender, identifications, and identities: Dialogues at the edges.* London*:* Routledge.

Winnicott, D. W. (1971). *Playing and reality.* London: Tavistock.

12 Adolescence in a digital age—developmental challenges, risk behavior, and potential space

Line Indrevoll Stänicke

Adolescence: a transformative life period[1]

Adolescence (11–18 years of age) is a transformative life period characterized by cognitive, neuro-biological, emotional, psychological, and social changes (Thapar et al., 2015). For the adolescent, emotional arousal, difficult feelings, and interpersonal stress are often felt as overwhelming with an urgent need for discharge. In this period, contact with friends and peers become important for sharing good and difficult experiences, feelings of belonging, and getting to know oneself and others' feelings and thoughts, and possibility for role exploration, creativity, and identity formation (Erikson, 1968; Fonagy et al., 2019). Adolescence may be described as the "second chance" of separation (Blos, 1967) and as a transition between childhood and adulthood. Over time, the young person may develop an increased capacity for problem-solving, affect regulation, and mentalization (Fonagy et al., 2019), which increases autonomy (Gullestad, 1993) and a stable self-identity (Erikson, 1968).

Today, the internet and social media are integrated parts of young people's social lives and identity from an early age. In addition to social exploration, online engagement enables different self-experiences, boosts self-esteem, and offers information (Livingstone et al., 2022). During adolescence, when the focus of attention is directed toward friends and peers for social guidance, engagement in social media may be understood as an extended peer arena for role exploration and self-identity formation (Stänicke, 2022).

Risk behavior and self-harm in adolescence—offline and online

Importantly, during adolescence, risk behavior such as alcohol or drug abuse, driving too fast, sexual risk behavior, or self-harming in general is not uncommon. Self-harm refers to inflicting pain on one's body (such as cutting or burning) with or without suicide intentions and is associated with several mental disorders and an increased risk of death (Witt et al., 2021). Recent data suggest that 17% of typical 12–18-year-olds engage in

DOI: 10.4324/9781003565284-16

self-harm, and the numbers are higher for girls struggling with psychological issues (Farkas et al., 2024). Self-harm is usually initiated early in adolescence and reaches its apex around 15 years of age.

The worrisome and rising numbers of adolescents who intentionally inflict pain on their bodies have prompted researchers to point to the possible influence of digital risks like engagement in self-harm content (like pictures, texts, or videos) in social media (like TikTok, Instagram, or Snapchat) (Susi et al., 2023). Approximately 8%–17% of European adolescents are exposed to self-harm or suicide content online (Smahel et al., 2020). Frequent online use and repeated search for self-harm content online correlates with higher levels of social-psychological distress, unmet need for mental health support, and thoughts of self-harm and suicide. Qualitative reviews underline how young people experience engagement in self-harm content online as enabling a social community and support but lowering the threshold for destructive behavior (Stänicke et al., 2023). Those at risk online seem to be at risk offline.

How can we understand young people's engagement in self-harm and self-harm content online? Further, what does the digital arena add to risk engagement? In the following, I will present knowledge on the function of self-harm and findings from a multiple case interview study of young people (*n* = 20), interviewed first as adolescents (12–18 years of age) and then after five years (18–23 years of age). All self-harmed and were engaged in self-harm content online during adolescence. By presenting three cases, I want to illustrate how self-harming and engagement in self-harm content online may serve different functions and seem closely related to self-experience and self-identity formation during adolescence. I will argue that even though digital risk engagement comes with a risk of increased mental health difficulties, the activity can have transitional qualities, enabling an intermediate area between the inner and outer world (Winnicott, 1953/1971). Following this, engagement in self-harm content online may serve as a transitional object for illusions, play, and relational and personal exploration.

The function of self-harm

Today, several reviews proclaim that self-harm has an affect regulating function—the action *regulates* difficult feelings, the person gets a sense of *control,* and achieves something good—a *relief* (Klonsky, 2007; Miller et al., 2019). In addition, a neuro-biological perspective highlights increased response to stress and differences in the threshold of pain, and a behavior perspective highlights how self-harm can be reinforced by inner emotional states like good feelings or by enabling social attention. Importantly, in general case studies and qualitative studies are seldom included in reviews because of the lack of statistical power. In this way, knowledge of *why* people harm themselves is mostly offered at a group level without context-sensitive descriptions. Further, developmental, socio-cultural, psychodynamic, and relational perspectives are seldom represented.

From early on in his writings, Freud (1901) underlined the necessity of understanding the function of *irrational symptoms* by exploring the individual's inner psychic reality, including motivations and phantasies. In his writing, he discussed human activities that may seem irrational, like self-mutilation. The symptom could establish an inner psychic balance or be motivated by an underlying psychic *conflict* between sexual drives. Later, he wrote that self-mutilation was an expression of a compulsion to *repeat* and *process* earlier trauma (Freud, 1914) or could be understood as *anger directed toward self* (Freud, 1917). Later, Pao (1969) and Kafka (1969), who was inspired by Winnicott's thinking and the relational turn in psychoanalysis, argued that self-harm is a sign of developmental problems and should be understood as *nonverbal communication* of unrepresented feelings like anger in the relationship with the mother. Self-harm was discussed as a concrete *exploration* of the borders between an inner and outer world through the body and, more specifically, a concrete attempt to *separate* from the mother. In this way, the body could be an object for self-development. Several authors have been inspired by this perspective, metaphorically described self-harm as "the voice of the skin" (McLane, 1996), as psychic pain "written on the body" (Ashead, 2016), or how "the body becomes a canvas" for mental pain (Lemma, 2010).

In 2018, we did a meta-analysis of 21 qualitative studies of adolescents' experience of self-harm, to bring empirical data from the youth perspective (Stänicke et al., 2018). We found that adolescents described self-harm as an attempt *to obtain release from* and *to control difficult feelings*, thus supporting that self-harm is experienced as having an affect regulation function. However, adolescents also emphasized self-harm as a way *to represent unacceptable feelings* and *to connect with others*. In this way, self-harm may also be an attempt to communicate without words. Today, as mentioned, this perspective is not listed in reviews because of a lack of evidence from quantitative studies.

Furthermore, it was striking how many of the adolescents described self-harm in a relational context—they harmed themselves *to protect someone* from difficult or conflicting feelings. By using their body, they handled difficult experiences in a self-sufficient manner. This may be understandable in regard to important developmental challenges during adolescence—like reaching independence and autonomy. Adolescents need to develop their ways of regulating and handling difficulties. Still, adolescents' voices highlight how they stand in a conflict between attempts to protect their caregivers from difficult self-experiences—like being angry or vulnerable—in order to get sufficient support and comfort. In this way, self-harm should be understood *in* a relational context and according to developmental knowledge. This finding is in line with authors who highlight that self-harm has an outreaching and sharing function—self-harm is understood as "a cry for help" (Kwawer, 1980), it "cuts the silence" (Brady, 2014) and may bring "a sign of hope" (Motz, 2010).

Young people's experience of self-harm content online

Findings from a multiple case study that involved interviewing 20 adolescents between 12 and 18 years of age in a clinical setting highlight how self-harm is closely related to the self (Stänicke et al., 2019). As the adolescents' describe it, they started to harm themselves because of relational and emotional difficulties, getting the idea from friends, peers, or internet content. They were ambivalent about treatment and how to end self-harm—they had finally found a way to support themselves and avoid being overwhelmed. Self-harm was embedded in their experience of themselves—they harmed themselves to *punish* themselves, to *get rid of unwanted* experiences of themselves, or to *express* earlier trauma. Further, diversities in the form and semantic content of their meaning-making of self-harm brought information about specific self-representations—"the punished self", "the unknown self", and "the harmed self" (Stänicke, 2021).

Five years after the first interviews, I interviewed 15 of them once more (Stänicke, 2022)[2]. The now young adults, 18–23 years of age, reflected on how they handled difficulties today, if they had developed alternative ways of coping, and their lived experience of being engaged in self-harm content online. At the time of the interviews, 2/3 of the participants had ended self-harming and struggled less with mental health problems. However, 1/3 harmed themselves occasionally or in more indirect ways—such as using drugs, having risky sex with strangers, being in violent relationships, or eating too little.

First, many of the participants described how they felt *a solitude during adolescence, they felt like an outsider and searched for a place to fit in*. One of the girls, Carolyn, said: "I felt that I didn't" fit in with normal people ... And when you are 14 ... All you want is to fit in». Carolyn did not share her problems with her parents—she was afraid of being a burden (1.1.1)—and searched extensively online for information: "I searched for everything ... including mental illnesses, suicide methods, and self-harm". She looked at others' posts, and even though she never shared personal content, she *felt understood* and not alone: "When you're feeling alone as a 15-year-old, and you think there is something wrong with you, and you discover ... here are 1,000...peers who have ... gone through a lot of the same".

Another girl, Elly, described how she was bullied in elementary school and felt that her teacher and mother did not understand her difficulties. She longed for a peer community. She heard about a girl at school who self-harmed and started to share pictures and texts on an Instagram account to get in contact with her: "It helps to find another place to fit in ... you get a kind of satisfaction", Elly said. Reading and sharing content online became a way to connect—she *felt noticed*.

A third girl, Anna, described how she, from she was 12 years of age, had several online accounts for sharing personal texts about mental health problems. Her parents were in a big conflict, she felt criticized by her mother about her weight and, in addition, a friend had spread rumors about her. She experienced that several young people contacted her online, and she and a friend established an online group to offer advice and information about places to get help: "It was a community for lost and lonely people. I wanted to be of help". By supporting others, she *felt useful*.

Second, young people described the activity of looking at or sharing self-harm content online as *tempting and fascinating* and, at the same time, *dangerous and addictive*. Carolyn became *preoccupied*: "I could just sit there and read for hours … then I had something to do … and to look forward to… even if I actually did feel like shit". She lacked the energy to do anything else, and online involvement became a kind of distraction and all-consuming playful activity. Carolyn understood others' suicide posts as a need for contact and not as a wish to die but was still *triggered* by the content: "So I think it's more about getting contact—not ending the game, in a way. (…) But a lot of blogs and books were EXTREMELY triggering and set me off on a really bad path".

Elly found the activity *absorbing*: "Because a big part of it was the excitement … I LOVED it" (Elly). She got an intense online friendship with the girl: "It was just the two of us. Every day, we supported each other.—Oh god, so insanely dangerous! I was completely fixated". She noticed online warnings of triggering content as a sign of something tempting to tune into:

I chose the bad because the bad is very good when you are bad (…) It is really romanticized in those pictures … to be ill, miserable and depressed … it's a sort of beautiful depression look pretty girl, with mascara on her face … and very thin.

After some time, the online friendship became very *competitive*:

Every morning we sent each other messages (laughing) about how much we weighed … and had eaten … It was just INSANELY dangerous and exciting … It was like a struggle of who had it the worst or was thinnest.

(laughing a little)

Anna felt *responsible* for doing something to help those who wrote to her:

When a guy is sitting there with a razorblade and saying, "I'm going to commit suicide—I can't take it anymore". If I sent him a text and said "hey, please don't do this", … I could help him. It was a good feeling.

The online involvement lowered the threshold to sharing problems and being supportive to each other. At the same time, Anna felt *helpless*: "People sharing pictures of self-harm and the best way to die … I became mentally exhausted by being there for everybody".

Third, engaging in self-harm content online was described as helpful in handling and accept personal problems and increased self-understanding—through the online activity, they seemed *to search for and explore themselves*. Carolyn said: "To look at black and white pictures of sad girls with wounds, scars, and blood … it put me in a vulnerable position. But it felt good to be able to relate to something". She felt a *relief*—both calming and comforting. The online content confirmed an inner state and became a way to relate to herself—*something to identify with*:

> I actively searched for it. To choose to be sad. I got very used to liv-ing in that misery. It actually was uncomfortable to go OUT of it. This was my comfort zone … it doesn't work to read about happy people because you can't relate to it.

Elly read and reposted others' self-harm content online as a way to *express difficult feelings*:

> It has been my way of venting my sadness … I "bi-blogged" it instead of writing it down in a book … If I had a bad time, I put on some sad music, searched for and reposted sad pictures … I wanted to be in my bubble.

Elly described the online activity as an online diary documenting her development:

> it was me and my diary … It went through all of my phases … If you scroll from when I was 12 and up through the years, it was SUPER SAD and … "I will kill myself" and "I am depressed" … to flowers and coffee cups in the sun.

Anna described the accounts as an important part of her *life history*: "Oh God, what have I spent my life on! Still, I haven't deleted all of them. It feels like telling a story … I am not a part of that story anymore. But it is me". Anna highlighted how the involvement made her see something beautiful in her suffering: "Even if it was not helpful … you make your own sadness into something esthetical".

Finally, the participants described how they were alone in dealing with online difficulties—adults could not understand, and *it was no one in charge* to help them. In the follow-up interview, Carolyn, now herself an adult, thought adults would be traumatized by seeing pictures of children with open wounds. In addition, she thought they would be overlooked, avoided, or not trusted if they tried to help. Carolyn could still search for triggering content like posts on suicide: "In my bad periods, I don't have the energy to do the things that I would rather be doing, and then I end up there". But she noticed how the activity confirmed her problems: "you can end up in a kind of hole where you just read about exactly the same as what you're going through—it makes it worse".

Retrospectively, Elly thought she could have ended the activity earlier:

> If someone had told my mom about the account, then my mom would have monitored my cell phone—And not let me do it (…) Then I think it wouldn't have gone that far … at some point I WANTED her to SEE it… and to say it without saying it.

Elly made a choice: "I actually HAVE thought about it… but I choose NOT to do it. Earlier—it was not a choice".

In Anna's opinion, it could have been helpful if some adults with passive accounts contacted persons with suicidal content:

> Maybe a professional could find out who they are and just say: "Hi, I saw that you have an account!"… not that I would have realized then that "oh, that was stupid" because you already know that … But you don't dare to continue.

Anna also decided to end the accounts: "It gets overwhelming to see others suicide notes when you have your own problems to struggle with".

With this as a background, I will now return to the question of how to understand engagement in self-harm content online. Is this engagement related to developmental challenges during adolescence, such as self-identity formation? And if so, what does the digital arena add to the process of identity formation?

Engagement in self-harm content online during adolescence—social belonging, playfulness, and exploration of self

Young people's experience of engagement in social content online highlight how social media may provide youths with a place to belong, to get support, and to express difficult parts of their self. These qualitative findings lend additional empirical support to the notion that engagement is a "double-edged sword" (Lewis & Seko, 2015). Social media networks may serve as a *community* for vulnerable youths and cover a need to belong (Stänicke, 2022). They may find a *place to fit in* and a peer community with "like-minded" peers as a way out of solitude. Peers and friends are important during adolescence to get to know others' perspectives, feelings, and thoughts (Erikson, 1968). In this way, social media may be understood as an *extended peer arena* for social exploration, learning, and coping (Stänicke,

2022). Those who harm themselves and search for self-harm content online, share their problems, and the engagement may support them during crisis. Still, the activity may also lower the threshold for self-harm (Susi et al., 2023). Paradoxically, the participants seldom know where to get professional help, and some adolescents may search for information about self-harm online to find help and support.

Interestingly, the participants emphasized a kind of *playfulness* in the activity, how the involvement was "like a game that never should end". The online posts with suicide content were described as "not real suicide letters" but as a need for contact. It was easier to ask for help online, and the online sphere seemed to lower the threshold for sharing problems. For some, to show a picture was easier than to describe their pain in words. In addition, it was described as "safer" to talk to someone they did not know instead of their parents or therapist, who—we might infer—could reduce access to their telephone or computer or increase weight control if they knew about their online activity. Winnicott wrote that it is only through playing that the child can *discover the self* (Winnicott, 1953/1971, p. 144). He also stated that it is only through playing that friendships can emerge that enable a person to be different and separate. In this way, both playing and friendships may have transitional qualities important for self-development. The children may play to master anxiety or difficult feelings like anger or losing control. In friendship, difficult feelings may be shared and tolerated.

The participants also valued how the online activity could bring *relief* or a way to *express* difficult self-experiences like negative self-thoughts, fantasies, or mental health problems. The content may show their personal life story as an online diary. Some experienced increased acceptance of their problems and described a possibility of seeing something beautiful in their suffering. The self-harm content online may represent self-destructive impulses, and, in this way, the online community may also be something to identify with. Further, the engagement may enable exploration of the borders between "me" and "not me"—keeping a distance *and* a kind of privacy. In this way, the present results underline how digital engagement with self-harm content online was closely related to the young person's *developmental processes of identity formation*.

Psychic reality and the outer world: the role of illusion and disillusion

In Freud's (1901) writing, several concepts point to *the relationship* between our inner and the outer world. He wrote about "psychic reality" *as different from* external reality and highlighted how subjectively we may experience an outer world. For example, we may defend ourselves and *project* mental content that we cannot accept as our own into qualities of other people or as part of an outer world. He also wrote about how human activities— like art—can be important for our inner psychic balance and an *important channel* for expressing destructivity and discontent that must be denied because we need to be part of a social group (Freud, 1927).

According to Jan Abram (2007), before 1953, the year Winnicott published the paper "Transitional Objects and Transitional Phenomenon", there was "no accounting for the space *between* inside and outside in the psychoanalytic literature" (p. 312). Winnicott's (1953/1971) concept of *transitional phenomenon* points to *an intermediate area* and a dimension of living, neither completely subjective or internal nor completely objective or external, but a place that both connects and separates inner and outer. Winnicott also used the term "the potential space" when referring to this in-between area of living. In his perspective on development, the transitional phenomenon occurs from the beginning, even before birth, in the mother-infant dyad. Winnicott emphasized that the infant needs the mother to let him/her be in a necessary *illusion of omnipotence* and to feel like the world is his/her creation because separation is not yet tolerable. Then, to develop a sense of self and to establish borders between the inner and outer reality, the mother needs to facilitate a gradual *disillusionment*. As the infant begins to separate Me from not-Me, going from absolute dependence into the stage of relative dependency, the baby makes us of the "transitional object", which—in the long run—leads to the use of illusion and symbols (Abram, 2007, p. 311). Winnicott (1953/1971) underlined how transitional phenomena are intrinsically linked with being, playing, creativity, and culture.

Self-identity formation in a digital age—digital activity as a transitional phenomenon

Inspired by Winnicott's (1953/1971) concepts of "transitional phenomena", we may understand digital activity as having a transitional quality—an intermediate area in between the inner and outer world. Winnicott writes that "the transitional object and transitional phenomenon start each human being off with what will always be important for them" (p. 239). The transitional phenomena represent the early stages of "the use of illusion". The intermediate area is in direct continuity with the area of the small child who is lost in play (Winnicott, 1953/ 1971, p. 241). For lonely adolescents, self-harm networks online may represent a place to belong and to get support. In addition, the engagement in self-harm content online may be understood as a transitional object—bridging the inner and outer world, enabling both relational *and* personal exploration and development of illusions. The difficult, bad, non-accepted, or unknown self-experiences can be represented and integrated into a more stable self-identity. However, the engagement comes with a risk of increased self-harm and mental health difficulties.

Online involvement with self-harm content serves a *variety of functions* for young people. We may say that the adolescent's inner world and everyday life of being in the world influence their experiences of their online world.

Carolyn lacked closeness to her parents and friends but felt she gained knowledge about difficult issues in life and *felt understood* through her digital involvement. Elly had no friends, and being online was an important way *to connect* with others and to share problems. Anna felt criticized by her mother. When she supported others online, she *felt useful.* Maybe she helped others in a way she needed herself. We may ask if their experiences reflect personal and relational needs according to their relational context. The importance of feeling understood, seen, and useful may express basic psychological relational needs for a young person growing up. The digital arena is a place to search for psychological and existential meaning.

Interestingly, knowledge of adolescents' reasons for self-harm underlines how this behavior may be an attempt to get *relief* and *control* as well as an attempt to *express* or *share* overwhelming feelings (Stänicke et al., 2018). By using the body in a concrete and harmful way, the young person may transform overwhelming inner suffering into a physical pain, and at the same time, they express and represent conflictual, unknown feelings, and vulnerability (Stänicke, 2021). The motivation for exploring self-harm content online may be more outwardly oriented than self-harming, which is directed toward one's body. Importantly, the digital arena is *both* private and social—the representation and exploration of self-experiences through online engagement become public—a process which may be metaphorically described as "an online diary".

As mentioned earlier, oppositional behavior, testing of social norms, and risk-taking behavior, such as drug or alcohol abuse, driving too fast, or self-harming, are not uncommon during adolescence (Thapar et al., 2015). My study underlines how digital involvement was experienced by adolescents as *risky*, both for themselves and others. Importantly, despite the negative consequences, the involvement was fascinating, engaging, tempting, and exciting *at the same time.* Even when they saw trigger warnings, they chose to continue. In this way, online involvement with digital risks may serve as a "transitional" or "potential area" of experiencing and experimental interaction that is "in-between" reality and fiction—without doing it for real and with less responsibility (Winnicott, 1953/1971). Offline and online risk behavior may be understood as *a way to test* social norms and borders between what is 'accepted' and "unacceptable", pain and pleasure, and self and others.

Importantly, over time, the game-like and exciting experiences increased self-harm and mental problems, competition, normalizing and social modeling of non-adaptive problem solving, and exhaustive support of others. The adolescents experienced that the engagement triggered self-harm, suicide ideation, and mental health problems. They felt addicted, afraid of losing their online friends and community, and *struggled to end the involvement.* Digital exploration may both be a rescue and serve a developmental function and, at the same time, increase vulnerability. The results underline how they experienced a lack of "someone" responsible who could act when needed. There was no one in charge. In the developmental process of autonomy, youths may appreciate digital exploration and, at the same time, need some guidance.

Closing remark

Psychoanalysis has a rich repertoire of theories on the human mind and its function. Still, new cultural expressions provoke a need to test analytic theories and nuance them according to current cultural phenomena. Self-harm is probably a human activity from the beginning of time, but engagement in self-harm content online is new to us. In this chapter, I have aimed to demonstrate how the psychoanalytic concept of "transitional phenomenon" in Winnicott's thinking is highly relevant for understanding a new phenomenon like digital activity. Engagement in self-harm content online may serve as a transitional object for illusions, play, and relational and personal exploration. The digital arena may also provide as a substitute for the lack of social support offline. Further, I argue that engagement in self-harm content online highlight how transference phenomenon also can include to represent and integrate destructive impulses as part of self.

However, both self-harm and online engagement come with a risk of increased mental health difficulties. Maybe we may even call the engagement as "a digital self-harming"? Further, an adolescent—as the small child—is still *challenged to develop borders* between an inner and outer world, to be disillusioned, and to embrace vulnerability, helplessness, aggression and destructive impulses as part of themselves. Furthermore, a developmental task is to develop less destructive affect regulation strategies. Digital experiences may facilitate illusion, but digital risks may also have a role in disillusion. Maybe the digital risk experiences, in the long run, represent a possibility for experiencing a border between the omnipotent illusion and reality—*a digital disillusion.*

Notes

1 This paper was presented at the European Psychoanalytic Conference in Cannes, 2023.
2 The Norwegian Regional Committees for Medical and Health Research Ethics (REK) approved the study (2014/832). Data is anonymized. The results are earlier presented in Stänicke, 2022.

References

Abram, J. (2007). *The language of winnicott: A dictionary of winnicott's use of words*. UK: Karnac.
Ashead, G. (2016). Written in the Body: Deliberate Self-Harm and Violence. In E. Weldon & C. Van Velsen (eds.), *A practical guide to forensic psychotherapy*. London: Jessica Kingsley Publishers.

Blos, P. (1967). The second individuation process of adolescence. *Psychoanalytic Study of the Child*, 5(22), 162–186.

Brady, M. T. (2014). Cutting the silence: Initial, impulsive self-cutting in adolescence. *International Journal of Child Psychotherapy*, 40, 287–301. https://doi.org/10.1080/0075417X.2014.965430

Erikson, E. H. (1968). *Identity: Youth and crisis*. New York: Norton.

Farkas, B. F., Takacs, Z. K., Kollárovics, N., & Balázs, J. (2024). The prevalence of self-injury in adolescence: A systematic review and meta-analysis. *European Child Adolescent Psychiatry*, 33(10), 3439–3458. doi: 10.1007/s00787-023-02264-y.

Fonagy, P., Luyten, P., Allison, E., & Campbell, C. (2019). Mentalizing, epistemic trust and the phenomenology of psychotherapy. *Psychopathology*, 52(2), 94–103. https://doi.org/10.1159/000501526

Freud, S. (1901). *The psychopathology of everyday life. Standard edition of the complete psychological works of Sigmund Freud, 6, 1–239*. Translated by J. Strachey. London: Vintage & Hogarth Press.

Freud, S. (1914). *Remembering, repeating and working-through (Further recommendations on the technique of psycho-analysis II)*. Standard edition of the complete psychological works of Sigmund Freud, 12,146–156. Translated by J. Strachey. London: Vintage & Hogarth Press.

Freud, S. (1917). *Mourning and melancholia. Standard edition of the complete psychological works of Sigmund Freud, 14, 239–259*. Translated by J. Strachey. London: Vintage & Hogarth Press.

Freud, S. (1927). *The future for an illusion. Standard edition of the complete psychological works of Sigmund Freud, 21, 1–56*. Translated by J. Strachey. London: Vintage & Hogarth Press.

Gullestad, S. E. (1993). A contribution to the psychoanalytic concept of autonomy. *The Scandinavian Psychoanalytic Review*, 16(1), 22–34. https://doi.org/10.1080/01062301.1993.10592286.

Jan Abram (2007). The Language of Winnicott: A Dictionary of Winnicott's Use of Words. 2nd Edition.

Kafka, J. S. (1969). The body as transitional object: A psychoanalytic study of a self-mutilating patient. *British Journal of Medical Psychology*, 42, 207–212. https://doi.org/10.1111/j.2044-8341.1969.tb02072.x

Klonsky, E. D. (2007). The functions of deliberate self-injury: A review of the evidence. *Clinical Psychology Review*, 27, 226–239. https://doi.org/10.1016/j.cpr.2006.08.002

Kwawer, J. S. (1980). Some interpersonal aspects of self-mutilation in a borderline patient. *Journal of American Academy of Psychoanalysis*, 8(2), 203–216. PMID: 7358536

Lemma, A. (2010). *Under the skin. A psychoanalytic study of body modification*. London: Routledge.

Lewis, S. P., & Seko, Y. (2015). A double-edged sword: A review of benefits and risks of online nonsuicidal self-injury activities. *Journal of Clinical Psychology*, 72(3), 249–262. https://doi.org/10.1002/jclp.22242

Livingstone, S., Stoilova, M., Stänicke, L. I., Jessen, R. S., Graham, R., Staksrud, E., & Jensen, T. K. (2022). *Young people experiencing internet-related mental health difficulties: The benefits and risks of digital skills*. An empirical study. KU Leuven: ySKILLS.

McLane, J. (1996). The voice on the skin: Self-mutilation and Merleau-Ponty's theory of language. *Hypatia*, 11, 107–118. https://doi.org/10.1111/j.1527-2001.1996.tb01038.x

Miller, A. B., Massing-Schaffer, M., Owens, S., & Prinstein, M. J. (2019). Nonsuicidal Self- Injury Among Youth. In T. H. Ollendick, S. W. White, & B. A. White (eds.), *The oxford handbook of clinical child and adolescent psychology*. Oxford: Oxford University Press. https://doi.org/10.1093/oxfordhb/9780190634841.013.34

Motz, A. (2010). Self-harm as a sign of hope. *Psychoanalytic Psychotherapy*, 24, 81–92. https://doi.org/10.1080/02668731003707527

Pao, P.-N. (1969). The syndrome of delicate self-cutting. *British Journal of Medical Psychology*, 42, 195–206. https://doi.org/10.1111/j.2044-8341.1969.tb02071.x

Smahel, D., MacHackova, H., Mascheroni, G., Dedkova, L., Staksrud, E., Olafsson, K., Livingstone, S., & Hasebrink, U. (2020). EU Kids Online 2020: Survey results from 19 countries. *EU Kids Online*. https://doi. org/10.21953/lse.47fdeqj01ofo

Stänicke, L. I. (2021). The punished self, the unknown self, and the harmed self—toward a more nuanced understanding of self-harm among adolescents. *Frontiers of Psychology*, 12, 543303. https://doi.org/10.3389/fpsyg.2021.543303

Stänicke, L. I. (2022). 'I chose the bad': Youth's meaning making of being involved in self-harm content online during adolescence. *Child & Family Social Work*, 1–11. https://doi.org/10.1111/cfs.12950

Stänicke, L. I., Haavind, H., & Gullestad, S. E. (2018). How do young people understand their own self-harm? A meta-synthesis of adolescents' subjective experience of self-harm. *Adolescent Research Review*. https://doi.org/10.1007/s40894-018-0080-9

Stänicke, L. I., Haavind, H., Rø, F. G., & Gullestad, S. E. (2019). Discovering one's own way: Adolescent girls' different pathways into and out of self-harm. *Journal of Adolescent Research*, 1–30. https://doi.org/10.1177/0743558419883360

Stänicke, L. I., Hermansen, M. H., & Halvorsen, M. S. (2023). A transitional object for relatedness and self-development—A meta-synthesis of youths' experience of engagement in self-harm content online. *Child & Family Social Work*. https://doi.org/10.1111/cfs.13058.

Susi, K., Glover-Ford, F., Stewart, A., Knowles Bevis, R., & Hawton, K. (2023). Research review: Viewing self-harm images on the internet and social media platforms: Systematic review of the impact and associated psychological mechanisms. *Journal of Child Psychology and Psychiatry, and Allied Disciplines*, 64(8), 1115–1139. https://doi.org/10. 1111/jcpp.13754

Thapar, A., Pine, D. S., Leckman, J. F., Scott, S., Snowling, M. J., & Taylor, E. (2015). *Child and adolescent psychology*. Sixth edition. West Sussex: John Wiley and Sons, Ltd.

Winnicott, D. W. (1953/1971). Transitional Phenomenon and Transitional Object—A Study of the First Not-Me Possessions. In D. W. Winnicott (ed.) *Playing and reality*. London: Routledge.

Witt, K. G., Hetrick, S. E., Rajaram, G., Hazell, P., Taylor Salisbury, T. L., Townsend, E., & Hawton, K. (2021). Interventions for self-harm in children and adolescents. *Cochrane Database of Systematic Reviews*, 2021(3), CD013667. https://doi.org/10.1001/14651858

13 Narcissism in "emerging adulthood"

Chances and risks

Inge Seiffge-Krenke

Introduction

We are increasingly encountering emerging adults as patients in clinical settings, many of whom exhibit narcissistic disorders. It is particularly important to clinically differentiate narcissistic disorders from normal developmental phenomena during this age phase. We must face the reality that we are no longer dealing with concepts that were valid in previous decades, but with something new that also requires a new therapeutic approach. We can no longer refer to "arrested adulthood" (Côté, 2000) or "prolonged adolescence" (Blos, 1954); instead we should recognize a phase of emerging adulthood, which is characterized by distinctive features, among which extreme self-focus is particularly prominent. In addition, three developmental tasks (restructuring identity, achieving autonomy from parents, finding a partner, and choosing a career) are crucial to navigate (Miller, 2017; Seiffge-Krenke, 2019). These tasks require considerable narcissistic self-regulation as well as internal shifts and reorganizations of both past and present experiences. Early on, Anna Freud (1958) pointed to the threat of regression to early ties and the uncertainty of commitment to new ones. This phenomenon is actually one of the main symptoms seen in emerging adult patients today, often accompanied by narcissistic withdrawal and casual, uncommitted relationships. This contribution briefly summarizes research on normal young adults and their increasing narcissism, followed by an analysis of the social and familial dynamic changes that may have contributed to increased narcissism. It concludes with a brief outlook on treatment techniques for patients of this age group.

The developmental dynamics in emerging adulthood and their clinical significance

Based on the theory of Jeff Arnett (2000), who coined the term "emerging adulthood" for the intermediate stage between adolescence and adulthood (ages 18–30), numerous empirical studies have analyzed the specific characteristics of this new developmental phase. The classic criteria for adulthood

DOI: 10.4324/9781003565284-17

(career entry, stable partner relationship, starting a family, financial independence, and independent living) no longer apply to this age group but shifted into the third decade of life. Furthermore, the development of identity had lengthened and changed qualitatively (Kroger et al., 2010; Seiffge-Krenke, 2022a). Many young people live semi-autonomously and remain dependent on their parents for financial support (Seiffge-Krenke, 2013). Additionally, the number of "nestlings" (young adults living with their parents) and returnees has significantly increased in many countries, partly due to the pandemic (Seiffge-Krenke, 2016).

Extreme self-focus

In addition, five features characterize this developmental phase, among which extreme self-focus stands out. These characteristics have been identified in numerous studies of normal, non-clinically conspicuous young people across a large number of industrialized countries (Arnett, 2015; Seiffge-Krenke & Lübke, 2025).

From Arnett's perspective (2000), the central characteristic of emerging adulthood, the phase between 18 to 30 years, is the *exploration of one's identity*, particularly in the areas of partnership and profession. Identity formation begins in adolescence, but it is intensified by the opportunities and developments in the following years. Since emerging adults are still free from the typical obligations of being an adult, such as work and childcare, this form of independence offers a unique opportunity to explore, discover, and test their own possibilities and goals, ultimately shaping their sense of self. Another defining feature is the "age of feeling in-between". Although individuals from the age of 18 are legally considered adults, they only partially fulfill this role. They can make autonomous decisions largely independent of social norms and financial restrictions. Differences in professional and partnership status, living situations, and values contribute to significant *diversity* with work status and ethnic origin influencing these processes. Instability is another characteristic, evident in professional transitions and relocations. This instability is not surprising, given that studying, separation from parents, forming partnerships, and starting a career are central tasks in the transition to adulthood (Seiffge-Krenke & Gelhaar, 2008), often necessitating changes in residence. The majority of young professionals give up their employment within a year, averaging seven job changes in the first ten years of employment. There are also many changes in the living situation; the number of "nestlings" have increased internationally (Seiffge-Krenke, 2016), and many young adults find themselves returning to their children's rooms due to the impacts of COVID-19. Instability is also evident in romantic relationships, with 43% of young people experiencing at least one breakup within the last year, and 24% at least two (Shulman et al., 2017).

Possibly due to the many changes in the areas of partnership, occupation and residence, there is clear evidence of a *strong self-focus among emerging adults*. Greater autonomy, combined with less responsibility for financial support, provides young people with the space to concentrate on their own development. This intensive examination of the self leads to an increase in narcissism; however, there is often no meaningful reference to others. The identity-forming search for social resonance in new media, characterized by social comparison of a large number of "friends" (Manago et al., 2012), further amplifies self-focusing and narcissistic tendencies. In our study involving 3,000 young people (Seiffge-Krenke, 2017), we found the five characteristic features identified by Arnett to be clearly present. However, professional status (employed, studying, job-seeking, or in training) influenced these characteristics. The finding of extreme self-focus and narcissism among students of the same age is of clinical significance, as students comprise a considerable part of our clientele in psychotherapeutic practices. In contrast, emerging adults of the same age who were already employed were significantly less self-focused, explored significantly less, felt more grown-up and were much more related to others. Difficulties in realizing one's own identity, as well as work and relationships-related challenges, were associated with internalizing symptoms in this large sample of emerging adults (Seiffge-Krenke & Lübke, 2025).

Identity development and narcissism

Self and identity are concepts with a long and controversial history in psychoanalysis. I have used Erikson's definition here, which sees identity in the tension between the needs and wishes of the individual and the constantly changing demands of the social environment throughout development. He defines identity as a "subjective feeling of sameness and continuity across times and contexts" Erikson (1959, p.21). Identity development is a lifelong task that becomes even more pressing at the end of life. However, at the time Erikson wrote, he located the decisive impulses for identity development primarily in adolescence, between the poles of identity synthesis and identity confusion, postulating that failure to navigate this stage would impair subsequent developmental tasks, such as intimacy and generativity.

Based on Erikson's (1959) work, many empirical studies have been carried out in North America and Europe over the last two decades, yielding very coherent findings. They all used an operationalization of Erikson's theory with the components of exploration and commitment in the domains of values, love, and work, as well as a form of maladaptive exploration, called ruminative exploration. The meta-analysis by Kroger et al. (2010), which included 650 studies utilizing identity status diagnostics, found that only 17% of the 18-year-olds had achieved identity (commitment following sufficient exploration). A considerably larger percentage were in a moratorium or a diffuse state of identity. The foreclosure stage was relatively uncommon, as it requires an early commitment in a specific domain. Increases in achieved identity were noted with age: by age 22, about 34% of emerging adults had an achieved identity status, and by age 30, this figure rose to

47%, indicating they showed some form of commitment to values, partnerships, or professions after a phase of exploration. On the basis of 120 longitudinal studies, Kroger et al. (2010) further demonstrate that the identity formation process is far from complete. In the following years, most emerging adults developed "achieved" forms of identity. At the same time, compared to previous decades, the percentage of young people who currently possess a foreclosure identity, i.e. an identity adopted without exploration, has decreased.

Several authors have emphasized that contemporary Western societies have become increasingly individualistic. Societal changes, such as a broader range of career options and greater uncertainty in career planning, may have contributed to more exploration and less commitment in the domains of love and work. Too many different identity options in Western industrialized countries is often cited as a reason why young people struggle to form a coherent identity, resulting in quite high rates of ruminative exploration. Notably, only ruminative exploration in identity has been associated with psychopathology (Klimstra & Denissen, 2017). In addition, permanent comparison in social media and the trend toward optimization may contribute to and reinforce narcissistic tendencies. Experiences like internships in Manila, PJs (professional jobs) in Colombo and BA courses in Hong Kong satisfy needs for grandiosity and excessive admiration, which are often showcased on social media accordingly.

Family influences: narcissistic "abuse" by parents, parental
separation anxiety and excessive support

The prolonged dependence of emerging adults creates new emotional, social, and financial obligations for parents that were not present in previous generations. At the same time, parents themselves are affected by identity insecurities and upheavals (such as separation or unemployment) in ways that did not apply to earlier generations of parents. There is also evidence that certain parental upbringing styles and attachment patterns can impair children's self- and identity development. Our own longitudinal studies show that insecure attachment patterns and excessive parental support lead to children becoming "nesters" or late movers (von Irmer & Seiffge-Krenke, 2008). Studies have shown that parents often provide support for their "children" for too long, accompanying them into adulthood with anxious monitoring (Kins et al., 2013). In recent years, manipulative strategies and psychological control as parenting practices have increased significantly, with detrimental effects on identity development (Barber et al., 2005). These parents put pressure on the "child" by inducing feelings of guilt or by using manipulative tactics to get the "child" to develop a certain identity concept or development that aligns with their own preferences. However, this interferes with the development of an independent identity and autonomous functioning. When "children" in emerging adulthood increasingly explore what is appropriate for them, parents may respond by increasing psychological control (Luyckx et al., 2007). These changes go hand in hand with the fact that children have become crucial for the parents' narcissistic self-esteem, and this self-object is not easily relinquished. Both parents, mothers and fathers, increasingly attempt to restore closeness to their "child" through psychological control. Parental separation anxiety (Kins, Soenens & Beyers, 2011) has been shown to contribute to the rise in parental psychological control, preventing the "child" from exploring an independent identity and gaining autonomy. From a psychoanalytic perspective, intrusive parental behavior and parental separation anxiety have traditionally been described in relation to clinical patients (Mahler, 1985). Meanwhile, these unfavorable parental behaviors are now also observed in clinically normal families (Seiffge-Krenke & Escher, 2018), where they delay identity development and compromise the mental health of the offspring (Klimstra & Denissen, 2017). Since all findings mentioned above relate to clinically inconspicuous emerging adults and their families, the boundaries between normality and pathology seem difficult to discern—an important question for psychoanalysts.

Strong self-focus and the escape from intimacy

Many emerging adult patients come to therapy with questions like "Who am I?", "I don't want to be who I am", "Why am I not able to have a relationship?" Emerging adults' quality of romantic relationships is reminiscent of narcissistic relationship building in patients. In the initial conversations, it is not uncommon for us to identify a transgenerational link, in which the "child" plays an significant role for the parents, as the following case sample illustrates. The patient is diagnosed with depression, requiring us to also consider aspects of both narcissism and depression (see Marianne Leuzinger-Bohleber's contribution in this book).

> Sidonie is a capable 22-year-old medical student whose studies are devalued by her parents. She is expected to fail her exams, just like her father, who never graduated. In the meantime, the patient has had massive problems to keep up with her studies. She has work problems, procrastinates her upcoming exam preparations, and has come to the initial interview worried that she may not be able to complete her studies fearing that she will have to give up like her father. All of her attempts at autonomy are undermined, with her parents insisting she spend weekends with them in their sleepy village 20 km away. When Sidonie mentions buying a new bed, it sparks a heated discussion in the family. The parents insisted she continue sleeping in her narrow young girl's bed, instead of supporting her choice, buy her a television for her student apartment. The patient is visibly annoyed and expects support from the therapist in order to free herself from the

intrusively close and controlling relationship with her parents, especially the father. He still seems to be very attached to his daughter,
although he constantly criticizes her career plans. He seems to struggle with separation and even sleeps in her bed in her room whenever
the daughter is at her place of study. Holidays are also planned with
the "child"; where Sidonie was surprised to learn she was expected to
sleep in her parents' bedroom at the holiday destination. When Sidonie refused, the parents went on the trip alone but argued throughout the entire holiday. When asked about her love relationships, the
patient becomes very hesitant; she obviously keeps men at a distance
and admits that she doesn't want a relationship. She does it so that
when she feels like it, she calls one of her acquaintances or friends.
They will then come over and they will have sex. Beyond that, she
feels she cannot handle more at the moment.

From a psychodynamic point of view, it is obvious that the patient remains
strongly attached to her parents, though with growing ambivalence, and
the generational boundaries are not clear. The father's intrusive behavior,
such as sleeping in her bed during her absence, stimulates oedipal fantasies
in the daughter, who increasingly tries to "free herself from her parents",
at least on an external level. However, the latent pull and the possibly still
unresolved oedipal theme act as a barrier in her search for a non-incestuous
love object.

Moreover, Sidonie's narcissistic self-regulation seems to have been
impaired from an early age. Probably, the father was an idealized object
early on. He failed professionally and constantly devalued his daughter,
who repeated his career path and wanted to bring it to a successful end.
This puts the daughter's narcissistic self-regulation during the phase of
emerging adulthood with its many challenges to a severe test. While she
strives to successfully complete her medical studies, she simultaneously
fears public failure and feels worthless and incapable. Possibly, the devalued fantasies of the "bad parent" have been introjected into her ego and the
internal maternal object is too weak to support and stabilize her. According to Sidney Blatt (2004), the patient appears to suffer from a depression
of the *introjective type,* characterized by a strict, punitive superego and ego
ideal, self-criticism, low self-esteem, and basic feelings of failure, shame,
and guilt. Blatt (2004) also suggests that oedipal conflicts and fantasies are
particularly influential in the genesis of the introjective type of depression
and lead to impairments in partner relationships (Blatt & Blass, 1996). Sidonie concentrates entirely on her career and avoids the dangerous terrain of
romantic relations. *Disobjectification* through detachment, as described by
Leuzinger-Bohleber in a chapter of this volume, is evident in her case.

In this case, the function of the child as a self-object of the parents is also
obvious; the patient has the function to neutralize or stabilize the parents'

broken marriage. It is understandable that she is extremely cautious about entering into relationships given her intrusive and controlling experiences in her parents' home. In addition to these obstacles, we have to reflect on the delay in identity development and its consequences for forming romantic relationships. According to Erikson (1968), the ability to have intimate relationships follows the development of a more secure sense of identity, as one is then better equipped for relationships. Consequently, delayed identity development can hinder the establishment of close partner relationships.

As we were able to show in a longitudinal study (Beyers & Seiffge-Krenke, 2010), a mature identity (achieved identity) is still the prerequisite for successful, intimate partnerships. However, this was true for only a small proportion of the emerging adults examined. Most of them had unstable, non-committed relationships with frequently changing partners. Fulfilling sexual needs took precedence and couple bonds were not yet intended. "Non-relationships" were the prevailing relationship type in emerging adults. The meta-analysis by James-Kangal and Whitton (2019) further showed that 70% of emerging adults are hesitant to form close bonds with partners. Casual, non-committed short-term relationships, such as hookups, are common (Claxton & van Dulmen, 2013). The fact that many emerging adults are often "on the run from intimacy" (Seiffge-Krenke, 2021) is also relevant for psychoanalytic treatment.

New chances: opportunities or risks?

One might ask whether the emergence of "emerging adulthood", a phase between adolescence and adulthood now observed as a phenomenon in many Western industrialized countries, is truly something new or if it has always existed—albeit mainly for the privileged upper class.

From a privilege for the few to an opportunity for the many Historically, there have always been individuals who have had an extreme self-focus, who have fulfilled their narcissistic needs and "used" and even exploited their families. Two examples are Aby Warburg and Marcel Proust.

Aby Warburg, the eldest of five brothers of a wealthy Jewish banking family in Hamburg, gave up his birthright on the condition that his brothers would support him and his studies for the rest of his life. Aby Warburg is considered the founder of cultural history and iconography and was one of the first to understand how to integrate interdisciplinary approaches at a high scientific level. His brothers supported him generously. Even as a student, he spent enormous sums of money on buying books. The vast library, containing 18,000 volumes, was transferred to London in 1933. The brothers also paid for the living expenses of his family of five as well as for his stays in places like Florence and New Mexico.

Another example of someone who lived as he wished and took the freedom to pursue his interests while relying on family support was Marcel Proust.

> Born in 1871, Proust lived at nearly the same time as Aby Warburg. His father, a famous professor of medicine, and his brother, who was two years younger, also became a doctor. Marcel, however, developed asthma early in life and maintained a very close relationship with his mother. The beginning of this famous work, *In Search of Lost Time,* which comprises seven volumes, is directly related to the death of his beloved mother. Proust did not undertake any professional training, but devoted himself entirely to observation and writing. This was made possible by the enormous wealth his mother brought into the family. For the last 15 years of his life, Proust lived completely withdrawn from the outside world in a large apartment on Boulevard Haussmann in Paris, and devoted himself exclusively to writing. He was supported by numerous helpers, including his chauffeur and his housekeeper, who had to travel through bomb-damaged Paris to get food that Proust remembered from his childhood.

The freedom to narcissistically realize one's own identity was therefore tied to a very specific upper-middle-class financial background and to the tolerance of the family to support these ideas and life plans—and no coincidence: these are men's fates. It is, of course, no coincidence that these biographies of the two men, who were almost the same age, are also very similar in the external conditions for their respective identity designs, namely a wealthy parental home and the privilege of pursuing one's own interests. In Proust's case, the secondary benefit of illness was also very strong and he understood that the illness enabled him to live, and that without it, it would not have been possible to devote himself entirely to his work, writing and observing.

Erikson, born in 1902, whose theory of life cycles was so influential, also came to psychoanalysis and his theory of identity only after a long period of wandering and personal searching (Roazen, 1976). Erikson came into contact with psychoanalysis through his work as a private tutor and began therapy with Anna Freud. In 1933, he emigrated to the USA via Denmark. Through his field research on Native Americans, he realized how much danger there is of absolutizing one's own culture. Of outstanding importance for his theory— and in doing so he went beyond the one-person psychology that was still very popular at the time—was his view of the social determination of identity development. "Identity is the intersection between what a person wants to be and what the environment allows him to be" (Erikson, 1959, p.56).

How the "age of narcissism" contributes to increased self-focus
and delayed identity development

This societal perspective is important in our consideration of the extreme self-focus already seen in young, non-clinically emerging adults. According to Christopher Lasch, we live in a so-called narcissistic age. Today's times place great demands on the stable development of narcissistic self-regulation. Many people are extremely concerned with themselves and use selfies and social media to confirm their existence, so some suspect that our society is producing more narcissistic personality disorders than ever before (see contribution of Stephan Doering in this volume). Does our consumer and performance-oriented society encourage such self-centeredness? And does this ultimately have an impact on the reconstruction of young people's identities and their increasing self-focus? The prolonged identity exploration, the lack of commitment, the strong self-focus, and the amount of narcissism found in 18 to 30 year olds in many Western industrial nations represent a cultural and contemporary rather than a national phenomenon. In fact, since the 1980s, there has been evidence of an increase in narcissism in the younger generation, and it has been referred to as a "narcissistic age" (Bohleber & Leuzinger, 1981).

In and of themselves, many changes in the last decades are to be viewed as predominantly positive. These include emancipatory developments (e.g. breaking away from the classic division of roles between men and women), sexual revolutions (e.g. more tolerant sexual morals and acceptance of premarital sexual experiences) and the spread of individualistic value systems (e.g. importance of self-realization, see also the contribution of Siri Erika Gullestad in this volume). Added to this are factors such as longer school and training periods, but also the need to protect oneself from unemployment in economically uncertain times by obtaining multiple qualifications, a perspective that emerging adults are frequently thinking about. This makes the development of self-coherence difficult for them, and the imponderables of their future life situation, which they can only partially influence, also impair self-agency. An analysis by Malkin (2013) shows that in all Western industrialized nations, there is a need for excessive admiration, a lack of empathy, feelings of grandeur in relation to one's own importance, fantasies of unlimited success, power, beauty or ideal love, and the belief that one is "special" and "unique". Young people in Western industrial societies are currently growing up in this societal trend toward excessive preoccupation with one's own self. They are therefore surrounded by models of the self in which egocentrism and orientation toward one's own narcissistic interests have become the social norm. Seeing and experiencing oneself in the mirror of others creates coherence, and this is where the new media have an important function that one also has to be seen critically of (Altmeyer, 2019).

Second window of vulnerability: higher symptom burden or better health?

Empirically, there is not only evidence of "fun and exploration", but also that emerging adulthood—after adolescence being the first one—is a second window of vulnerability. Young adults aged 18 to 29 have the highest 12-month prevalence of mental illness across all age groups (Lambert et al.,

2013). The increases are particularly strong among female students. Studies conducted during the COVID-19 epidemic showed a sharp increase in anxiety and depression, but also loneliness (Tsiouris et al., 2023). Additionally, there are findings showing a decline in symptomatology and increased well-being, which is associated with more freedom and increased options in this developmental phase. In longitudinal studies, Schulenberg and Zarrett (2006) found a continuous increase in well-being from the ages of 18 to 26. Galambos et al. (2006) also demonstrated this increase longitudinally, with a simultaneous reduction in depressive affects. Anxiety symptoms decreased and the prevalence of phobias decreased. On the other hand, it was shown that some emerging adults have fears about the new challenges and are unsettled by the instability (Arnett, 2015). In the longitudinal study by Salmela-Aro, Aunola and Nurmi (2008), in which university students were followed over a period of ten years, 16% of young adults showed a high and increasing level of depression.

Emerging adults in many countries, including Germany, are under strong identity-related stress, which is related to the discrepancy between a low level of development and high goals against the background of unpredictable professional opportunities (Skaletz & Seiffge-Krenke, 2010). The failure of developmental tasks (such as restructuring of identity, autonomy from parents, finding a partner, and choosing a career) has significant health consequences such as physical complaints (Seiffge-Krenke & Sattel, 2024), anxiety and depression (Klimstra & Denissen, 2017; Seiffge-Krenke & Lübke, 2025). The association between problems in identity development and various indicators of psychopathology is even more evident in patients than in clinically normal emerging adults (Seiffge-Krenke & Escher, 2018).

The association with typical developmental demands in this age phase and psychopathology was also recently demonstrated in our large sample of over 3,000 young adults (Seiffge-Krenke & Lübke, 2025). In this three-year longitudinal study, health, identity, profession, and romantic relationships were examined with regard to the manifestation and prediction of internalizing symptoms. One striking feature is the relatively high level of life satisfaction among students, while at the same time, compared to other work status groups, they have high levels of internalizing symptoms. This actually seems to confirm the contradictory picture described in international research.

Final remarks on psychoanalytic technique of emerging adult' patients

As far as the origin of narcissism as a clinical picture is concerned, the controversy between two models is well known in psychoanalysis: On the one hand, the self-psychological approach followed by Kohut (1977), which held that a coherent self is formed through a sensitive mirroring of the child's statements by the caregiver (see also introduction to this volume). The grandiose self is therefore a healthy structure that should be tempered by gradual frustration. On the other hand, there is Kernberg's object-relationship theory approach (see Otto Kernberg's chapter in this book). He held that pathological narcissism develops as a reaction to cold and indifferent caregivers. The frustration of basic oral needs leads to hatred, anger and envy, which are compensated for by the creation of grandiose self-parts. It is suggested that they describe different types. Kohut's descriptions are more typical for the vulnerable narcissism, while Kernberg's concepts are more likely to be assigned to the type of grandiose narcissism.

Kohut (1977) endeavored to integrate normal and pathological phenomena of narcissism. He took the view that narcissistic feelings occupy objects that are experienced as an extension of the self; he called these self-objects. Kohut conceived his own line of development of narcissism (or of the self and its self-objects) independently of the drive- and object relationship-development and described that self-love persists alongside object love. In the course of the consolidation of the self, the need for merging fades into the background, but needs for mirroring, idealization, and equality remain for a long time.

This chapter adds a new perspective of developmental findings, based on large investigations on non-clinical samples in many countries. The narcissistic phenomena are largely temporary, as they often resolve with the transition to adulthood and the assumption of adult roles and tasks. However, there are some new aspects: It has actually been shown that some phenomena that we previously attributed to clinically conspicuous patients can now also be found in the normal population. In the developmental phase of emerging adults examined here, these include extreme self-focus, more narcissistic partnership forms, intrusive parental relationships, unresolved oedipal bonds with strong separation anxiety—to name just a few phenomena. Narcissistic patients are certainly characterized by other, special characteristics – as mentioned there are two models in psychoanalysis with very different explanations of clinical narcissism. Nevertheless, in conclusion, we will briefly discuss some of the special features of treatment that could apply to patients in this age group—regardless of the diagnosis—and that can be partly derived from the already clearly modified developmental dynamics (see, for more details, Seiffge-Krenke, 2022b).

In integrating psychodynamic and developmental perspectives, this contribution reflects on emerging adults, who are "in between" adolescents and adult patients when it comes to technique. There are many clinical contributions in this book (see also Abend, 1987; Escoll, 1987; Fingert Chused, 1987), so I can be brief here. The high mobility of the patients makes adjustments in the frame and in the indication necessary, and analysts need to reflect on the flexibility and stability of the frame. Identity problems occur frequently, but a distinction must be made between intrapsychic identity conflicts that may inhibit development, and structural deficits such as identity diffusion. Structural deficits often include low empathy for others and insufficient self-object differentiation, which need to be addressed. Since autonomy from parents is another central topic, the guilt of autonomy and conflicts of loyalty must also be dealt with, potentially including accompanying work with parents in case of parental separation anxiety. A great deal of empathy and caution is necessary when working with patients, as many of them have experienced intrusive parent objects and are hesitant to engage in such an intimate process with an analyst. Due to parental over-overprotection, it is likely that patients will also develop rescue fantasies toward us and expect us to solve their problems. We have to reflect whether too much support from the therapist may continue a parental pattern. Among the issues that need to be addressed, then, is that not everything is possible and makes sense, and so renunciation and mourning are also called for The analytical task is to develop a trusting patient-therapist relationship together in which it becomes possible to understand which obstacles prevent commitment in a certain area, which function the "escape from intimacy" had in the context of earlier parent-child relationships, for example. Jointly analyzing the obstacles that prevent patients from making decisions or committing to work and love or limiting distressing, unproductive rumination can be very helpful in the process of becoming an adult.

References

Abend, S. (1987). Evaluating young adults for analysis. *Psychoanalytic Inquiry 7*, 31–38.

Altmeyer, M. (2019). *Ich werde gesehen, also bin ich. Psychoanalyse und die neuen Medien*. Göttingen: Vandenhoeck & Ruprecht.

Arnett, J. J. (2000). Emerging adulthood: A theory of development from the late teens through the twenties. *American Psychologist, 55*, 469–480.

Arnett, J. J. (2015). *Emerging adulthood: The winding road from the late teens through the twenties*. New York: Oxford University Press.

Barber, B. K., Stolz, H. E. E., Olsen, J. A. A., Collins, A., & Burchinal, M. (2005). Parental support, psychological control, and behavioral control: Assessing relevance across time, method, and culture. In *Monographs of the Society for Research in Child Development, 70*, (pp. 1–13).

Beyers, W., & Seiffge-Krenke, I. (2010). Does identity precede intimacy? Testing Erikson's theory on romantic development in emerging adults of the 21st century. *Journal of Adolescent Research, 25*, 387–415.

Blatt, S. J. (2004). *Experiences with depression: Theoretical, clinical, and research perspectives*. New York: Am Psychol Assoc.

Blatt, S. J., & Blass, R. (1996). Relatedness and self-definition: A dialectic model of personality development. In edited by Gil G. Noam & Kurt W (eds.), *Development and vulnerability in close relationships*, (p. 309–338). Fischer. Mahwah, NJ: Lawrence Erlbaum.

Blos, P. (1954). Prolonged adolescence: The formulation of a syndrome and its therapeutic implications. *American Journal of Orthopsychiatry, 24*, 733–742.

Bohleber, W., & Leuzinger, M. (1981). Narzissmus und Adoleszenz. In Psychoanalytisches Seminar Zürich (Hg.), *Die neuen Narzissmustheorien. Zurück ins Paradies?* (pp. 117–131). Frankfurt a.M.: Syndikat,.

Claxton, S. E., & van Dulmen, M. H. (2013). Casual sexual relationships and experiences in emerging adulthood. *Emerging Adulthood, 1*, 138–150.

Côté, J. E. (2000). *Arrested adulthood*. New York: NYU Press.

Erikson, E. H. (1959). *Identity and the life cycle*. New York: W. W. Norton. [Deutsch (1971): *Identität und Lebenszyklus*. Frankfurt: Suhrkamp.

Erikson, E. H. (1968). *Identity, youth and crisis*. New York: W. W. Norton.

Escoll, P. (1987). Psychoanalysis of young adults: An overview. *Psychoanalytic Inquiry, 7*, 5–30.

Fingert Chused, J. (1987). Idealization of the analyst by the young adult. *Journal of the American Psychoanalytic Association, 35*, 839–859.

Freud, A. (1958). Adolescence. In *The writings of Anna Freud*. Vol. 5, (pp. 136–166). New York: International Universities Press.

Galambos, N. L., Barker, E. T., & Krahn, H. J. (2006). Depression, anger, and self-esteem in emerging adulthood: Seven-year trajectories. *Developmental Psychology, 42*, 350–365.

James-Kangal, N., & Whitton, S. W. (2019). Conflict management in emerging adults' "nonrelationships." *Couple and Family Psychology: Research and Practice, 8*, 63–76.

Kins, E., Soenens, B., & Beyers, W. (2011). "Why do they have to grow up so fast?" Parental separation anxiety and emerging adults' pathology of separation-individuation. *Journal of Clinical Psychology, 67*, 647–664.

Kins, E., Soenens, B., & Beyers, W. (2013). Separation anxiety in families with emerging adults. *Journal of Family Psychology, 27*(3), 495–505.

Klimstra, T., & Denissen, J. J. A. (2017). A theoretical framework for the association between identity and psychopathology. *Developmental Psychology, 53*, 2052–2065.

Kohut, H. (1977). *Narzißmus. Eine Theorie der psychoanalytischen Behandlung narzisstischer Persönlichkeitsstörungen. [Narcissims: A theory of psychoanalytic treatment of narcissistic personality disorders]*. Frankfurt/M.: Suhrkamp.

Kroger, J., Martinussen, M., & Marcia, J. E. (2010). Identity status change during adolescence and young adulthood: A meta-analysis. *Journal of Adolescence, 33*, 683–698.

Lambert, M., Bock, T., Naber, D., Löwe, B., Schulte-Markwart, M., Schäfer, I., Gumz, A., Degkwitz, P., Schulte, B., König, H. H., Konnopka, A., Bauer, M., Bechdolf, A., Correll, C., Juckel, G., Klosterkötter, J., Leopold, K., Pfennig, A., & Karow, A. (2013). Die psychische Gesundheit von Kindern, Jugendlichen und jungen Erwachsenen – Teil 1: Häufigkeit, Störungspersistenz, Belastungsfaktoren, Service-Inanspruchnahme und Behandlungsverzögerung mit Konsequenzen. *Fortschritte der Neurologie & Psychiatrie, 81*, 614–627.

Luyckx, K., Soenens, B., Vansteenkiste, M., Goossens, L., & Berzonsky, M. D. (2007). Parental psychological control and dimensions of identity formation in emerging adulthood. *Journal of Family Psychology, 21*, 546–550.

Mahler, M. S. (1985). *Studien über die ersten drei Lebensjahre*. Stuttgart: Klett-Cotta.

Malkin, M. L. (2013). The view from the looking glass. How are narcissistic individuals perceived by others. *Journal of Personality, 81*, 1–15.

Manago, A. M., Taylor, T., & Greenfield, P. M. (2012). Me and my 400 friends: The anatomy of college students' facebook networks, their communication patterns, and well-being. *Developmental Psychology*. Advance online publication. doi: 10.1037/a0026338

Miller, J. M. (2017). Young or emerging adulthood: A psychoanalytic view. *Psychoanalytic Study of the Child, 70*, 8–21.

Roazen, P. (1976). Erik H. Erikson. *The power and limits of a vision.* New York: The Free Press.

Salmela-Aro, K., Aunola, K., & Nurmi, J. E. (2008). Trajectories of depressive symptoms during emerging adulthood: Antecedents and consequences. *European Journal of Developmental Psychology, 5,* 439–465.

Schulenberg, J. E., & Zarrett, N. R. (2006). Mental health during emerging adulthood: Continuity and discontinuity in courses, causes, and functions. In J. J. Arnett & J. L. Tanner (eds.), *Emerging adults in America: Coming of age in the 21st century* (pp. 135–172). Washington, DC: APA Books.

Seiffge-Krenke, I. (2013). "She's leaving home…" Antecedents, consequences, and cultural patterns in the leaving home process. *Emerging Adulthood, 1,* 4–24.

Seiffge-Krenke, I. (2016). Leaving home: Antecedents, consequences and cultural patterns in Arnett, J. J. (ed.), *The Oxford handbook of emerging adulthood.* (pp. 177–190). New York: Oxford University Press.

Seiffge-Krenke, I. (2017). Studierende als Prototyp der "emerging adults". Verzögerte Identitätsentwicklung, Entwicklungsdruck und hohe Symptombelastung. [Students as prototype of emerging adults: Delayed identity, developmental pressure and high psychopathology.] *Psychotherapeut, 62,* 403–410.

Seiffge-Krenke, I. (2019). Die neue Entwicklungsphase des "emerging adulthood". Typische Störungen und Entwicklungsrisiken und Ansätze der psychotherapeutischen Versorgung [The new development phase of "Emerging Adulthood" typical disorders and development risks and approaches to psychotherapeutic care]. *Psychodynamische Psychotherapie, 3,* 176–192.

Seiffge-Krenke, I. (2021). Sex ja Liebe nein? Entwicklungspsychologische und therapeutische Perspektiven von Partnerbeziehungen im jungen Erwachsenenalter. [Sex yes love no? Developmental psychological and therapeutic perspectives of partner relationships in young adulthood]. *Psychodynamische Psychotherapie, 4,* 347–360.

Seiffge-Krenke, I. (2022a). *Therapieziel Identität. Veränderte Beziehungen, Krankheitsbilder und Therapie. [Therapy goal identity: Changing relationships, clinical pictures and therapy.]* (2. Aktualisierte Auflage) Stuttgart: Klett-Cotta.

Seiffge-Krenke, I. (2022b). Psychodynamische Psychotherapie mit jungen Erwachsenen. [Psychodynamic psychotherapy with emerging adults] Stuttgart: Kohlhammer.

Seiffge-Krenke, I., & Escher, F. J. (2018). Was ist noch "normal"? Mütterliches Erziehungsverhalten als Puffer und Risikofaktor für das Auftreten von psychischen Störungen und Identitätsdiffusion. [What else is "normal"? Maternal parenting behavior as a buffer and risk factor for the occurrence of mental disorders and identity diffusion]. *Zeitschrift für Psychosomatik Medizin und Psychotherapie, 64,* 128–143.

Seiffge-Krenke, I., & Gelhaar, T. (2008). Does successful attainment of developmental tasks lead to happiness and success in later developmental tasks? A test of Havighurst's (1948) theses. *Journal of Adolescence, 31,* 33–52.

Seiffge-Krenke, I., & Lübke, L. (2025). "Emerging adults" in Deutschland: Differentielle Unterschiede in Bezug auf Identität, Beruf und Partnerschaft und deren Zusammenhänge mit internalisierenden Symptomen. *Zeitschrift für Psychosomatische Medizin und Psychotherapie* (in Press).

Seiffge-Krenke, I., & Sattel, H. (2024). How personality factors, coping with identity-stress, and parental rearing styles contribute to the expression of somatic complaints in emerging adults in seven countries. *Front Psychiatry, 15*(15), 1257403.

Shulman, S., Seiffge-Krenke, I., Scharf, M., Boingiu, S. B., & Tregubenko, V. (2017). The diversity of romantic pathways during emerging adulthood and their developmental antecedents. *International Journal of Behavioral Development, 26,* 1–8.

Skaletz, C., & Seiffge-Krenke, I. (2010). Models of developmental regulation in emerging adulthood and links to symptomatology. In S. Shulman & J.- E. Nurmi (eds.), The role of goals in navigating individual lives during emerging adulthood. *New Directions for Child and Adolescent Development, 130,* 71–82.

Tsiouris, A., Werner, A. M., Tibubos, A. N., Mülder, L. M., Reichel, J. L., Heller, S., et al. (2023). Mental health state and its determinants in German university students across the COVID-19 pandemic: findings from three repeated cross-sectional surveys between 2019 and 2021. *Front. Public Health, 11,* 23–51.

Von Irmer, J., & Seiffge-Krenke, I. (2008). Der Einfluss des Familienklimas und der Bindungsrepräsentation auf den Auszug aus dem Elternhaus. *Zeitschrift für Entwicklungspsychologie und Pädagogische Psychologie, 40,* 69–78.

14 Narcissism, trauma and depression

Clinical observations from the MODE study[1]

Marianne Leuzinger-Bohleber

Introduction

Artists of all times have been aware of the unconscious connection between narcissism, trauma, and depression, just think of the famous painting by Albrecht Dürer *Melencolia* (1514) or its modern variant *Melancholia* (1989) by Fernando Botero. He paints a man in a colorful frilled, female dress looking in a mirror seemingly being in love with himself. If you look closely at the painting, you will notice the man's frozen face, which reveals that he is a traumatized person. In many of Botero's other paintings, the victims of individual and collective traumatization are also impressively depicted (see e.g. Leuzinger-Bohleber & von Hoff, 2004).

Our research group came across the long-term consequences of collective trauma for the first time in an empirical psychoanalysis study, the Follow-Up study of the German Psychoanalytic Association (DPV). Completely unexpected at that time, we discovered that 62% of the 402 patients in our study of our sample were traumatized children of the Second World War. These patients all had been in psychoanalyses with analysts of the DPV in the 1980th. Many of them had suffered from severe depression throughout their lives (Leuzinger-Bohleber, 2003). We made analogous observations in the LAC Depression Study:[2] 84% of the 252 chronically depressed patients who were undergoing long-term psychoanalytic and behavioural therapy had experienced severe early childhood trauma[3] (cf. Negele et al., 2015; Krakau et al., 2024). As will be discussed below, we have similar first findings in the currently ongoing MODE study.[4] It is striking that 42% of the patients included in the study are between 20 and 30 years old, i.e. in the developmental phase of so-called *emerging adulthood* (see chapter by Seiffge-Krenke in this volume). As illustrated below using two brief case examples, adolescence, with its changes in the body and the self as well as the inner and outer separation from primary objects, combined with traumatic experiences of loss, plunged these patients into severe crises: The vulnerable self and narcissistic self-regulation collapsed. This adolescent breakdown paved the way for chronic depression with serious consequences for the further development of these young people.

DOI: 10.4324/9781003565284-18

Trauma and narcissistic depression

Breakdown of narcissistic self-regulation due to severe traumatization

According to current psychoanalytic studies, the experience of extreme helplessness and powerlessness is at the centre of both chronic depression and severe traumatization (Leuzinger-Bohleber, 2021, 2022, 2022a; Leuzinger-Bohleber & Ambresin, 2024). In a traumatic experience, the physiological protection shield against stimuli is disrupted by a sudden, unforeseen extreme experience. The self is exposed to unbearable powerlessness and an inability to control the situation. It is flooded with panic and extreme physiological reactions. This flooding of the self leads to a state of psychic and physiological shock (cf. also the definition of psychological trauma by Cooper, 1986). As Bohleber (2000) has shown recurring to Ferenczi and Balint, this economic explanation of trauma must be supplemented by object-relational perspectives.

> Traumatic reality destroys the empathic shield formed by the internalized primary object and destroys the trust in the continuous presence of good objects and the expectability of human empathy, namely that others recognize and respond to basic needs. In trauma, the inner good object is silenced as an empathic mediator between self and environment.
>
> (Bohleber, 2000, p.821)

All of this has serious consequences. It is now undisputed that traumatic experiences, even after the acute danger has been overcome, can lead to great narcissistic vulnerability in those traumatized and result in severe depression, even in individuals who lack the now proven genetic and neurobiological vulnerability for depression (overview in Salazar & Zambrano, 2021; Böker, 2011; Xu et al., 2016). This applies to those affected themselves, but tragically often also to their children or even their children's children (cf. e.g. Bohleber, 2010, 2012; Leuzinger-Bohleber, 2003, 2022a). The connection between narcissistic vulnerability, trauma and depression focussed on here can be observed particularly impressively in these families.

For example, many patients in the MODE study are children of severely traumatized mothers (Leuzinger-Bohleber, 2022, 2022a; Leuzinger-Bohleber & Ambresin, 2024). To shortly summarize our clinical observations: Due to their traumatization, the mothers of these patients had probably not been able to hold and contain their infants in their early, extreme affective and physiological states in a good enough way. Therefore, they extensively exposed their babies to early trauma, as Winnicott (1949) impressively described: In a mental state of total dependency, the infants were flooded with unbearable physical pain, affects and impulses: they fell into nothingness. This primary traumatization (Winnicott) had been preserved in the unconscious as expectations of catastrophes, fear of death and annihilation, combined with the unconscious belief that, as a self, they had no influence on coping with catastrophes in the external reality of life and were completely alone, without a helping object (cf. Abram, 2021, p.784ff.). These early object relational experiences also had a decisive influence on the development of the self and the narcissistic self-regulation.

On so-called narcissistic depression

In his initial paper on psychoanalytical depression research, *Mourning and Melancholia* (1917), Freud already focussed on the role of narcissism in the development of depression when he discussed that melancholia is caused by an incapability to mourn: The melancholic refuses to psychically accept the loss of the object and instead identifies with the lost, idealized object.

Since Freud, psychoanalytic theories of depression have added further psychodynamic considerations, as I have illustrated in two reviews based on Hugo Bleichmar's papers (Bleichmar, 1996, 2010). There are various psychodynamic pathways that lead to depression (Leuzinger-Bohleber, 2022, 2022a). Depending on which of the pathways dominates in a particular patient, we speak of *guilt depression, narcissistic depression, psychotic depression* or *depression that is* predominantly *caused by traumatization*. Narcissistic self-regulation plays a decisive role in all of these forms of depression. However, it is at the centre of so-called *narcissistic depression*.

Edith Jacobson (1971) describes a basic conflict that can be found in all depressive states, but which stands out in narcissistic depression: if the ego cannot achieve the satisfaction it desires and cannot use its aggression to actively realize its desires, then it turns its aggressive impulses against the self. A narcissistic conflict arises between the desired, idealized self-representation and the representation of the failing, devalued real self. New narcissistic wounds lead to a devaluation of the love object. In order to bear these injuries and make amends, glorified grandiose fantasies of the love objects (idealized objects) are introjected into the superego, while the devalued fantasies of a bad parent (devalued objects) are introjected into the ego. In this way, the child can hold on to the hope of love in the future, but from now on is exposed to the massive criticism and hostility of its own idealized unconscious fantasies and evaluations (cf. also Rado, 1928; Bibring, 1952. At the same time, the narcissistic self-regulation of the ego is permanently damaged.

Wolfgang Loch (1967) and Herbert Will and colleagues (2008) also speak *of narcissistic depression* in view of the underlying tensions *between ego and ego ideal*. Here, it is not feelings of guilt fueled by aggression and self-hatred that dominate, but *shame and humiliation as well as feelings of abandonment and helplessness*.[5] In 1965, Joffe and Sandler described the loss of narcissistic integrity as the central cause of the depressive reaction. The focus is not so much on the loss of a love object, but on the loss of one's own well-being, which is inextricably linked to it. It is the *feeling of* having been robbed of *an ideal psychological state.*

Kohut (1973) placed the normal and pathological development of narcissism at the centre of his work. He postulated a line of development in the area of narcissistic self-regulation that was independent of drive development. In relation to the grandiose self, he outlined a line from the archaic world of the grandiose self to a mature narcissistic self-regulation, i.e. a mature form of self-esteem and a supporting self-confidence. In the realm of the grandiose object, he spoke of an idealized, omnipotent object that transforms into a mature form of admiration of others (cf. Kohut, 1973, Table, p. 26).

As is well known, Otto Kernberg (2014) in particular has contradicted this view (see his chapter in this volume). For him, there is no narcissistic line of development that is independent of object relationships. Rather, the development of narcissism is inextricably linked to experiences of object relations and, in particular, to the role of destructive aggressive impulses, archaic envy and fantasies of omnipotence (see also Klein, 1957). Pathological object relationships lead to various forms of narcissistic or borderline personality disorders. It seems to me that Kernberg's conceptualizations have prevailed in the Anglo-Saxon psychoanalytic community: Most contemporary psychoanalysts hardly speak of an independent developmental line of narcissism, but rather of the destructive quality of inner object relations and their devastating effects on the self and its narcissistic cathexis.

Sidney Blatt (2004), one of the best-known psychoanalytic depression researchers, has also inextricably linked narcissistic pathology in depressives with the development of object-relations. On the basis of many empirical studies, he characterized two different organizations of depression: the *anaclitic type,* which focuses on interpersonal factors such as narcissistic depletion through dependence on an idealized object, helplessness, feelings of loss and abandonment. Early traumatic experiences of object relations (often in the first year of life) play a decisive role in its development. In contrast, the *introjective type* shows a strict, punitive superego and ego ideal, self-criticism, low self-esteem, basic feelings of failure and guilt as well as pronounced experiences of shame. Oedipal conflicts and fantasies are particularly influential in the genesis of the introjective type of depression. In both types of depression, the pathological object relationships also determine the damaged narcissistic development.

In contrast to this object-relations theory view of narcissism and depression, André Green (1998, 2001, 2007) has presented his very own theory of narcissism, in which he refers, among other things, to Freud's drive dualism between the life and death drives. According to this, Eros is always directed towards the object, towards attachment, towards *objectification,* whereas the death drive strives for the greatest possible fulfilment of a *disobjectification function* through detachment (Green, 2001, p.874). Green derives his concept of *negative narcissism* from these considerations, with which he succeeds in explaining the most severe depressive states. This concept proved to be helpful in several psychoanalyses in the MODE study. We were able to observe that some of the early traumatized patients not only withdrew into a chronic state of dissociation, but also disobjectified their objects, themselves and even all attachment desires and libidinal and aggressive impulses in threatening states of suicidality. Such an extreme withdrawal of cathexis corresponds to negative narcissism according to Green (for further details see Green, 2001). The following clinical observations may illustrate this:

Mrs C. (23 years old) was referred to the MODE study after a serious suicide attempt. During the assessment interviews, she told us that she had always suffered from depression and was convinced that she had no place in this world. Her father had left her mother even before she was born. The severely traumatized mother, daughter of two German war refugees from the Second World War, reacted extremely to the loss of her partner and suffered from massive depression throughout the first year of Mrs C.'s life. As a single mother, she was also overwhelmed in the following years: Violence and emotional neglect ensued. Mrs C. developed into a quiet, withdrawn child.

A disappointment in love during adolescence led to a mental breakdown with two serious suicide attempts and an extreme withdrawal. Until she graduated from high school, she had hardly any close friends and almost only had contact with her mother.

Her chronic depression and the inner states associated with it became directly observable after just eight therapy sessions in a severe suicidal crisis in psychoanalysis: In the last analytical session before the Christmas break, I was very worried because I could hardly reach Mrs C. emotionally. She seemed completely withdrawn into herself and her world. When I finally asked her directly about suicidal fantasies, she confirmed them to me with the words: "It's the only solution. It's the only good thing I can do: to free the world from me and myself from the world…"—Extremely worried, I said with great emotion: "You are completely immersed in your world and probably don't realize that you are throwing everything at my feet…". Mrs C. looked at me in astonishment and seemed emotionally available to me for the first time in the session. Nevertheless, I was worried that she might hurt herself during the Christmas break and was very relieved when she returned to the sessions after the break.

In retrospect, Mrs C.'s condition at the time reminds me of André Green's concept of negative narcissism mentioned above: Mrs C. seemed to have given up any cathexis with her objects, herself but also with potential future attachment desires and to be unaware of the extreme destructiveness associated with this.

It seems to me that I mobilized intensive emotions—completely unconsciously at the time—against the patient's extreme withdrawal (Green would probably speak of Eros as the antagonist of Thanatos). I myself was astonished by the passionate intensity with which I tried to reach Mrs C. emotionally and in some way establish a bond with her. In later phases of psychoanalysis we returned to this interaction several times. In the fourth year of psychoanalysis, Mrs C. remembered this scene again and said thoughtfully: "We must have been very lucky together: you really did bring me back to earth from outer space ..."

André Green's concept of *narcissistic moralism* also proved to be of clinical interest for the psychoanalyses in the MODE study. Patients with this pathology rely on moral principles to free themselves from the vicissitudes of attachment to the object and to achieve liberation from the shackles attached to the object relationship, allowing the id and ego to be loved by a demanding superego and a tyrannical ego ideal (Green, 2005). This leads to an ascetic pride and triumph over the object, but also over one's own body and the unbearable experiences of powerlessness and helplessness associated with it.

22-year-old Mr E. described his childhood as "very happy", but he fell into a severe crisis in adolescence. He lost the ground beneath his feet and was suicidal for a long time. "At that time, I wished every morning not to wake up again, as I thought it would be a relief for everyone ...". He also suffered from severe fears, e.g. that black spiders were hiding in his room. He had to spend hours searching every corner of the house and could hardly sleep...Mr E. didn't understand why he had fallen into such a severe adolescent crisis.

In psychoanalysis, it gradually became clear that the changes in the male body caused by puberty had made Mr E. extremely insecure. Impressive dreams led to associations with his parents' stories about his behavior as a premature baby in an incubator. He had struggled to survive for weeks and obviously reacted to being separated from his parents. A nurse had told the parents that the baby always began to cry desperately when they left for their lunch break. Many observations in psychoanalysis indicated that the uncontrollable changes in his pubescent body revived embodied memories of these early states of extreme helplessness and powerlessness (cf. *Leuzinger-Bohleber & Pfeifer, 2002*)[6]. In addition, his parents were going through a serious marital crisis at this time and a separation was imminent, which was threatening for Mr E. not only in the current reality, but also in relation to his inner object world, as the impending loss of his real parents was psychologically associated with the early fears of separation just outlined. In addition, the quarrelling parents shattered his idealized object representations of "peace-loving, Christian parents" and led to an abrupt loss of his ideals. One consequence of this was that the narcissistic self-regulation that he had developed during latency collapsed (cf. e.g. *Bohleber, 2017*). Mr E. became acutely suicidal. He lost his adolescent sense of self and the support of a stable, inner object world. This led to an extreme withdrawal from his inner and outer objects, his self and his body. "My body became my enemy…" he once said in his psychoanalysis.

It was impressive that the 15-year-old E. tried to solve his adolescent crisis by joining a religious youth group. In the sense of projective identifications, he developed an archaic-rigid, sadistic ego ideal and superego, combined with a subjugation of his self and his drive impulses, which he experienced as aggressive and destructive. This allowed him a certain separation from his parental home and the subjective experience of being independent of relationships through his very own inner value space. He thus demonstrated a psychodynamic that is reminiscent of André Green's concept of moral narcissism outlined above. E. saw himself as a future monk. His great role model was Brother Roger of the Taizé religious community.

But in emerging adulthood, this defense gradually collapsed. He made a serious suicide attempt, which ultimately motivated him to undergo psychoanalysis.

Breakdown of narcissistic self-regulation in emerging adulthood.

Initial clinical observations of the MODE study show that many of the early traumatized patients in this study show similar psychodynamic conflicts and fantasies as the one's just summarized of Mrs C. and Mr E.

The MODE study only included chronically depressed patients who had experienced early traumatization (cf. Ambresin et al., 2023). The psychoanalyses revealed that the vast majority of them had experienced a severe adolescent crisis and a breakdown in emerging adulthood because they were unable to cope with the developmental tasks of this phase of life. These clinical-psychoanalytical observations are further empirically verified using all the data from the study and compared with social science findings on young adulthood in Western societies (cf. Seiffge-Krenke, 2015; Leuzinger-Bohleber, 2021a, see chapter by Seiffge-Krenke in this volume).

Over the last few decades, psychological and social science researchers have studied this stage of life in detail, a stage of life that they characterize in a new way in view of today's social realities. Psychologist Jeffrey Arnett (2000) has labeled this new developmental phase *emerging adulthood*. In his view, it is the most volatile phase in human life, characterized by enormous diversity, complexity and susceptibility to disruption. Young adults today are no longer guided by an image of adulthood that is defined by the completion of an education, career planning or marriage and parenthood, but rather by certain character traits. For them, adulthood means: (1) taking responsibility for themselves and (2) being able to make independent decisions.

Arnett describes five typical characteristics of the associated development processes: Self-focussing, identity delay, instability, feeling in-between, and diversity. They have now been found in numerous studies with young people in many Western industrialized nations (Arnett, 2000, 2014, Seiffge-Krenke in this volume). This makes it clear that identity formation has become the central task of this developmental phase and has thus shifted from the period of late adolescence to the period of young adulthood (see also Bohleber, 2017; Bohleber & Leuzinger-Bohleber 1981, 2016; Seiffge-Krenke, 2015; Leuzinger-Bohleber, 2015a, 2016, 2021; Leuzinger-Bohleber et al., 2022, 2022a).

We have discussed these concepts in detail in two other papers and illustrated them using detailed reports from psychoanalyses of the MODE study, so we can refer to them here (Leuzinger-Bohleber, 2023; Leuzinger-Bohleber & Ambresin, 2024[7]; Krakau et al., 2024). In the context of this chapter, we would merely like to note that the process of separation from the primary object, the psychic integration of the idiosyncratic body representations and their own trauma history into a stable sense of self and the finding and stabilization of their own social, professional and sexual identity was psychically unmanageable for Ms C. and Mr E. For them and other MODE patients, this development had come to a complete standstill. Their depressive withdrawal often had the effect of a reversal of the passively feared into something actively brought about: the patients made their self disappear, withdrew into their cocoon and subjected themselves to the powerful (real and inner) objects or their reflection in the ego ideal and superego.

In this chapter, I tried to show that narcissism plays a decisive role in this developmental stagnation.

> If the self cannot free itself from the sphere of influence of its primary object representation, the ego ideal often remains stuck on a wish-fulfilling level of an ideal self. The inner exchange between a delineated self and a reality-focussed ego ideal, which is so important for development during this time, does not take place; instead, vague illusionary visions of the future prevail, which have no relation to real self-representations
>
> (Bohleber, 2017, p.11)

(see also Blos, 1979; Seiffge-Krenke, 2015, and in this volume).

Summary and discussion

In this chapter, we started from the current psychoanalytic view that experiences of powerlessness and helplessness are at the centre of the subjective experience of both depressed and traumatized individuals. We discussed the fact that this always involves a violation of the basic sense of self, which is one reason why narcissism, trauma and depression are so closely intertwined.

From a psychoanalytical perspective, depressive disorders are usually determined simultaneously by the current personal, institutional and/or social situation as well as by embodied memories of *primary traumatization according to Winnicott* (cf. Abram, 2021), which—from an anthropological and evolutionary-biological perspective—we have all experienced as psychophysiological premature births, albeit to varying degrees. With regard to the connection between narcissism, trauma and depression focused on here, I would therefore like to summarize somewhat simplified: If early good enough object-relation experiences in the biologically determined, extremely vulnerable period of the first months and years of life enabled the development of a stable emerging self (Daniel Stern) combined with a basic epistemic trust (Fonagy), individuals are more likely able to endure the actualizations of basic human experiences of powerlessness and dependence on others in the present, e.g. the unavoidable, often daily confrontation with individual and collective traumatization. They unconsciously associate memories of early and earliest experiences with the fact that someone is always there to empathize with them in this situation. This enables them to refrain from a narcissistic, omnipotent defense against the unbearable powerlessness and instead to react *adequately* to depression, i.e. to pause, reflect and look for room for coping and solving current societal problems with others. If, on the other hand, the early object relationships were not good enough to cope with powerlessness, panic and fear of death, there is a lack of adequate narcissistic self-regulation, a basic trust in a helping other and the ability of the self to actively defend itself. It is very likely that individuals like Ms C. and Mr E. are flooded with embodied memories of early traumatization and the experience of complete loneliness and helplessness in current situations of powerlessness. This usually leads to a severe depressive breakdown, a state of psychic shock, social withdrawal and passive, self-destructive resignation or an omnipotent, narcissistic defense.

In this sense, narcissistic problems are always part of the picture of chronic depression and can be described in clinical detail through various psychodynamic processes. In all our empirical outcome studies, the DPV-Follow-UP study, the LAC-Depression study and now also in the MODE study, the close connection between narcissism, depression and trauma as well as their transgenerative dimension can also be demonstrated empirically.

Further empirical analyses will follow in the MODE study in order to investigate in more detail how traumatic early object-relations experiences hinder the development of a stable self with an adequate narcissistic self-regulation and lead to chronic depressive disorders. At this stage, I had to limit myself to presenting some initial results of the *clinical-psychoanalytical research of the* MODE study.[8]

A Most of the patients in the MODE study had experienced a narcissistic breakdown of their vulnerable self due to the reactivation of their early trauma through renewed experiences of loss in adolescence and subsequently developed chronic depression. Between the ages of 20 and 30, i.e. in the developmental phase of so-called *emerging adulthood*, their depression led them into a dead-end street, often accompanied by suicide attempts, which ultimately led them into psychoanalytical treatment

The study shows a broad spectrum of different depressive courses (cf. also Gullestad, 2003): Mr E. had withdrawn into a traditionalist inner and outer world in the sense of A. Green's moral narcissism. Unconsciously, she despised her body, her peers, the internet, social media and other forms of digital communication. Psychoanalysis revealed that she had taken refuge in a regressive world of fantasies of merging with the primary object and associated fantasies of grandiosity and omnipotence. Far more common, however, were withdrawals such as those briefly outlined in relation to the psychoanalysis with Mrs C.: She lived in a "bubble" in her room, connected to the outside world only via the internet. Real relationships were avoided, additionally favoured by the pandemic and fears about the extremely uncertain future of humanity due to the climate change. These clinical observations are still being systematically analysed in the entire MODE study sample.

B Forty-two percent of the patients in the MODE study sample were between 20 and 30 years old. Many of them were still living at home. This was often attributed to economic constraints, but the analytical work made it clear that there were also powerful inner sources that favoured developmental blockages in young adulthood (cf. Leuzinger-Bohleber, 2023, 2024).[9]

Traumatized mothers seem to be blind to the incestuous dimension of their close, often sexualized relationship with their sons. For young depressive patients, this is one of the unconscious sources of their massive conflicts of loyalty, their overstimulated aggressive-destructive impulses and fantasies, but also a massive temptation to return to the womb of childhood. In Bion's terminology: these patients had no (internalized) good object, either in external or in psychic reality, to use the experience of separation for productive, independent thinking, i.e. for the development of alpha functions. Instead, the sensory experiences of traumatic separation remained unchanged, undigested, and were experienced as *things in themselves,* as beta elements, i.e. as something that could not be perceived and thought about. These indigestible beta elements therefore favoured projective identifications through which their real mothers took on traits of Jocasta, the narcissistically deluded mother of Oedipus, in the patients' perception, a fantasy world that was often also reflected in life-threatening, suicidal productions.

C In this group of early traumatized, depressed MODE patients, the developmental processes of *emerging adulthood* seemed to have come to an almost complete standstill. In the best-case scenario, it may be possible to break through the knot of developmental stagnation by working through the archaic destructive-aggressive fantasies and conflicts in the transference and bring the analysands back onto the path of their age-appropriate psychological and psychosocial development (cf. detailed case description in Leuzinger-Bohleber, 2023). Brief therapies or less intensive psychotherapies, which primarily teach techniques for coping with depressive symptoms, forego the opportunity to understand the unconscious sources of psychic and psychosocial withdrawal, dissociations, negative or moral narcissism or identity diffusions in the therapeutic relationship and to perceive and work through the associated wishes and conflicts in the professional analytical relationship.[10] Without intensive work with transference and the security of a professional relationship, it seems hardly possible to open a door to the depressive crypt into which severely traumatized patients have withdrawn (cf. e.g. Yassa, 2002).

In summary, these initial results of clinical psychoanalytic research in the MODE study suggest that for these severely ill chronically depressed patients in so-called emerging adulthood, as members of the Internet generation and a digital world, the intensity and professionalism of the (real) analytic (transference) relationship can be a great opportunity. Within the reliable framework of psychoanalysis, they can try to understand the withdrawal of their libidinal cathexis not only from the world of inner and outer objects but also from their self and their body, and venture a journey into their unconscious world of fantasy and conflict. The security and intensity of a professional relationship seems to be a prerequisite for deciphering and psychoanalytically processing the complex and often fatal processes of individuation and separation from their primary objects in the transference relationship.

Notes

1 A modified version of this chapter has been published in German in the journal *PTT* "Persönlichkeitsstörungen: Theorie und Therapie".

2 LAC is the abbreviation for *results of psychoanalytical and cognitive behavioural long-term psychotherapies for chronically depressed patients* (cf. Leuzinger-Bohleber et al., 2019a,b)

3 Interestingly, statistically significant differences between psychoanalytic and behavioural therapy treatments were found in this group of patients in particular (Krakau et al., 2024).

4 Multilevel Outcome Study of Psychoanalyses of Chronically Depressed Patients with Early Trauma ("MODE") (cf. Ambresin et al., 2023).

5 It is interesting that the French sociologist Alain Ehrenberg (2016) has taken up this understanding of psychodynamics again. In his study, he declares *the exhausted self to be a disease of today's society*, whose behavioural norms are no longer based on guilt and discipline, but above all on responsibility and initiative. The late bourgeois individual seems to have been replaced by an individual who has the idea that *anything is possible* and is characterized by a fear of self-realization, which can easily escalate into a feeling of exhaustion. The pressure to individualize is reflected in feelings of failure, shame and inadequacy and ultimately in depressive symptoms. For Ehrenberg, neurosis is the illness of the individual who is torn apart by the conflict between what is permitted and what is forbidden. Depression, on the other hand, he describes as the illness of the individual who is inhibited and exhausted by the tension between the possible and the impossible. Depression thus becomes a tragedy of inadequacy (on the role of social and cultural factors in depression, see also Jiménez et al., 2021).

6 In this context, I cannot list the clinical observations that supported these speculative hypotheses. It was clear that working through these hypotheses analytically gradually changed Mr E.'s body representation. He developed a new perception of his male body. A number of diffuse psychosomatic symptoms were alleviated and in some cases disappeared completely. At the same time, his ego ideal and superego changed. Mr E. developed a more differentiated inner value space in which, among other things, ambivalences towards himself, his own drive desires, but also towards the analyst and his new attachment figures could be accepted and endured. It was also impressive that he was gradually able to understand his extreme need for control as a defense against feelings of powerlessness and helplessness, a prerequisite for being able to increasingly do without it and to begin to rebuild trust in his own agency and a helpful object (cf. Leuzinger-Bohleber, 2024).

7 We must also refer to these two studies when discussing the relevant question of resilient factors in this patient group.

8 As 112 chronically depressed, early traumatized patients are undergoing psychoanalysis as part of the MODE study, this represents a great opportunity for systematic clinical psychoanalytic research. I would like to thank these patients and the 62 experienced, committed colleagues for their creative co-operation in the study.

9 Within this framework, it was not possible to address the effects of other facets of the current social situation on adolescent development processes (cf. Seiffge-Krenke, 2015, among others). For example, Tylim (2017) discusses how adolescents use new media for their narcissistic regression in order to deny the grieving process of childhood.

10 These clinical-psychoanalytical observations remind me of the characteristics of psychoanalysis, which Habermas described as early as 1968 as an *emancipatory interest in knowledge* in contrast to the *technical interest in knowledge of* behavioural therapy. Felsch (2024) reminds us of this when he writes: "In contrast to hermeneutics, which uncovers the buried meaning of historical documents, therapeutic practice (of psychoanalysis, MLB) aims to trigger a process of self-reflection in patients, which should enable them to recover "a piece of lost life history". In this context, Habermas also spoke of the "continuation of an interrupted, neurotically inhibited educational process made possible by reflective insight" (Habermas, 1968, p.51).

References

Abram, J. (2021). On Winnicott's concept of trauma. *The International Journal of Psychoanalysis, 102*(4), 778–793.

Ambresin, G., Leuzinger-Bohleber, M., Fischmann, T., Axmacher, N., Hattingen, E., Bansal, R. & Peterson, B. (2023). The Multi-Level Outcome Study of Psychoanalyses for Chronic Depressed Patients with Early Trauma (MODE). *Rationale and Design of an International Multicenter Randomised Controlled Trial.* Accepted for publication, *BMC Psychiat, 23*, 844. https://doi.org/10.1186/s12888-023-05287-6

Arnett, J. J. (2000). Emerging adulthood: A theory of development from the late teens through the twenties. *American Psychologist, 55*(5), 469–480.

Arnett, J. J. (2014). *Emerging Adulthood: The winding road from the late teens through the twenties.* Oxford: Oxford University Press.

Bibring, E. (1952). The problem of depression. *Psyche–Z Psychoanal, 6*, 81–101.

Blatt, S. J. (2004). *Experiences with depression: Theoretical, clinical, and research perspectives.* Am Psychol Assoc.

Bleichmar, H. (2010). Rethinking pathological grief: Different types and therapeutic approaches. *The Psychoanalytic Quarterly, 79*, 71–94.

Bleichmar, H. B. (1996). Some subtypes of depression and their significance for psychoanalytic treatment. *The International Journal of Psychoanalysis, 77*, 935–961.

Blos, P. (1979). *The adolescent passage. developmental issues.* New York: International University Press.

Böker, H. (2011). *Psychotherapy of depression.* Bern: Huber.

Bohleber, W. (2000). The development of trauma theory in psychoanalysis. *Psyche–Z Psychoanal, 54*(9–10), 797–839.

Bohleber, W. (2010). *Destructiveness, intersubjectivity and trauma: The identity crisis of modern psychoanalysis.* London: Karnac.

Bohleber, W. (2012). *What psychoanalysis does today. Identity and intersubjectivity, trauma and therapy, violence and society.* Stuttgart: Klett-Cotta.

Bohleber, W. (2017). *Late adolescence and young adulthood in the modern era. Conceptual and therapeutic considerations.* Unpublished paper presented at the Joseph Sandler Research Conference 3–5 March 2017 in Frankfurt am Main.

Bohleber, W., & Leuzinger, M. (1981). Narcissism and adolescence. In: Psychoanalytic Seminar Zurich (eds.), *The new theories of narcissism. Back to paradise?* Frankfurt a. M: Syndikat, 117–131.

Bohleber, W., & Leuzinger-Bohleber, M. (2016). The special problem of interpretation in the treatment of traumatised patients. *Psychoanalytic Inquiry, 36*, 60–76.

Cooper, A. (1986). Toward a limited definition of psychic trauma. In: A. Rothstein (eds.),*The reconstruction of trauma. its significance in clinical work,* Madison, CT: International Universities Press, 41–56.

Ehrenberg, A. (2016). *The weariness of the self: Diagnosing the history of depression in the contemporary age.* McGill-Queen's Press-MQUP.

Felsch, Ph. (2024). *The philosopher habermas and We.* Berlin: Ullstein.

Freud, S. (1917). *Mourning and Melancholia* (Collected Works). Vol. XII, p.428, Frankfurt a.M.: Fischer.

Green, A. (1998). The moral narcissism. *Psyche–Z Psychoanal, 52*(5), 415–449.

Green, A. (2001). Death drive, negative narcissism, desobjectalisation function. *Psyche–Z Psychoanal, 55*(9–10), 869–877.

Green, A. (2005). Chapter 13 *The Work of the Negative*. Key Ideas for a Contemporary Psychoanalysis: *Misrecognition and Recognition of the Unconscious, 49*, 212–226.

Green, A. (2007). Pulsions de destruction et maladies somatiques. *Revue française de Psychosomatique*, (2), 45–70.

Gullestad, S. E. (2003). One depression or many? The *Scand Psychoanal Z, 26*(2), 123–130.

Habermas, J. (1968). *Cognition and interest*. Frankfurt: Suhrkamp.

Jacobson, E. (1971). *On the psychoanalytic theory of affects. Depression: Comparative studies of normal, neurotic and psychotic states*. New York: International Universities Press, 3–41.

Jiménez, J. P., Botto, A., & Fonagy, P. (eds.) (2021). *Depression and personality. Etiopathogenetic theories and models of depression*. Berlin: Springer Nature Switzerland.

Joffe, W. G., & Sandler, J. (1965). Notes on pain, depression and individuation. *Psychoanal Study of the Child, 20*(1), 394–424.

Kernberg, O. F. (2014). An overview of the treatment of severe narcissistic pathology. *The International Journal of Psychoanalysis, 95*(5), 865–888.

Klein, M. (1957). Envy and gratitude. *Psyche–Z Psychoanal, 11*(5), 241–255.

Kohut, H. (1973). *Narcissism*. Frankfurt: Suhrkamp.

Krakau, L., Ernst, M., Hautzinger, M., Beutel, M., & Leuzinger-Bohleber, M. (2024): Childhood trauma and differential response to long-term psychoanalytic versus cognitive-behavioural therapy for chronic depression in adults. *British Journal of Psychiatry, 2024*, 1–8, doi.10.1192/bip.2024.112

Leuzinger-Bohleber, M. (2003). The long shadows of war and persecution: War children in psychoanalysis. Observations and reports from the DPV catamnesis study. *Psyche–Z Psychoanal, 57*, 982–1016.

Leuzinger-Bohleber, M. (2015a). Working with severely traumatised, chronically depressed analysands. *The International Journal of Psychoanalysis, 96*, 611–636.

Leuzinger-Bohleber, M. (2016). 4 Radicalisation processes in adolescence—an indicator of failed integration? 51 *Migration, early parenthood and the transmission of traumatisation: The integration project "FIRST STEPS"*, 171.

Leuzinger-Bohleber, M. (2021). The pandemic as a developmental risk. A psychoanalytic essay. *Child and Adolescent Psychotherapy, 191*(52), 403–421.

Leuzinger-Bohleber, M. (2021a). Contemporary psychodynamic theories of depression. In J. P. Jiménez, A. Botto, & P. Fonagy (eds.), Aetiopathogenetic theories and models of depression, Cham, Switzerland: Springer, 78–104.

Leuzinger-Bohleber, M. (2021b). Psychoanalysis as a plural science of the unconscious. *General Journal of Philosophy*, (46).2/2021, 253–267.

Leuzinger-Bohleber, M. (2022). "… I feel very alone and forever a stranger in this world …" (Susan Taubes). Depression—a disease of ideals and trauma. Lecture at the EPF conference in Vienna, 16 July 2022 (published in the EPF Bulletin).

Leuzinger-Bohleber, M. (2022a). Depression and Generativity—Where do we stand today after 30 years of psychoanalytic research? Sigmund Freud Lecture, 2022, video recording on the website of the Sigmund Freud Foundation.

Leuzinger-Bohleber, M. (2023). "Il fili di ragno lo circondavano" Lánalisi 'ad alte frequenza' è una buona scelta per gli arresti evolutivi nello "stato adulto emergente"? *Rivista di Psicoanalisi, LXIX*, 2, 1–26.

Leuzinger-Bohleber, M. (2024). *Depression. A contemporary introduction*. London: Routledge.

Leuzinger-Bohleber, M., & Ambresin, G. (2024). Clinical outcome and process research in the MODE study; from the psychoanalysis of a young man in emerging adulthood. In S. Gullestad, E. Stänicke, & M. Leuzinger-Bohleber (eds.), Psychoanalytic studies of change. an integrative perspective. London: Routledge, 24–39.

Leuzinger-Bohleber, M., & Hoff, D. v. (2004). Unheimliche weiblichkeit—moderne varianten eines alten themas oder travestie des unheimlichen in gemälden von fernando botero. *Free Association, 7*(1), 109–121.

Leuzinger-Bohleber, M., & Pfeifer, R. (2002), Memory of a depressive primary object? Memory in the dialogue between psychoanalysis and cognitive science. *The International Journal of Psychoanalysis, 83*, 3–33.

Leuzinger-Bohleber, M., Beutel, M. E., & Fischmann, T. (2022). Chronic depression. Psychoanalytic long-term therapy. Series: Praxis der psychodynamischen Psychotherapie—analytische und tiefenpsychologisch fundierte Psychotherapie, Vol. 12. Göttingen: Hogrefe Verlag.

Leuzinger-Bohleber, M., Ambresin, G., Fischmann, T., & M. Solms (eds.) (2022a). *On the Dark Side. Understanding the subjective experience of patients with chronic depression: psychoanalytic, neurobiological and sociocultural perspectives.* London: Routledge.

Leuzinger-Bohleber, M., Hautzinger, M., Fiedler, G., Keller, W., Bahrke, U., Kallenbach, L., … & Küchenhoff, H. (2019a). Outcome of long-term psychoanalytic and cognitive-behavioural therapy in chronically depressed patients: A controlled trial with preferential and randomised allocation. *The Canadian Journal of Psychiatry, 64*(1), 47–58.

Leuzinger-Bohleber, M., Kaufhold, J., Kallenbach, L., Negele, A., Ernst, M., Keller, W., … & Beutel, M. (2019b). Measuring sustainable psychological changes in the long-term treatment of chronically depressed patients: Symptomatic and structural changes in the LAC Depression Study on the outcome of long-term cognitive-behavioural and psychoanalytic treatments. *The International Journal of Psychoanalysis, 100*(1), 99–127.

Loch, W. (1967). Psychoanalytic aspects of the pathogenesis and structure of depressive-psychotic states. *Psyche–Z Psychoanal, 21*, 758–779.

Negele, A., Kaufhold, J., Kallenbach, L., & Leuzinger-Bohleber, M. (2015). Childhood trauma and its relation to chronic depression in adulthood. *Depression Research and Treatment, 2015*, Article ID 650804, 2–11.

Rado, S. (1928). The problem of melancholia. *The International Journal of Psychoanalysis, 9*, 420–438.

Salazar, L. A., & Zambrano, T. (2021). Genetic and epigenetic determinants of depression. From basic research to translational medicine. In J. P. Jiménez, A. Botto, & P. Fonagy (eds.), *Depression and personality, etiopathetic theories and models in depression*, 146–162.

Seiffge-Krenke, I. (2015). "Emerging Adulthood": Research findings on objective markers, developmental tasks and developmental risks. *Journal of Psychiatry, Psychology and Psychotherapy*.

Tylim, I. (2017). Adolescent narcissism in the age of cyberspace. *The Psychoanalytic Study of the Child, 70*(1), 130–134.

Winnicott, D. W. (1949). 1958 Collected Papers: From Paediatrics to Psychoanalysis. 1st ed. London: Tavistock (cited in Abram, 2021).

Will, H., Grabenstedt, Y., Banck, G., & Völkl, G. (2008). *Depression: Psychodynamics and therapy*. Stuttgart: W. Kohlhammer Verlag.

Xu, Y., Hackett, M., Carter, G., Loo, C., Gálvez, V, Glozier, N., Glue, P., Lapidus, K., McGirr, A., Somogyi, A. A., Mitchell, P. B., & Rodgers, A. (2016). Effects of low-dose and very low-dose ketamine among patients with major depression: A systematic review and metaanalysis. *International Journal of Neuropsychipharmacology, 19*(4), 1–15.

Yassa, M. (2002). Nicolas Abraham and Maria Torok—the inner crypt. *The Scandinavian Psychoanalytic Journal, 25*(2), 82–91.

15 Changes in dreams in psychoanalyses of chronic depressed patients in a narcissistic psychic retreat

Clinical research in the MODE study

Tamara Fischmann, Gilles Ambresin,
and Marianne Leuzinger-Bohleber

Introduction

As discussed in various chapters in this volume, narcissistic personality disorders are considered difficult to treat psychoanalytically. However, if the narcissistic disorder of self-regulation does not completely dominate the inner object world of the patient, but occurs in combination with chronic depression and early traumatization, the chances of treatment are better (Leuzinger-Bohleber in this volume). We would like to demonstrate this clinical finding in the following on the basis of a single case study. We focus on the changes in the manifest dreams. As we have discussed in other papers, we interpret the changes in dreams as an indicator of transformations in the inner object world of our patients. Probably the most sophisticated method for analyzing manifest dreams is the Zurich Dream Process Coding System (ZDPCS), developed by Ulrich Moser and his research group and now used by various research groups (Ambresin et al., 2022; Ambresin & Leuzinger-Bohleber, 2024; Fischmann & Leuzinger-Bohleber, 2018; Fischmann et al., 2021; Leuzinger-Bohleber, Donié, Wichelmann).

(1) We begin with a relatively detailed case example of a psychoanalysis with a 24-year-old female patient in the MODE study (2). In a third chapter, we summarize the ZDPCS (3). We then examine four dreams of the patient (4) and, in the discussion, contrast the results of clinical-psychoanalytic research with the extra clinical dream research (5).

"It is the only good thing I can do: to free the world from me and myself from the world" (Mrs C.). From psychoanalysis with an early traumatized patient with narcissistic depression[1]

(by Marianne Leuzinger-Bohleber)

DOI: 10.4324/9781003565284-19

Mrs C. is a tall, handsome, leptosome-looking 24-year-old student. She is referred to the outpatient clinic of our institute by her roommate in a shared flat after a serious suicide attempt. Already during the assessment interviews, she tells me that she, the youngest of four sisters, was an "accident": her father left her mother shortly before her birth for another woman. Her mother was overtaxed as a single parent working fulltime. Mrs C. developed into a shy, low-maintenance child. As long as she can remember, she always suffered from depression. However, her suicidal fantasies and impulses intensified from the age of 13, after the death of her beloved grandmother who had become demented.

As part of the MODE study, she begins a one-session per week psychoanalytic treatment, which she changes after a year at her own request first to a three-session and then to a four-session psychoanalysis. Only in the course of psychoanalysis does she casually relate that she suffered from colitis ulcerosa at the age of 15. At 19, she had to undergo emergency surgery and narrowly escaped death.

Two months after the beginning of the treatment, before the Christmas break, a severe suicidal crisis occurs after only eight analytical sessions. I have summarized this clinically significant event in my chapter in this volume:

> In the last analytical session before the Christmas break, I was very worried because I could hardly reach Mrs C. emotionally. She seemed completely withdrawn into herself and her world. When I finally asked her directly about suicidal fantasies, she confirmed them to me with the words: "It's the only solution. It's the only good thing I can do: to free the world from me and myself from the world ..."— Extremely worried, I said with great emotion: "You are completely immersed in your world and probably don't realize that you are throwing everything at my feet ..."[2]. Mrs C. looked at me in astonishment and seemed emotionally available to me for the first time in the session. Nevertheless, I was worried that she might hurt herself during the Christmas break and was very relieved when she returned to the sessions after the break.
>
> In retrospect, Mrs C.'s condition at the time reminds me of André Green's concept of negative narcissism: Mrs C. seemed to have given up any cathexis with her objects, herself but also with potential future attachment desires and to be unaware of the extreme destructiveness associated with this.
>
> It seems to me that I mobilized intensive emotions—completely unconsciously at the time—against the patient's extreme withdrawal (Green would probably speak of Eros as the antagonist of Thanatos). I myself was astonished by the passionate intensity with which I tried to reach Mrs C. emotionally and in some way establish a bond with

her. In later phases of psychoanalysis, we returned to this interaction several times. In the fourth year of psychoanalysis, Mrs C. remembered this scene again and said thoughtfully: "We must have been very lucky together: you really did bring me back to earth from outer space".

(Leuzinger-Bohleber, chapter in this volume)

During the first year of psychoanalysis, Mrs C. becomes increasingly emotionally involved in the treatment. She misses practically no therapy session. Nevertheless, my basic feeling remains that I have to be very careful with her. Mrs C. seems to be afraid that I will overwhelm her and erase her fragile self. The main unconscious fantasies revolve around an archaic fear of destroying her objects or being destroyed in relationships herself. All of this is connected with the unconscious conviction that a devastating catastrophe could occur at any time. She hardly remembers dreams. Before the first summer break, after six months of low-frequency psychoanalysis, she recounts the following dream:

> I meet Y (a friend who studies with her) in a dream again after 15 years. He is in a bad psychic condition because a life dream, falafel stand at a fair with the great sauce of his father did not work out. Thus his life dream collapsed. This makes me very sorry but cannot do anything about it. I cry hard and wake up crying.

The associations lead to the patient's central feeling of being completely powerless and helpless at all times, exposed to catastrophes and cannot even stop crying. She can't protect her boyfriend or herself. "Y cannot use his father's inheritance". In the manifest dream, Mrs C. does not appear as an acting subject, but passively watches the events from the outside.

Through the four-session psychoanalysis she requested, the psychoanalytic process is intensified in the second year of treatment. The central unconscious fantasies can now be worked on directly in the transference relationship.

Shortly before the summer vacations, she asks for an additional analytic session for the first time and then recounts the following *nightmare*:

> I was on vacation with my family, in South America. The first part was not a nightmare. My father and sisters were in the hotel in the city. I myself was staying with mother in another hotel, on the beach. We were going to do nice things, boating, etc. Suddenly I was sad because I thought I won't have the time to do everything I wanted to do which is nice. Then suddenly there were a lot of people. It was a kind of war, a war of liberation. Military people said I had to go back to hotel. I passed by street barricades, a burning car ... I fled towards the hotel, but I knew that tourists were being taken hostage there.

I escaped over three barricades. Finally, I climbed on a roof and tried to save myself on a metal bar. Below me was the abyss. I knew that if I was discovered, I would have to jump, otherwise I would be decapitated or tortured. A terrorist then came. He held a chopped off head in front of my face. I knew I now had to jump into the abyss. It took forever. Then I woke up in a panic.

Her boyfriend, who she had found after the first year of analysis, was with her. He woke her up because she was screaming and took her in his arms.

The associations lead to the process of separation from the mother, which is experienced as fatal.

In the dream, she kills herself to escape from the regressive wishes of letting her mother fulfill her longings. "My childish self still allows itself to be seduced, but then apparently has to fall into the abyss". In the next analytic session, Mrs C. reports that after the last session she thought, "I don't want to be so passive … But then I heard that other voice again right away: 'But you are just lazy … My mother's voice is probably still very present'". Analyst:

> How important that you noticed this!—As bad and devaluing as this voice is for your self-esteem, by paying attention to it, we can see that it prevents you from getting out of passivity and taking personal responsibility. Moreover- as we have seen in the first part of your dream—it seems tempting to hand over the inner responsibility, your life, to your mother ….

The realization that there is also a secondary gain of illness in the passive withdrawal of depression, a seduction to fall into the arms of the primary object and to refuse to actively grieve for the lost childhood, is a recurring topic in the second year of analysis. It touches on one of the central challenges of treatment, namely to bring the depressed patients out of their psychic and social withdrawal and to help them regain a basic feeling of self-agency as well as the desire to take responsibility for their own lives in order to be able to gradually renounce the satisfaction of passive infantile drive wishes and longings. Of course, this analytical work always aims at strengthening the patient's narcissistic self-regulation.

The following dream from the third year of analysis may give an insight into the inner processes involved. Object-relational experiences, drives and longings as well as narcissistic needs and conflicts are intertwined in a complex way:

> I now remember a dream, only fragments, it was not a nightmare, but a terrible content …
>
> I was chased by a couple in a forest area. It was an atmosphere like in a movie, not like in a nightmare … I killed them several times, but

that didn't help. They were still after me. I had to use extreme methods to defend myself. In the end, there was only one person left, the woman. I had to cut her open and chop off all parts of her body. It was cruel, but I knew it was right, that it had to be done.

She associates: "Strange, somehow the dream was abstract, this knowledge that it was right, although it was so brutal. I was a perpetrator for the first time in a dream—it was the woman I had to chop up".

A.: "It has been a lot about women here lately, about me, but also about your mother. Yesterday you told me about her suicide threats that made you so powerless and angry". We talk again about her colitis ulcerosa, which started in adolescence. She remembers that after a conflict with a boy at school, whom she had insulted and who had massively shamed her afterward, she consciously decided: "I don't want to be such a nasty, disgusting person anymore, but I want to take myself back and become a calm, empathetic woman"—I have to think of her (murderous) separation conflicts with her mother during that time and say:

And with that you made your 'nasty', seemingly 'unbearable' and 'indigestible' parts of your personality disappear. It is impressive that your body has then produced a symptom that is about what the body cannot take into itself because it is 'indigestible' and 'harmful' to it—a symptomatology that is so much connected with disgust and shame ....

We came back to this dream again and again in our psychoanalytic work in the coming weeks. I think the dream shows, among other things, in an impressive way that the individuation and separation process had a murderous quality for Mrs C. and made it difficult, or almost impossible, for her to master the necessary separation aggression and—in the sense of symbolic matricide—to distinguish reality from fantasy. I lack the space here to illustrate how central the working through of these unconscious phantasies was in the transference, also because the inner and outer separation and individuation process was repeatedly further complicated by her mother's behavior in reality. For example, in these weeks, she again directly threatens her with suicide if she refuses to go on vacation with her and prefers her boyfriend.

For the first time, I learned more about the mother's trauma history in this context. She comes from a traumatized German refugee family from the East. In extreme poverty, six family members lived in a single room for years. In addition, Mrs C.'s grandfather experienced a psychotic breakdown when her mother moved out at age 15.[3] Therefore, we suspect that the mother, due to her traumatization and severe postpartum depression, triggered or intensified by abandonment by her husband, could not psychically hold and contain Mrs C.'s early destructive impulses and fantasies well enough, probably one of the reasons why the analysand "had already experienced the catastrophe" (Winnicott) and could hardly psychologically integrate her early passionate libidinous and aggressive destructive impulses and fantasies. They had been preserved, among other things, in catastrophic expectations in her unconscious.

In many loops of analytical understanding and working through, it became comprehensible to Mrs C. what serious consequences this inner (unconscious) fantasy and longing world had both for her narcissistic self-regulation and for the formation of a mature self-ideal. Successively she dared to come out of her extreme social isolation and extreme psychic retreat, "her bubble" as she called it, and to participate actively in "real life" again. Above all, the fact that she dared to reject the real demands of her mother, to openly express the age-appropriate separation aggression and to take up a love relationship, but also her real successes in her resumed studies, were absolutely decisive. The real experienced narcissistic satisfactions allowed her successively to renounce her fantasies of grandiosity and omnipotence, respectively to integrate them psychically into her narcissistic self-regulation. This was connected with processes of a modification of her ego ideal and superego, which served her as a new, self-chosen, stable inner orientation and allowed a basal feeling to grow in her that she had become "masteress in her own house" (see e.g. Bleichmar, 1996; Diamond, 2015; Winston, 2017).

These inner transformations become clear in the last dream that she tells in the penultimate analysis session:

> I want to go to the analytic session with X. (her boyfriend). Somehow, he comes with me. It was good that way. We set off without rushing. Everything is fine. But then suddenly there is a terrible storm. We get soaking wet, there is water everywhere, there is lightning and thunder. I try to get through and say I really want to try… but at some point it was no longer possible, we had to turn back. I am sad when we get home. But then I think, "I really tried everything. It's not my fault!" and then I think, "It's all about me …" and call you.

The associations revolve mainly around her inner struggle to gain confidence in the new object (the analyst) who understands and accepts the fact, that she tried everything to link her own desires (to come to analysis) with those of the analyst. At the same time, she confirms herself in the manifest dream that in new object relations (to the analyst, to her boyfriend) "It's all about me" and not about submission to the desires and wishes of the object. In this way, she refers to a central thread of psychoanalysis: her traumatized mother "abused" her as a self-object: she was unable to support the patient's early and adolescent separation and individuation in a good enough way. These object relation experiences became mixed up with the patient's unconscious fantasies that separation and individuation are associated with homicidal dangers in which neither the object nor the self survives.

This brief summary of our clinical work with dreams may illustrate how closely narcissism, depression and trauma were intertwined in the patient's internal world of objects.

In the next two sections, we are aiming to "triangulate" the just mentioned clinical psychoanalytic hypothesis by systematic analyses with the help of the ZDPCS, in other words with an approach investigating clinical material after the psychoanalytic sessions. We have characterized this kind of research as "extra-clinical psychoanalytic research" (see e.g. Leuzinger-Bohleber, 2021).

ZDPCS: the "dream-generation-model" by Moser and von Zeppelin—an attempt to integrate psychoanalytical and interdisciplinary knowledge on dreams[4]

Moser and von Zeppelin (1996) consider the sleep dream as a simulated micro-world. The simulation is driven by affectivity, leading in the end to images of entities involved (subject, object and things) and relationships linking them. A dream is triggered by events of the previous day or night. This event reactivates unresolved conflicts and problems (current concern). The dream has the function of retrospective problem solving. While in the waking state, in contrast to the dream state, we react immediately to our environment and by that consolidate information into our memory, there is often a restriction of consolidation processes in the waking state due to capacity restrictions of the memory system, so that consolidation cannot take place immediately and need to be deferred for later processing. In this context, it is interesting to note that these consolidation processes also take place during sleep in a so-called off-line mode. This is how new information is then integrated into long-term memory during sleep and dreaming after having been deferred due to capacity restrictions in the waking state. As the dream is looking for a solution of reactivated conflicts and problems the action and expression components of the affects are inhibited in the dream state as representation of the inner life dominates. But the range of affect modulation is significantly larger than in the micro-worlds of the waking state and stress is absorbed via imagination and via cognition. Affects may nevertheless become too strong and will lead to interruptions of the dream—so-called interrupts—and might even cause waking-up, so that the dream microworld contains situation sequences (Sit) with "interrupts" separating these from one another. The dream is not involved in regulating concrete-real object relationships but rather works with memories and with acquired solution and defense strategies [called self- and object-models and generalized interaction-representations (RIGs),[5] or, on a different level of observation, rather prototypical affective microprocesses (PAMs).[6] According to this@@ dream-generation-model, dreams often start with a positioning field (PF) without interactions. What appears in this PF is regulated by a security principle, which prevents the emergence of threatening affects by means of distance relations. Once the affective cathexis of the microworld is very strong, the dream narrative initiates an interactive field of interactions (IAF), where the PF is still there "by default" as a background presence. The dream contains procedures of approaching and distancing from the intended wish fulfillment (i.e., problem solving) via regulation of involvement and commitment as well as via interactive procedures of shaping its security regulation. Via a feedback-loop (reentry), the dream may be interrupted, if the affectivity gets too unbearable, and a new PF is created, thus increasing safety for the next situation. Every dream sequence contains a PF, which includes, always per situation, all mentioned elements: subject, objects, inanimate things, often summarized in a PLACE, which is a kind of spatial micro-world. Within the micro-world dream, which is considered to be an affective-cognitive bundle, initiated by current concerns, a "dream complex" can be seen as a template that enables the dream to be organized accordingly. Thus, a "dream complex" can be assumed to consist of one or more complexes that have their origin in conflictual and/or traumatic experiences stored in non-declarative long-term memory. These complexes have ultimately found their condensates in introjects, i.e., affective-cognitive templates of conflictual or traumatizing memory traces. When these introjects are triggered by closely related current concerns from the outside, these "dream complexes" may be considered structurally like stored situations of the introjected complex, and a dream emerges in search for resolving the complex. The memory traces of such complexes are characterized by invariant intense, unbearable affects connected by so-called k-lines and are stored isolated from memories with relational reality.

Each of these isolated complexes contain unbound affective information and represent links between self- and object-models and generalized interaction-representations (PAMs), which are accompanied by convictions and a hope for wish-fulfillment (i.e., problem-solving). They have a repetitive character (W), as they are in constant search for a solution in order to get rid of the disturbing unbound affects. Another way of saying this—referring to the terminology of attachment research—is as follows: An internal working model (IWM) of the social world is created in childhood. In the case of abuse/neglect, the IWM is well adapted to the abusive context, but then is maladaptive later in life outside the family of origin. The IWM generates predictions that don't conform to the social reality. Thus, there are major prediction errors. These prediction errors result in affective responses. They are "unbound" in the sense of being activated and not resolved via an updated prediction or a change in circumstances/sensory input that conform to prediction. Perhaps the function of dreaming is to rework the RIG or IWM to minimize future prediction error. We cannot describe this elaborated dream-generation model and the coding system based on it in more detail here but hope that the following illustration (see Figure 15.1) may elucidate this model.

Outside the dream world, where the reality principle prevails, these conflictual or traumatic complexes cannot be thought of declaratively as they are being pushed into the unconscious[7] because of their intolerability. In the dream world, in which the pleasure principle prevails, the affective information comes more easily to the fore, and the "dream organizer" (i.e., the dreaming sleeper) seeks a solution by creating a tolerable micro-world in which the affective information suppressed or dissociated in the waking state can come "alive" and become solvable (cf. Figure 15.1). In other words, a function of dreaming is to establish a basis for the affect to become attached to meaning systems and become mentalizable. It could also be the case that this function during dreaming contributes to the encoding of memories along emotional lines such that in the future memories associated with a given emotional state are more easily accessible when in that emotional state. The "dreamlike" problem solution of such unbearable complexes is facilitated by balancing innate tendencies for security and the desire for involvement. Whenever this fails in a dream, the dream scene is interrupted and either a new one is created, or the dreamer wakes up in a state of panic. Thus, the number of "interrupts" of dream scenes within a dream may, according to our first empirical findings (Fischmann & Leuzinger-Bohleber, 2018; Fischmann, Russ, & Leuzinger-Bohleber, 2013), be considered one indicator for change. The less "interrupts" within a long dream the closer to the solution of the dream complex the dreamer is. Of course, in shorter dreams, we find less "interrupts": these dreams break off early.

Based on this dream-generation model, Moser and von Zeppelin (1996) have developed a coding system which can be used to analyze the manifest

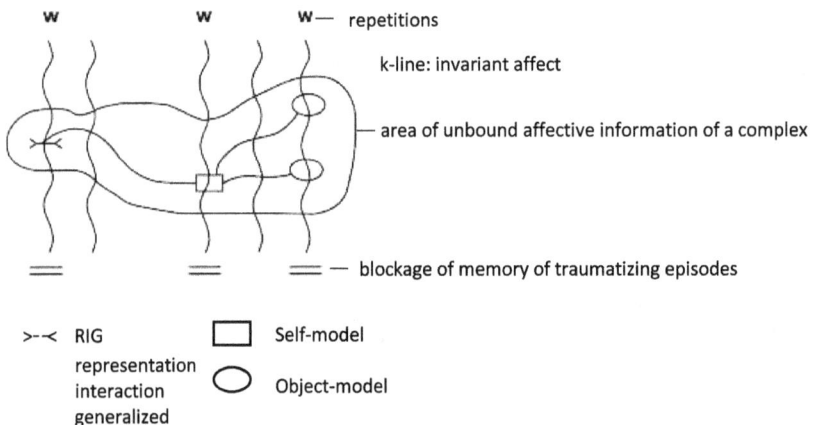

Figure 15.1 Memory model of conflictuous complexes according to moser and von zeppelin (1996)

dream content—the Zurich Dream Process Coding System (ZDPCS). It can be applied to investigate systematic changes in the manifest dream content for instance of dreams of analysands during their psychoanalyses, as was done in the LAC depression study.

Transformations in the manifest dreams: Indicators of transformations in the inner object-world and the narcissistic self-regulation?

In the following the dreams of Mrs C. are analyzed with and interpreted according the ZDPCS.

Interpretation

This dream is a nightmare as Mrs C. experiences intense anxiety in this dream and wakes up from it. What is also recognizable is that Mrs C. is an observer in her dream, as she projects her own feelings of despair and loss (bad; sorry) onto her friend (Y) and is left behind with a feeling of helplessness (cannot do anything). These are both indicators of traumatic dreams where the self is rendered helpless and withdraws—fearing to get involved, becoming an observer of his insufferable emotions.

Table 15.1 Dream of first year (low-frequency psychoanalysis)

Dream narrative	Sit	PF	LTM	IAF	VR	CP/AFF R
I meet Y (a friend who studied with her) in a dream again after 15 years	S1	SP OP$_1$ (friend Y) BEK PLACE (dream)		IRC RES (meet)		
He is in a bad psychic condition because a life dream, falafel stand at a fair with the great sauce of his father did not work out. Thus his life dream collapsed	S2	OP$_1$ (friend Y) IMPLW CEU (falafel stand at fair) CEU (sauce) ATTR (great)		IRD NPR ((IRS OP)) [bad psychic condition; life dream collapsed]		AFF R (bad)
This makes me very sorry but cannot do anything about it	S3	SP OP$_1$		IRC constr (cannot do anything about it)		EX AFF R (sorry)
I cry hard and wake up crying...	---					EX AFF R (cry hard)

Note: Sit.= situation sequences; PF= positioning field; LTM=locotime motion; IAF= interactive field of interactions; VR=verbal relation; CP/AFF R=cognitive process/affective reaction

Table 15.2 Dream of second year (high-frequency sessions)

Dream narrative	Sit	PF	LTM	IAF	VR	CP/AFF R
I am on vacation with my family, in South America	S1	SP PLACE (South America) OP-G$_1$ (family) BEK (my) SOC SETT (on vacation)				
The first part was not a nightmare	CC					CC (not a nightmare)
My father and sisters are in the hotel in the city	S2	SP OP$_2$ (father) BEK (my) OP$_3$ (sisters) BEK (my) PLACE (hotel) POS REL (in city)				
I myself am staying with mother in another hotel, on the beach. We were going to do nice things, boating, etc.	S3	SP OP$_4$ (mother) BEK (my) PLACE (hotel) POS REL (on the beach)		IRC pot (going to do)		
Suddenly I am sad because I think I won't have the time to do everything I want to do, which is nice	—	SP				EX AFF R (sad)
Then suddenly there are a lot of people. It is a kind of war, a war of liberation	S4	SP OP-G (people) IMPLW (war of liberation)				
Military people say I have to go back to hotel.	S5	SP OP (people) ATTR (military) PLACE (hotel)			VR (say I have to go back)	
I pass by street barricades, a burning car …	S6	SP CEU (barricades) CEU (car) ATTR (burning)	SP^t (I pass)			

Dream narrative	Sit	PF	LTM	IAF	VR	CP/AFF R
I flee toward the hotel, I know that tourists are being taken hostage there	S7	SP PLACE (hotel) POS REL (toward) IMPLW (know tourists are taken hostage there)		IRC (I flee)		
I escape over three barricades	S8	SP CEU (barricades) ATTR (three) POS REL (over)		IRC (escape)		
Finally I climb on a roof and try to save myself on a metal bar. Below me is the abyss. I know that if I am discovered, I will have to jump, otherwise I will be decapitated or tortured	S9	SP PLACE (roof) POSE REL (on) CEU (metal bar) PLACE (abyss) POS REL (below) IMPLW (I know...)		IRC pot (have to jump; decapitated; tortured)		
A terrorist then comes	S10	OP (terrorist)	OP^t			
He holds a chopped off head in front of my face	S11	SP PART OF (face) OP (terrorist) CEU (chopped off head) POS REL (in front)		IRC (OP holds...)		
I know I now have to jump into the abyss. It takes forever	S12	SP PLACE (abyss) IMPLW (know have to jump)		IRC (jump takes forever)		
Then I wake up in a panic	--	SP				EX AFF R (panic)

Note: Sit.= situation sequences; PF= positioning field; LTM=locotime motion; IAF= interactive field of interactions; VR=verbal relation; CP/AFF R=cognitive process/affective reaction

Interpretation 1

Again, this dream is a nightmare with intense anxiety (panic) and waking from it in panic. The dream is frequently interrupted—there being altogether 12 situations is an indicator for the necessity to amend the dream scenes (situations) in such a way that Mrs C. can bear her intolerable feelings of sadness. She has to populate her dream-scenes anew (add or drop elements in the positioning field) whenever the emotional temperature rises too high for her to bear them. Another indicator for her struggling is that she does not dare to get involved (no IAF coding) in the first half of the dream (Sit. 1–6), except for one potentially happy one (S3), where she is sad that it might not happen. The affective processes in the dream are mostly characterized by sadness, helplessness or panic. Her microworld (MW) dream is populated by security-threatening objects (OP) and *cognitive* elements. The PF is amply endowed (and thus holds potential INVOLVEMENT possibilities), but these are mostly threatening. The OPs are either absent (mother) and not interactive or threatening and pursuing (terrorists). The MW dream depicts a scenario of attack and threat from which she implicitly knows she must escape (IMPLW). The leap into the abyss takes forever and it is unclear whether she will succeed. There are no helpful others available to help her; she is on her own.

Interpretation 2

This dream is not a nightmare although it is characterized by intense fear of persecution, but without waking up from it. There are still relatively many INTERRUPTS (5 situations), but the dreamer is actively involved from the outset (IAF); she actively defends herself and by this conveys self-agency. Still there are no helpful others (OPs); she is on her own—being isolated in a narcissistic bubble. In this dream—in her third year of analysis—she tries something new: from a possible insight from her psychoanalysis, she dares (as being "offline" in the MW dream) to engage herself in a cruel and attacking manner, knowing this is necessary in order to defend herself. This seems to be a progress leading out of helplessness (CP: knows it is right; had to be done) by getting involved, thereby trying to catapult herself out of her narcissistic bubble.

Interpretation 3

In this dream from the end of therapy, we can see that the quality of a nightmare has disappeared. This dream is possibly not even an anxiety dream. There are a range of affects: joy and happiness (that she is not alone, that the friend accompanies her to her last analytic session), anxiety (storm), disgust (mud), sadness (that she cannot reach the analyst) and confidence, even pride (that she manages to call the analyst, knowing that she will understand

Table 15.3 Dream of third year (high-frequency sessions)

Dream narrative	Sit	PF	LTM	IAF	VR	CP/AFF R

I am chased by a couple in a forest area. It was an atmosphere like in a movie, not like in a nightmare....	S1	SP
		  PLACE (forest)
		  OP$_1$ (couple)
		SOC SETT (in movie)
				IRC RESP		CC (not a nightmare)

I killed them several times, but that didn't help	S2	SP OP$_1$ (couple)		IRC fail (kill; failed)		
They were still after me. I had to use extreme methods to defend myself	S3	SP OP$_1$ (couple)		IRC TRI connecting (still after me) IRS (SP) (extreme methods to defend myself)		
In the end, there was only one person left, the woman	S4	SP DROP PART OF OP$_1$ OP$_2$ (woman)				
I had to cut her open and chop off all parts of her body. It was cruel	S5	SP^2 OP$_2$ (woman) PART OF (parts of her body)		IRC KIN (cut her open) IRC KIN (chop off)		AFF R (cruel)
but I knew it was right, that it had to -- be done...						CP (knew it was right; had to be done)

Note: Sit.= situation sequences; PF= positioning field; LTM=locotime motion; IAF= interactive field of interactions; VR=verbal relation; CP/AFF R=cognitive process/affective reaction

Table 15.4 Dream of fourth year (high-frequency sessions)

Dream narrative	Sit	PF	LTM	IAF	VR	CP/AFF R
I want to go to the analytic session with X. (her boy friend). Somehow he comes with me. It was good that way. We set off without rushing. Everything is fine.	S1	SP OP_1 (boyfriend X) BEK SOC SETT (analytic session)		IRC pot (SP) (want to go) IRC RES LTM (we set out)		CC (everything is fine)
But then suddenly there is a terrible storm. We get soaking wet, there is water everywhere, there is lightning and thunder	S2	SP OP_1 (X) CEU stuff (storm; lightning, thunder) CEU stuff (water) POS REL (everywhere)		IRC RES (we get soaking)		
I try to get through and say I really want to try... but at some point it was no longer possible, we had to turn back	S3	SP OP_1 (X)		IRC fail (no longer possible) IRC TRI connecting (had to turn back)	VR (I really want to try to get through)	
I am sad when we get home	S4	SP OP_1 (X) PLACE (home)		IRC RES (we get home)		AFF R (sad)
But then I think, "I really tried everything. It's not my fault!" and then I think, "It's all about me".	--					CP (I think I really tried...; it's all about me)
And call you.	S5	SP OP_2 (analyst)		IRC (I call you)		

Note: Sit.= situation sequences; PF= positioning field; LTM=locotime motion; IAF= interactive field of interactions; VR=verbal relation; CP/AFF R=cognitive process/affective reaction

her). She is still struggling with her affect regulation, as can be seen by the still prominent number of interrupts between dream scenes (5 situations + 1 VR). But the dreamer (she) is actively involved from the outset (involvement). The involvement is mostly resonant (IRC RES) and triangulating (TRI connecting). She is no longer attacked by objects (OPs) but rather by nature elements (CEU stuff), that are not as threatening and from which she expects to more likely be able to save herself. The MW dream continues to be threatening, but now in a way that is not as self-destructive (annihilating the self) as when having been attacked by OPs. She feels more confident that when she seeks help, she will also get the help and that boosts her self-confidence in getting more involved, i.e. exiting her narcissistic bubble. She expressed her confidence that her analyst will understand her intentions and accepts deeply: "It's all about me"—in other words, that her self is in the center of her world and her interactions with (new) objects.

Summary of the extra-clinical ZDPCS findings

The dreams of the first two years of therapy (dream 1 and 2) are characteristic nightmares from which the dreamer wakes up in a panic. The first of these dreams is an observer-dream which is also characteristic for nightmares where the patient does not dare to get involved and rather observes others taking action. By observing she actually projects her own feelings onto others so as to not get too close to those unbearable feelings. Still this defense is not enough to get the rising panic under control, and she wakes up frightened. Dream 2 of the second year of treatment shows improvement—she is not an observer anymore, gets more involved. But she needs to amend the dream scenes constantly in order to keep the affective temperature at bay (12 different situations). Despite all these attempts at affect regulation, she wakes up in a panic. The two dreams of the third and fourth year of treatment are no longer typical nightmares. Although the third dream is characterized by intense fear of persecution, she does not wake up from it, i.e. not a nightmare. The rising anxiety in the dream asks for many interrupts (five situations), but she is able to get involved and conveys self-agency, which is a great improvement. In this third dream she tries to engage herself aggressively in order to leave her helplessness behind and by this to catapult herself out of her narcissistic bubble. In the fourth dream, the quality of a nightmare has disappeared altogether—it is not even an anxiety dream. The dream content is still threatening, but not in a self-destructive way anymore. She gained confidence and one might assume that she has exited her narcissistic bubble.

Discussion

One aim of this chapter was to illustrate that it is possible for patients with a severe disorder of narcissistic self-regulation with the main diagnoses of depression and trauma to achieve a transformation in their inner object world through psychoanalysis. As we have described in a relatively detailed summary of the analytic process with Mrs C., her suicidal fantasies at the beginning of the analysis showed how much she had withdrawn into a narcissistic bubble and was therefore unconsciously convinced that the only solution was "to free the world from me and myself from the world". As discussed, the analyst succeeded in reaching the patient's withdrawn self with a passionate emotional response, metaphorically mobilizing Eros and literally forcing the patient to look her in the eyes and, at that very moment, to abandon the defense of extreme withdrawal of cathexis from all her objects as well as from herself (according to André Green). Much later in psychoanalysis, it was possible to understand further unconscious fantasies and beliefs that had been activated in this core clinical scene: (a) the belief that the object had to be relieved of the self, which had been stimulated by the narratives concerning the patient's first months of life (her father had left the mother before her birth, the mother was presumably flooded by her traumatic fears of loss and sank into a severe postpartum depression with the well-known consequences for the early interaction with her baby); (b) the archaic fantasy that separation and individuation represented a mortal danger for the self and/or the object (suicidal fantasies, countertransference fantasies of the analyst), and; (c) the extreme denial of one's own aggressive impulses ("You probably don't realize that you are throwing everything at my feet …").

In order to describe the transformations through psychoanalysis in this single case, we focused on the change of the manifest dreams and the work with the latent dream contents in the psychoanalytic situation with the help of the patient's associations.

Using the four dreams listed, we replicated observations on the change in manifest dream content in successful psychoanalyses, which Leuzinger-Bohleber (Leuzinger-Bohleber, 1989) already described and which our research group is currently investigating further using a new dream scale, the DREAM-C (cf. Leuzinger-Bohleber et al., 2023; Leuzinger-Bohleber & Ambresin, 2024). According to this, manifest dream contents in "good enough" psychoanalyses change as follows:

1 Nightmares are becoming rarer
2 Dreams in which the dream subject is in the observer position are less frequent
3 More object relationships emerge
4 Increasingly, problem solving succeeds in dreams
5 The affective spectrum is expanded.

We have described these changes both clinically and analyzed them "extra-clinically" with the help of the ZDPCS:

Ad 1: Nightmares are becoming rarer

In nightmares, the dream subject is flooded with fear of death and panic and therefore wakes up. As we have discussed in detail in other papers, we recognize embodied memories of traumatic experiences in the unbearable affects in dreams that evoke a waking up of the patient (cf. psychoanalytical definition of trauma) (see e.g. Bohleber & Leuzinger-Bohleber, 2016) The self-agency and the basic trust in a helping object collapse.

Both clinically and with the help of the ZDPCS, we were able to observe that Mrs C.'s nightmares were indeed decreasing. It is interesting that in the first dream the early traumatization of the father leaving the family, combined with the extreme feelings of powerlessness and helplessness in the sense of "embodied memories", also appears in terms of content (the friend in the dream cannot guarantee the connection to his father (falafel stall), the patient breaks out in "endless crying"). Compared to this, the last dream shows clear changes: although a storm tries to prevent her from doing so, the patient finally manages to make contact with the analyst by telephone: She has sufficient self-agency and at the same time has regained trust in her object: she is convinced that the analyst will understand her and—in contrast to her traumatized mother—can accept that it is "about me", i.e. about the patient's self.

Ad 2: Dream subject is in the observer position

The first remembered dream, half a year after the beginning of the one-session psychoanalysis, already shows the first inner changes of the patient compared to the "suicide scene": the patient is no longer completely withdrawn into her narcissistic bubble but shows massive affects (crying), which, however, overwhelm her, an indicator of the traumatic quality of the experience. Her observer position is also an indication that embodied memories of traumatic experiences (with close relationships, boyfriend and father) are part of the latent dream: It is about catastrophes to which the patient is helplessly and powerlessly exposed. In the ZDPCS it becomes clear that the dreamer fears "to get involved, thus becoming an observer of his insufferable emotions".

The four dreams show in an impressive way that the dream self gradually gains activity despite the many interrupts (i.e. the massive inner conflicts that are activated in the dream), in other words the self-agency develops successively. This becomes particularly impressive in dream 3, in which the dream self-assures herself even in the manifest dream that the dream subject must be brutal, but at the same time "knew it was right, that it had to be done". The ZDPCS leads to similar insights: "There are still relatively many INTERRUPTS (5 situations), but the dreamer is actively involved from the outset (IAF); she actively defends herself and by this conveys self-agency".

Ad 3. More object relationships appear in the manifest dream

The four manifest dreams show that the dream self is successively more involved in interactions with objects: In the first dream, she still is in the observation position; in the second dream, the family reference persons as well as anonymous persons ("terrorists") appear, but they either seduce the dream self (mother), are absent (father and siblings) or pursue her (terrorists). In dream 3, the dream self is first pursued by a couple, then by a woman, from whom she must aggressively and destructively free herself. In contrast, in the last dream of the psychoanalysis, the dreamer is accompanied by her friend, who helps her to weather the storm, but does not manage to fight her way to the analyst. However, the dream self-subsequently confirms that she is able to establish a connection to the understanding object (analyst) on her own (through the telephone). The ZDPCS shows that the patient's fears of separation are still present (many interrupts): "but now in a way that is not as self-destructive (annihilating the self) as when having been attacked by OPs".

Ad 4: Increasingly, problem solving succeeds in dreams

Both the clinical-psychoanalytical observations and the ZDPCS analyses show that there is a great contrast between the first two and the last two dreams: the dream self has regained its self-agency and can use it to solve the problems that are dealt with in the dream (dream 3: freeing oneself from the persecuting woman, dream 4: making contact with the analyst in order to say goodbye to her in agreement in the last session of analysis).

Ad 5: The affective spectrum is expanded

The clinical analyses also agree with those of the ZDPCS with regard to this dimension of change. In the first dream, panic and uncontrollable sadness dominate. In the second dream, the affective spectrum is already broader (joy, surprise, panic). In the third dream, fear as well as aggression and inhibited pleasure appear. In the fourth dream, the affective spectrum is at its widest: happiness, anxiety, disgust, sadness, confidence, pride.

Within this limited framework, we hope to have given the reader an impression of the work of our research group, demonstrating that the change in dreams can prove to be an important indicator of the transformation of the patient's inner object world. We have also shown that the clinical and extra-clinical (ZPDCS) analyses lead to similar results, an important finding for psychoanalytic research. It has become clear how the two approaches to capturing psychic changes can complement, but also correct each other. While the clinical observations have the advantage of being placed in a rich psychoanalytic context (e.g. transference and countertransference phenomena, external object relations of the patient etc.) that is oriented toward therapeutic change, the ZDPCS offers the opportunity to train independent, blind raters and to assess the dream changes independently of the treating psychoanalyst. Furthermore, the reader will have noticed that the results of clinical and extra-clinical analyses are also qualitatively different.

We therefore consider the transformation of dreams, which for us still represents a via regia to the unconscious, to be a genuine psychoanalytic criterion for thinking critically about patients' transformations during their psychoanalyses.

Notes

1 I reported another version of this psychoanalysis in my keynote lecture at the EPF Congress in Vienna in July 2022 (Leuzinger-Bohleber, 2023). We have considered the rules for protecting the confidentiality of the patient.

2 I was extremely disturbed by Mrs C.'s condition and had to think of the concept of the death drive by André Green (Green, 2001), who writes, among other things: "The actual manifestation of the death drive, however, is the *withdrawal of cathexis*" (p.874). Mrs C. seemed to have withdrawn her libidinal and aggressive cathexis nearly completely from her self. In retrospect, it seems to me as if I—unconsciously at that time—desperately mobilized Eros in order to hold something against this death drive. I myself was frightened by the passionate vehemence with which I tried to reach Mrs C. emotionally (i.e., as Green describes it, to establish a bond with her). In later stages of analysis, we returned to the interaction at that time several times.

3 In many sessions, "embodied memories" of the mother's constant extreme inner tension and her extreme need to control her love objects can then be decoded and put into metaphors on the basis of detailed observations in the transference. Interestingly, her father tells her during these weeks that he left his wife at that time because he simply could not bear her constant tension, aggressiveness, catastrophe expectation as well as above all the aggressive-desperate atmosphere in the family as well as being controlled by his ex-wife any longer.

4 This section is based in a former publication Fischmann, Ambresin & Leuzinger-Bohleber, 2021.

5 Stern (2020) and his research group have developed the concept of RIGs (Representation Interaction Generalized) which had a great influence on empirical infant research. It is connected to the concept of schema or generalized cognitive-affective patterns which have been developed in the central early relationships and which determine mostly unconsciously the expectations to current relationships in the real world or in the transference.

6 Hortig and Moser (2012) rather speak in this later work of prototypical affective microprocesses (PAMs), which are defined as dyad-specific processes in affective relationship regulation (see also Bänninger-Huber, 1992). They are a product of both participants. In the case of mismatch, dysfunctional PAM structures are formed.

7 Lane (Lane, Ryan, Nadel, & Greenberg, 2015) comments that the emotional responses cannot be mentalized or mentally represented. They are not repressed. Dissociation can lead to lack of mental representation. I would also say that they are not "pushed into the unconscious" but rather that automatic emotional responses are too intense to be constructed as discrete, specific conceptualized experiences. In other words, they never made it into conscious awareness as discrete experiences.

References

Ambresin, G., Fischmann, T., & Leuzinger-Bohleber, M. (2022). Pluralism in psychoanalytic research. Conceptual framework of the MODE study. In M. Leuzinger-Bohleber, G. Ambresin, T. Fischmann, & M. Solms (eds.), *On the Dark Side of Chronic Depression. Psychoanalytic, Social-Cultural and Research Approaches.* London: Routledge, 121–132.

Ambresin, G., & Leuzinger-Bohleber, M. (2024). Changes in dreams. An indicator for transformation processes in psychoanalysis: Clinical outcome and process research in the MODE study. In S. E. Gullestad, E. Stänicke, & M. Leuzinger-Bohleber (eds.), *Psychoanalytic Studies of Change. An Integrative Perspective.* London: Routledge, 39–52.

Bohleber, W., & Leuzinger-Bohleber, M. (2016). The special problem of interpretation in the treatment of traumatized patients. *Psychoanalytic Inquiry, 36*(1), 60–76.

Bänninger-Huber, E. (1992). Prototypical affective microsequences in psychotherapeutic interaction. *Psychotherapy Research, 2*(4), 291–306.

Bleichmar, H. B. (1996). Some subtypes of depression and their implications for psychoanalytic treatment. *The International Journal of Psychoanalysis, 77*(5), 935.

Diamond, M. J. (2015). The elusiveness of masculinity: Primordial vulnerability, lack, and the challenges of male development. *The Psychoanalytic Quarterly, 84*(1), 47–102.

Fischmann, T., Ambresin, G., & Leuzinger-Bohleber, M. (2021). Dreams and Trauma Changes in the manifest dreams in psychoanalytic treatments—a psychoanalytic outcome measure. *Frontiers in Psychology, 12.* doi:10.3389/fpsyg.2021.678440

Fischmann, T., & Leuzinger-Bohleber, M. (2018). Traum und depression. In W. Berner, G. Amelung, A. Boll-Klatt, & U. Lamparter (eds.), *Von Irma Zu Amalie der Traum und Seine Psychoanalytische Bedeutung im Wandel Der Zeit.* Gießen: Psychosozial, 163–182.

Fischmann, T., Russ, M. O., & Leuzinger-Bohleber, M. (2013). Trauma, dream, and psychic change in psychoanalyses: A dialog between psychoanalysis and the neurosciences. *Frontiers in Human Neurosciens, 7,* 877. doi:10.3389/fnhum.2013.00877

Green, A. (2001). Todestrieb, negativer Narzißmus, Desobjektalisierungsfunktion. *55*(9–10), 869–877. Retrieved from https://elibrary.klett-cotta.de/article/99.120105/ps-55-9-869

Hortig, V., & Moser, U. (2012). Interferenzen neurotischer Prozesse und introjektiver Beziehungsmuster im Traum. *Psyche–Z Psychoanal, 66*(9–10), 889–916.

Lane, R. D., Ryan, L., Nadel, L., & Greenberg, L. (2015). Memory reconsolidation, emotional arousal, and the process of change in psychotherapy: New insights from brain science. *Behavioral and Brain Sciences, 38,* 1–64.

Leuzinger-Bohleber, M. (1989). *Veränderung kognitiver problemlösender Prozesse in Psychoanalysen.* Ulm: PSZ Verlag (Springer).

Leuzinger-Bohleber, M. (2021). Psychoanalyse als plurale wissenschaft des unbewussten. *Allgemeine Zeitschrift für Philosophie, 46*(2), 253–267.

Leuzinger-Bohleber, M. (2023). Depression—eine krankheit des ideals und des traumas. In *Psychoanalyse in Europa. Bulletin, Nr. 76,* 208–223 (in German, English, French).

Leuzinger-Bohleber, M., & Ambresin, G. (2024). Clinical outcome and process research in the MODE study: From the psychoanalysis of a young man in emerging adulthood. In S. E. Gullestad, E. Stänicke, & M. Leuzinger-Bohleber (eds.),

Psychoanalytic Studies of Change. An Integrative Perspective. London: Routledge, 24–38.

Leuzinger-Bohleber, M., Donié, M., Wichelmann, J., Ambresin, G., & Fischmann, T. (2023). Changes in dreams—the development of a dream—transformation scale in psychoanalyses with chronically depressed, early traumatized patients. *The Scandinavian Psychoanalytic Review, 46*(1–2), 82–93. doi:10.1080/01062301.2023.22 97116

Moser, U., & von Zeppelin, I. (1996). *Der geträumte Traum: wie Träume entstehen und sich verändern.* Stuttgart: Kohlhammer.

Stern, D. N. (2020). *The Motherhood Constellation: A Unified View of Parent-Infant Psychotherapy:* London: Routledge.

Winston, A. P. (2017). An island entire of itself: Narcissism in anorexia nervosa. In T. Wooldridge, (ed.), *Psychoanalytic Treatment of Eating Disorders.* London: Routledge, 70–82.

Index

Note: **Bold** page numbers refer to tables; *italic* page numbers refer to figures and page numbers followed by "n" denote endnotes.

For Product Safety Concerns and Information please contact our EU
representative GPSR@taylorandfrancis.com
Taylor & Francis Verlag GmbH, Kaufingerstraße 24, 80331 München, Germany